Prozac Backlash

Overcoming the Dangers of
Prozac, Zoloft, Paxil, and Other Antidepressants
with Safe, Effective Alternatives

JOSEPH GLENMULLEN, M.D.

Simon & Schuster
New York London Toronto Sydney Singapore

To
Muireann, Ciara, Peter, and Michael

Simon & Schuster
Rockefeller Center
1230 Avenue of the Americas
New York, NY 10020

Line art illustrations by Jackie Aher.

NOTE TO READERS
This publication contains the opinions and ideas of its author. It is intended to provide helpful and informative material on the subjects addressed in the publication. It is sold with the understanding that the author and publisher are not engaged in rendering medical, health, or any other kind of personal professional services in the book. The reader should consult his or her medical, health, or other competent professional before adopting any of the suggestions in this book or drawing inferences from it.
The author and publisher specifically disclaim all responsibility for any liability, loss, or risk, personal or otherwise, which is incurred as a consequence, directly or indirectly, of the use and application of any of the contents of this book.

The photomicrographs of the cerebral cortex of a monkey are from U. D. McCann, L. S. Seiden, L. Rubin, and G. Ricaurte, "Brain Serotonin Neurotoxicity and Primary Pulmonary Hypertension from Fenfluramine [Redux's parent compound] and Dexfenfluramine [Redux]." *Journal of the American Medical Association (JAMA)* 278 (August 27, 1997): 666–72.

Designed by Kyoko Watanabe

Manufactured in the United States of America

1   3   5   7   9   10   8   6   4   2

Library of Congress Cataloging-in-Publication Data
Glenmullen, Joseph, date.
Prozac backlash : overcoming the dangers of prozac, zoloft, paxil, and other antidepressants with safe, effective alternatives / Joseph Glenmullen.
p.   cm.
Includes bibliographical references and index.
1. Fluoxetine—Side effects.   2. Antidepressants—Side effects.   3. Depression, Mental—Alternative treatment.   I. Title.

RC483.5.F55 G56 2000
616.85'27061—dc21   99-059911

ISBN 0-684-86001-5

ACKNOWLEDGMENTS

Writing this book would not have been possible without the support and encouragement of my friends, colleagues, students, patients, and family. I am particularly appreciative of two Harvard colleagues, Drs. Joshua Sparrow and Elissa Kleinman, whose thoughtful comments on the manuscript greatly enriched it. Likewise, Thomas Moore at the George Washington University Medical Center provided invaluable commentary and tireless, sage advice. Individuals to whom I am indebted for reading portions of the manuscript in areas where they have specialized expertise include Professor Pavel Hrdina at the University of Ottawa; Dr. David Healy at the University of Wales College of Medicine; Professor Richard Lewontin at Harvard University; Dr. Maria Dorota Majewska at the National Institutes of Health; Professor Giovanni Fava at the University of Bologna; Professor Isaac Marks at the Institute of Psychiatry, University of London; Dr. Jerry Cott at the National Institute of Mental Health; Dr. Steven Bratman at Prima Health; and Professor Ivy Blackburn at the University of Northumberland at Newcastle upon Tyne. Many others gave generously of their time to speak with and send information to me on their research in areas covered in the book.

My agent Robert Lescher's early enthusiasm for the project is greatly appreciated. Another early enthusiast was my editor at Simon & Schuster, Fred Hills, who provided incisive commentary on the manuscript and its organization. Special thanks go to his assistant, Priscilla Holmes, for her astute editing, dedication, and care for the manuscript. I am also grateful to Veera Hiranandani for her help shepherding the book to completion. Indeed, I am grateful to everyone at Simon & Schuster for their extra effort, support, and enthusiasm.

Writing a book like this, one comes upon a new appreciation for the many libraries in the world, with their vast collections and their many dedicated, helpful librarians. I am particularly grateful to the librarians at Harvard's Countway Library of Medicine for their efforts at helping me track down publications from around the world. The former librarian to the Harvard University Health Services, Sylvia Gerhard, deserves special note for her assistance with literature searches.

I have been fortunate to work with wonderful colleagues for many years at the Harvard University Health Services. Special thanks go to Win Burr, his wife Barbara Burr, Ellen Kane, and Irving Allen for their humor, wisdom, and comradeship.

My psychiatric career has been enriched by teaching Harvard medical students, psychiatric residents, psychology fellows, and social work interns. Talented, challenging students have enriched my professional life and helped me clarify and hone my ideas.

I owe a special gratitude to my patients, who have really taught me what I know. They are the inspiration for the book. Many patients generously allowed me to include their stories. Of course, they have been disguised to protect their identities. Countless patients brought me articles from newspapers, magazines, and medical journals on subjects they knew are in the book. In a number of instances, key pieces of information were brought to my attention by patients. Their support and encouragement has been deeply appreciated.

Most of all, I wish to thank my wife and children, to whom the book is dedicated. From my wife's wisdom and unfailing support to my children's cartoons taped on the walls of my study to entertain me during the long hours working on the book—I could not have written it without them.

CONTENTS

The Prozac Phenomenon

Anne consulted with me during her first month at the Harvard Graduate School of Design. She had just moved to Cambridge from Chicago, where she had worked as an assistant in an architectural firm. Now Anne was embarking on becoming an architect herself.

"I'm on Zoloft. I came to see you because I'm running out of medication and need a new doctor here in Cambridge," she explained, with a straightforward, friendly smile.

Every fall, I see droves of new students like Anne on one of the popular Prozac-type antidepressants that boost the brain chemical serotonin: Prozac, Zoloft, Paxil, Luvox, and others. Instead of just renewing the serotonin booster, I first inquire about the patient's history: Why is she on the drug? What other treatment has she had? How long has she been on the medication? Has she tried going off it? As in Anne's case, the answers are often unsettling.

Anne had been on 150 milligrams a day of Zoloft for three years. Her primary-care doctor put her on a serotonin booster to give her a lift because Anne was "upset" over her boyfriend's breaking up with her. At the time she had relatively mild symptoms that would not qualify for a diagnosis of depression. She had been weepy and a little distracted for a week when her doctor gave her the initial prescription. Anne had not seen a psychiatrist, psychologist, or social worker for a psychological evaluation. Her primary-care doctor at her HMO simply prescribed Zoloft.

"Why 150 milligrams a day?" I inquired.

"Is that a high dose?" Anne asked, surprised.

I explained that in my experience most people only need 50 milligrams or 100 at most. The maximum dose is 200. Anything above 150 is usually reserved for people with severe symptoms, which she clearly had not had. Anne had no idea why she had been put on such a high dose.

"What happened with your ex-boyfriend?" I asked.

"We got back together a few months later. We've been married now for two years, quite happily."

"Did your doctor make any effort to see if you still needed the drug once the crisis had passed?"

"No."

"How often did you check in with him?"

"I didn't."

"You never saw him again?"

"No."

"How did you get more medication?"

"He gave me a prescription for a year. At the end of the year, I just telephoned his office and they called in another year's supply to the pharmacy."

I shook my head, unable to suppress my dismay at such cursory treatment. Unfortunately, stories like Anne's are quite common nowadays.

"You're not sure I need the Zoloft?"

I told Anne that at the time of the breakup, many doctors, including myself, would have recommended psychotherapy, which might well have seen her through the crisis given how mild her symptoms were and how quickly the crisis passed. I was especially concerned that no effort had been made to periodically reassess whether or not she needed the medication. Now Anne had had three years' exposure to a high dose of Zoloft.

"Three years' exposure . . . is that cause for concern?"

In recent years, the danger of long-term side effects has emerged in association with Prozac-type drugs, making it imperative to minimize one's exposure to them. Neurological disorders including disfiguring facial and whole body tics, indicating potential brain damage, are an increasing concern with patients on the drugs.[1] Withdrawal syndromes—which can be debilitating—are estimated to affect up to 50% of patients, depending on the particular drug.[2] Sexual dysfunction affects 60% of people.[3] Increasing reports are being made of people becoming dependent on the medications after chronic use.[4] With related drugs targeting serotonin, there is evidence that they may effect a "chemical lobotomy" by destroying the nerve endings that they target in the brain.[5] Prozac-type drugs are now wearing off in some 34% of patients who can suddenly find themselves with a return of dread symptoms.[6] And startling new information on Prozac's precipitating suicidal and violent behavior has come to light.[7]

"What do you recommend I do?" asked Anne as I described these dangers.

"I suggest we gradually lower your Zoloft dose to see if you can go off the medication. I suspect you don't need it."

"But I've just started this demanding degree program," Anne responded anxiously.

"We would reduce your dose slowly to see if you had a return of any symptoms."

Anne shook her head. "I'm afraid to make any changes right now. I just left my job and made this big move. Being in graduate school is a huge adjustment. My husband is just starting a new job in Boston. I feel there is too much at stake."

Many patients stay on their medication because they fear rocking the boat. In Anne's case, she was making a reasonable point; this was not the best time to experiment. Almost any other time in the three years she had been on it would have been better. Unfortunately, these earlier opportunities had been lost. Now she was faced with the difficult decision of lowering the dose at an inopportune time or extending her exposure to the drug another six months to a year.

After we discussed her situation at length, Anne's position remained unchanged. Before we ended the meeting, I gave her a month's prescription for Zoloft. It is a reflection of how seriously I take patients being on these drugs that I do not give people a year's supply. Instead, Anne and I made another appointment for the following month. Meeting with her monthly, I would get to know her better, hear about her progress in graduate school, and be better able to re-evaluate her medication needs by the end of her semester.

I have mixed feelings about writing prescriptions for people like Anne. Basing my judgment on experience with many patients, I thought she would have no trouble substantially reducing her dose. Once a Prozac-type drug is working, much lower doses are often sufficient to maintain its effects. In fact, I felt fairly confident that Anne could have stopped the medication altogether based on the trivial symptoms for which it was prescribed to her in the first place. Still, so long as patients are making informed choices, their wishes should be respected.

Two weeks later, Anne appeared in my office far sooner than expected. She looked exhausted and irritable. Tears welling in her eyes she said, "I went down to 100 milligrams of Zoloft and my symptoms have returned. In fact, I feel worse than when I went on the medication. I can't sleep. I can't concentrate."

"I thought you weren't going to reduce the dose."

"I had no idea Zoloft is so expensive."

"What do you mean?"

"The prescription you gave me cost over one hundred fifty dollars for a month!"

"How could you not have known? You've been on it for three years."

"My HMO gave it to me. I only made a ten-dollar copayment a month."

I suddenly remembered Anne had been working before she returned to school. Like most people with medical insurance through an employer, Anne's health care included medication coverage. By contrast, many student health plans, like Harvard's, do not cover medication.

"I can't afford this," said Anne. "I'm living on a student budget. Frankly, I couldn't have afforded it on my old job. But look at me. I desperately need it."

"When did you lower the dose?"

"Two days ago."

"Have you had any dizziness?"

"Not when I'm sitting still like this, but if I got up and moved around I would."

"What if you just turn your head?"

Anne turned slowly from left to right. "Yes," she said, surprised. "It feels like I have water sloshing around in my head. What does that mean?"

"This isn't a return of your symptoms. It's withdrawal from the Zoloft."

"It is?" said Anne, incredulous.

"The dizziness is the giveaway. And the fact that the symptoms appeared so quickly. Some people, after lowering their doses of these types of drugs, are unable to walk and have to take to bed because they are so unsteady. Others have electric shock–like sensations in their brains or visual hallucinations of flashing lights."

Anne winced at the prospect. Nevertheless, she decided to "tough it out," hoping she had already made it through the worst of the withdrawal.

Fortunately, Anne's withdrawal symptoms cleared within days. She felt completely back to normal, confirming that what she experienced was withdrawal and not a return of her original symptoms, which, in fact, had been far milder.

Now motivated not only by the cost but also by her distaste for a drug causing clear-cut withdrawal symptoms, Anne proceeded to taper off the Zoloft. Each time she reduced the dose, she again had a few days of mild withdrawal symptoms.

Although Anne did not develop tics on Zoloft, others of my patients have developed tics and twitches on Prozac-type antidepressants that persisted for months after the drug was stopped. The tics may be facial, like fly-catcher tongue darting or chewing-the-cud jawing, or involve the whole body, like involuntary pelvic thrusting. The tics are *the* dread side effect in psychiatry. With earlier classes of drugs that cause these kinds of tics, they are disfiguring, untreatable, and permanent in up to 50% of cases.[8]

These side effects raise concerns that patients may sustain silent brain damage that we have no way of assessing. Such damage could be compounded in the future by other medications, viruses, and toxins, which injure the involuntary motor system, and by the normal aging process, which causes a progressive loss of brain cells.[9] It could predispose patients later in life to prematurely develop senile tics, gait disturbances, and other neurological conditions that normally affect only the elderly.

After stopping Zoloft, Anne continued to check in with me periodically and did fine without medication. What if she hadn't come to Harvard and gotten a second opinion about being on the drug? Anne was unnecessarily exposed to the potential risks of Zoloft. In my experience, as many as 75% of patients are needlessly on these drugs for mild, even trivial, conditions.

The dangerous side effects discussed in the first half of this book have been the subject of intense research and discussion within psychiatry in recent years. Still, many doctors outside of academic medical centers are not adequately informed about them. Most patients are still unaware of the dangers.

In the December 1997 issue of the *Journal of Clinical Psychopharmacology,* Dr. Ronald Pies wrote an alert on the long-term risks of these serotonergic drugs.[10] Pies is on the faculty of both Harvard and Tufts Medical Schools. Commenting on the neurological side effects, including tic disorders, Pies wrote that "we simply do not know how many cases are being overlooked. Neither do we know how many cases will develop in patients taking these agents for 5, 10, 15, or more years." Because of the risks, Pies argued that Prozac-type drugs should not "be prescribed for the 'worried well' or for patients with mild depression, who respond favorably to psychotherapy alone."

For patients whose symptoms are more severe, the risk-benefit ratio of taking the drugs can be quite different. In these circumstances, I still recommend medication to patients. The risks of severe psychiatric syndromes can be worse than the risks of short-term use of the medication. Many patients with moderate to severe symptoms feel desperate for something to jump-start them back to normal life. By combining drugs with psychotherapy and other alternatives, one can usually minimize exposure to the drugs, keeping the dosage low and weaning off medication within six months to a year.

The 10-20-30 Year Pattern

Unfortunately, the dangerous side effects emerging with Prozac, Zoloft, Paxil, and other serotonin boosters are right on schedule, appearing like clockwork in a 10-20-30-year pattern characteristic of popular psychiatric drugs. The first potent antidepressants of the modern era were cocaine elixirs, introduced in the late 1800s. At the turn of the century cocaine elixirs were the most popular prescription medications, prescribed for everything from depression to shyness, just as the Prozac group are today.[11] Freud wrote three famous "cocaine papers" advocating the drug's use. Since cocaine elixirs, we have had numerous amphetamines, bromides, barbiturates, narcotics, and tranquilizers, all hailed as miracle cures until their dangerous side effects emerged.

Reviewing the history of these drugs, one finds a strikingly similar pattern: Initially, the drugs are aggressively marketed with claims that they are revolutionary breakthroughs, remarkable scientific advances over their predecessors. Early on, a few doctors champion their cause, becoming celebrities along with the drugs. Often, a handful of celebrities step forward to endorse the miracle cure. As they gain momentum, use of the drugs spreads beyond the confines of psychiatry and they are prescribed by general practitioners for everyday maladies. Indeed, the burgeoning list of "conditions" they are used to treat, including everyday life, is often one of the first clues that one is looking at a general mood brightener that provides a quick fix.

In the typical life span of the drugs, the earliest signs of problems appear about ten years after introduction. Pharmaceutical companies and drug proponents deny the problems, adopting the strategy of defending the medication to the last. As we lack serious long-term monitoring of drug side effects and rely almost entirely on spontaneous, voluntary reporting by doctors, it is typically only at the twenty-year mark that enough data has accrued for the problems to be undeniable and for a significant number of physicians to be sounding the alarm. Still another ten years or more elapse before professional organizations and regulatory agencies actively take steps to curtail overprescribing. Thus, the cycle from miracle to disaster typically takes thirty years or more. By then, even the most popular drugs are no longer covered by their patent and even their manufacturers have an incentive to abandon medications that have become passé and disreputable. Typically their energies are then focused on the next breakthrough: newly patented, more profitable agents, which can be promoted as "safer" because their hazards are not yet known.

The Prozac Group

Prozac and the other serotonin boosters—Zoloft, Paxil, and Luvox—have been the panaceas of the past decade. The pharmaceutical giant Eli Lilly marketed Prozac in the late 1980s as a dramatic new type of mood-altering drug, a designer medical bullet targeting serotonin. Lilly's sophisticated marketing made the new drug an instant success: In less than two years, Prozac was outselling all other antidepressants. In March 1990, the green-and-white Prozac capsule appeared on the cover of *Newsweek* under the banner "The Promise of Prozac."[12] The glowing cover story described Prozac as a medical "breakthrough" already being prescribed for so many conditions in addition to depression that "even healthy people have started asking for it." *New York* magazine called the novel pill a "wonder drug."[13] The *National Enquirer* described it as a miracle diet pill.

In 1993, psychiatrist Peter Kramer's enormously influential book *Listening to Prozac* made sensational claims that these new serotonergic agents not only treated serious depression but also cured a host of everyday maladies like timidity, shyness, sensitivity, lack of confidence, perfectionism, fastidiousness, fear of rejection, low self-esteem, competitiveness, jealousy, and fear of intimacy.[14]

Couched in a barrage of almost senseless data, which unfortunately looked like impregnable science to the lay reader, Kramer's endorsement of the drugs was so sweeping he even described them as making people feel "better than well."[15] His most astonishing claim was that the Prozac group could "transform" people by fundamentally altering their personalities. Coining the phrase "cosmetic psychopharmacology," Kramer proclaimed, "Some people might prefer pharmacologic to psychologic self-actualization. Psychic steroids for mental gymnastics, medicinal attacks on the humors, antiwallflower compound. . . . Since you only live once, why not do it as a blonde? Why not as a peppy blonde?"[16]

The general media had a feeding frenzy over Kramer's notion that these drugs could change personality, treating it as a historic breakthrough. The cover of *Newsweek* announced, "Beyond Prozac: How Science Will Let You Change Your Personality with a Pill."[17] Inside, the feature article was a minds-made-to-order scientific thriller asserting we would soon have many personalities-in-a-bottle to choose from. This was not the "one pill makes you larger, one pill makes you smaller" ode of the sixties counterculture but, seemingly, the voice of the scientific establishment.

As with earlier panaceas, celebrities came forward to endorse them. Television personality Mike Wallace testified, "I will take Zoloft every day for the rest of my life. And I'm quite content to do it."[18] "Serotonin boosters are extraordinary" was the impression given to the general public.

Indeed, the publicity made serotonin a household word. Droves of patients came into doctors' offices demanding one of the new pills. Coincidentally, it was at this time that managed care insurers began to exert increasing influence over doctors in their treatment plans for patients. In the area of mental health, this took the form of pressuring primary-care doctors to prescribe drugs rather than refer patients to specialists who might be able to treat them with more effective, safer alternatives. In the early 1990s, serotonin boosters became managed care's answer to the "problem" of more costly alternatives, with little thought given to the consequences for patients. This is why patients like Anne are prescribed one of the Prozac-type drugs for mild, often trivial conditions.

Soon primary-care doctors were writing 70% of prescriptions for Prozac, Zoloft, Paxil, and Luvox.[19] To the already long list of conditions treated with the drugs were added anxiety, obsessions, compulsions, eating disorders, headaches, back pain, impulsivity, drug and alcohol abuse, hair pulling, nail biting, upset stomach, irritability, sexual addictions, premature ejaculation, attention deficit disorder, and premenstrual syndrome. Diet centers began prescribing the Prozac group for weight loss.[20] Employee assistance programs began using them to prop up exhausted factory workers putting in grueling overtime shifts as a result of corporate downsizing.[21] Serotonin boosters are all-purpose psychoanalgesics, not just "antidepressants," which was merely the first application for which they were approved.

Early on, a few reasoned voices tried to introduce some skepticism and caution about the new drugs. *The New Yorker* described *Listening to Prozac* as "a love letter to the drug" and for months ran a series of satirical cartoons.[22] Among these was an illustration of three books with the titles *Listening to Tylenol, Listening to Tums,* and *Listening to Tic-Tacs.*[23] Its caption read, "Life's daily aches and pains need no longer be endured. Don't miss out." Another cartoon depicted Karl Marx, Dostoevsky, and Edgar Allan Poe gleefully on Prozac.[24] Proclaimed Marx, "Sure! Capitalism can work out its kinks!" Said Poe to a raven, "Hello, birdie!" Still another piece was entitled "Listening to Bourbon."[25]

The *New York Times Book Review* called Kramer's speculations "in the realm of science fiction."[26] The cover of *The New Republic* depicted a sporty, all-American couple smiling and waving under the headline "That Prozac Moment!"[27] Below was a surgeon general–style warning: "This drug may offer pseudo solutions to real problems." In the accompanying article, entitled "Shiny Happy People," David Rothman, a professor of social medicine and history at Columbia University, wrote a scathing critique of cosmetic psychopharmacology.

One of the most articulate critics of the hype surrounding serotonin boosters was Sherwin Nuland, a professor of surgery and historian of medicine at the Yale University School of Medicine, and the author of the acclaimed *How We Die*. Writing in *The New York Review of Books*, Nuland decried the public's being "subjected to the arguments of seemingly authoritative physicians and scientists who propose views that don't stand up to the scrutiny of trained professional eyes."[28] He called the pop psychopharmacology swirling around the serotonin boosters "preposterous," "unsubstantiated," and a "psychopharmacological fantasy." Noting that "it remains anything but certain that clinical depression is, in fact, caused by a decrease in serotonin," he denounced the junk science of serotonin deficiencies and biochemical imbalances as "uncertain gropings for proof of a fanciful theory."

Unfortunately, the din in the general media drowned out the few reasoned voices. As Prozac rocketed up the charts, it became the number-two best-selling drug in America. Zoloft and Paxil rank almost as high. More than 60 million prescriptions for the drugs were written in 1998. Annual sales of the three exceed $4 billion a year. Tens of millions of people, perhaps as many as 10% of the American population, have been exposed to serotonin boosters.[29] Half a million children are prescribed the drugs, with pediatric use one of the fastest-growing "markets."[30] This in spite of the fact that repeated studies have shown antidepressant drugs are no more effective in children than placebos.[31]

A particularly important element in the success of these medications has been the perception that they are safe and have virtually no side effects. Prescribed for everything from headaches to premenstrual syndrome, they may seem as safe as aspirin. Minimizing the drugs' risks, in *Listening to Prozac*, Peter Kramer declared, "There is no unhappy ending to this story. . . . the patient recovers and pays no price for the recovery."[32] Given the history of earlier miracle cures, one wonders at the wisdom of conveying this impression to the public.

Prozac Backlash

To understand the side effects of these drugs, one needs to know a few basic facts of brain chemistry. Brain chemicals are called neurotransmitters. Of the more than a hundred neurotransmitters now known, three are important for our purposes: serotonin, adrenaline, and dopamine, popularly referred to as the brain's "feel good" neurotransmitters.[33] Whereas earlier mood brighteners like cocaine and amphetamines boost all three of these neurotransmitters, the Prozac group were hailed as a breakthrough because they are "selective" for serotonin. This selectivity gives the impression that serotonin is localized in a depression center in the brain. If a depressed person's serotonin is low, the impression given is that the drugs top it up in a safe, targeted manner.

This impression does not match reality, however. Serotonin is one of the oldest neurotransmitters in the evolution of life forms. In humans only about 5% of serotonin is found in the brain. The other 95% is distributed throughout the rest of the body.[34] The majority is in the gastrointestinal tract, where serotonin modulates the rhythmic movements kneading food through the stomach.[35] In the cardiovascular system, serotonin helps regulate blood vessels to control the flow of blood. Serotonin is also found in blood cells and plays an important role in clotting. In the reproductive system, serotonin's influence on the genitals accounts for its sexual effects. Serotonin plays a significant role in controlling a host of hormones that regulate a panoply of physiologic processes.[36]

In the human brain, serotonin is one of the chemicals by which brain cells signal, or communicate with, one another. Serotonin nerves originate in the deepest, oldest part of the brain, called the brain stem. But while serotonin nerves originate here, they radiate diffusely, penetrating virtually every part of the brain. Efrain Azmitia, a professor of biology and psychiatry at New York University and one of the world's leading authorities on serotonin, says, "The brain serotonin system is the single largest brain system known and can be characterized as a 'giant' neuronal system."[37]

During gestation, this giant system orchestrates some of the development of the brain, regulating the maturation of the brain's architecture. No wonder this vast network then has global modulatory effects throughout the nervous system. Says Azmitia, "Serotonin has been implicated in sleep, aggression, sexual activity, appetite, learning, and memory to name but a few behaviors altered by serotonin drugs or damage to the 5-HT [serotonin nerve] fibers. . . . The broad range of functions complements the extensive anatomy of the serotonin neurons [brain cells]."

So while pharmaceutical companies have marketed Prozac, Zoloft, Paxil, and Luvox as "selective" for serotonin, serotonin is anything but selective in its widespread effects. There is, in fact, no known depression center in the brain. Rather, the drugs have global effects owing to serotonin's vast influence.

The illustrations on pages 18 and 19 show how Prozac-type drugs are thought to boost serotonin neurotransmission. Each serotonin nerve branches into a web of hundreds of thousands of delicate tentacles that reach out to communicate with other nerves. At the ends of these branches, the signaling nerve releases serotonin as a chemical messenger that travels across a microscopic space and attaches to receptors on the receiving nerve. The arrival of serotonin completes the signal to the receiving cell.

After a signal has been sent, the cell from which it originates cleans up unused serotonin by reabsorbing it in a process called "reuptake." Reuptake keeps signals crisp, terminating them in a timely fashion, which prevents lingering serotonin from continuing to stimulate the receiving cell. Prozac-type drugs inhibit—or block—reuptake, thereby boosting the level of serotonin, prolonging serotonin signals in the brain.

In the most cutting-edge research, the current and formerly popular antidepressants—including cocaine, amphetamines, and the Prozac group—appear to boost neurotransmitters beyond levels achieved under ordinary circumstances. Barry Jacobs, a professor of neuroscience at Princeton University, wrote in the December 1991 issue of the *Journal of Clinical Psychiatry* that most "external manipulation" of the system by drugs creates serotonin levels "beyond the physiological range achieved under [normal] environmental/biological conditions." Boosting serotonin to this degree "might more appropriately be considered *pathologic*, rather than reflective of the normal biological role of 5-HT [serotonin] [italics added]."[38]

Similarly, psychiatrist Steven Hyman, director of the National Institute of Mental Health, wrote in 1996, "Chronic administration of psychotropic drugs [i.e., drugs with psychological effects] creates perturbations [imbalances] in neurotransmitter function that likely exceed the strength and time course of almost any natural stimulus."[39] This "hyperstimulation" triggers "compensatory" reactions in the brain in its efforts to achieve "a new adapted state which may be qualitatively as well as quantitatively different from the normal state."

Most recently, neuroscientists have learned not only that the effects of a single neurotransmitter like serotonin are extremely widespread but that different neurotransmitters do not function independently of one another. Critical systems like serotonin, adrenaline, and dopamine are linked through

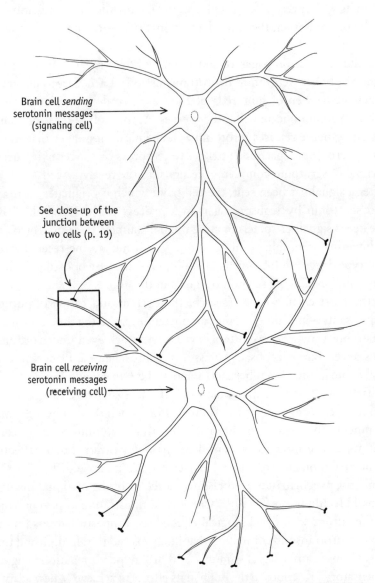

Brain cell *sending*
serotonin messages
(signaling cell)

See close-up of the
junction between
two cells (p. 19)

Brain cell *receiving*
serotonin messages
(receiving cell)

HOW PROZAC-TYPE DRUGS BOOST SEROTONIN NEUROTRANSMISSION

Serotonin brain cells are highly branching and form many connections, or junctions, with other cells. At these junctions, the cells do not actually touch. Instead they are separated by a small space across which serotonin travels as a messenger from one cell to the next. The illustrations on the facing page show close-ups of the junctions between cells with and without Prozac.

A.

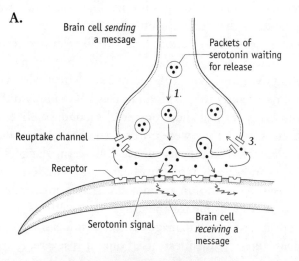

Brain cell *sending* a message

Packets of serotonin waiting for release

Reuptake channel

Receptor

Serotonin signal

Brain cell *receiving* a message

A SEROTONIN MESSAGE

The junction between two cells when Prozac is not present. 1. Packets of serotonin (represented by black dots) are released by the cell sending serotonin messages. 2. The serotonin travels across the space and attaches to receptors, sending a serotonin signal into the receiving cell. 3. After a signal has been sent, the cell from which it originated cleans up unused serotonin by reabsorbing it in a process called "reuptake." Reuptake keeps signals crisp, terminating them in a timely fashion, which prevents lingering serotonin from continuing to stimulate the receiving cell.

B.

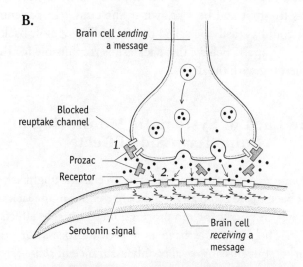

Brain cell *sending* a message

Blocked reuptake channel

Prozac

Receptor

Serotonin signal

Brain cell *receiving* a message

A SEROTONIN MESSAGE BOOSTED BY PROZAC

How Prozac boosts serotonin messages. 1. Prozac blocks the reuptake channels, inhibiting reuptake of serotonin back into the cell. 2. The result is more serotonin in the junction—with more serotonin attaching to more receptors—which creates prolonged serotonin signals in the brain.

complex circuitry. Dramatic changes in one, like boosting serotonin, can trigger compensatory changes in the others.

Chief among the brain's reactions to artificially elevated serotonin levels is a compensatory drop in dopamine.[40] Drugs producing a dopamine drop are well known to cause the dangerous side effects that are now appearing with Prozac and other drugs in its class. We simply did not know that serotonin boosters had these powerful secondary effects on other neurotransmitters when they were introduced. At the time they were an utterly new class of medications whose long-term dangers were unknown. Doctors and scientists are just beginning to understand the connections between the serotonin and dopamine systems in the brain that are thought to be responsible for the drugs' severe effects. But with earlier classes of drugs, the brain damage that can result is slowly progressive and often silent, and only manifests itself once it is severe. A critical variable determining the degree of damage appears to be total cumulative exposure to the drugs.

Thus, even the highly touted "selectivity" of the Prozac group is an illusion. In fact, the extreme emphasis these drugs place on serotonin may be a liability, because changes in serotonin levels can trigger secondary, or indirect, changes in dopamine. I call the compensatory reactions of the brain to these serotonergic drugs "Prozac backlash." Here I am using the word "Prozac" generically to stand for the whole group of closely related drugs, since Prozac is the first and best known in the class.[41] In patients on the other drugs, it could as easily be called by names like "Zoloft backlash" or "Paxil backlash." Experts believe this backlash is responsible for the severe side effects emerging with the drugs.

The Lack of Systematic Monitoring of Long-Term Side Effects

In light of the emergence of such serious side effects, one might ask why the public has not been made more aware. The answer lies in the lack of an adequate public health policy for monitoring long-term side effects of prescription drugs. The FDA does have an approval process for new drugs coming to market, but this approval is only assurance of *short-term* safety. Pharmaceutical companies are required to perform clinical studies of new psychiatric drugs in patients, but the tests typically last for only six to eight weeks, whereas the most serious, long-term side effects of drugs take years, sometimes decades, to emerge. Under these circumstances, prescribing an entirely new class of agents to millions of people is nothing short of an on-going human experiment.

"Man is becoming the primary guinea pig," says Ross Baldessarini, a professor of psychiatry and neuroscience at Harvard Medical School and one of the country's leading psychopharmacologists.[42] Psychopharmacology is the relatively new subspecialty of psychiatrists who only prescribe drugs and do not practice psychotherapy. Baldessarini made the sober comment at a Harvard conference on psychiatric drugs in the fall of 1998. "You really don't know what to expect," he said, when drugs are designed on the computer to target specific brain cells and receive only limited testing in laboratory animals before being prescribed to people.

But the even greater shortcoming in our public health monitoring system is what happens after new drugs have been introduced. A meager 4% of the FDA's budget is allocated to monitoring side effects after drugs are approved and being prescribed to millions of people. Each year the FDA reviews about 25 new drugs for approval. For this task, the agency has a professional staff of 1,500 doctors, scientists, toxicologists, and statisticians. But to monitor the safety of the more than 3,000 drugs already on the market and being prescribed to millions, the agency has a professional staff of just five doctors and one epidemiologist.[43] Because long-term monitoring is virtually nonexistent, in a 1993 article in the *Journal of the American Medical Association,* the then commissioner of the FDA, David Kessler, revealed that "only about 1% of serious events [side effects] are reported to the FDA."[44] The FDA itself is not responsible for this state of affairs, says Thomas Moore, a leading authority on drug side effects at the George Washington University Medical Center. The FDA's budget is set by Congress. In his 1998 book *Prescription for Disaster,* Moore details the intense pressure Congress is under from lobbyists for the pharmaceutical industry to weaken rather than strengthen drug testing and monitoring.[45]

In the absence of thorough follow-up, long-term drug effects only slowly come to light through random, spontaneous reports in obscure medical journals, which even most doctors do not read. This loose, word-of-mouth system takes years, often decades, to gain momentum around even common, dangerous effects. In *Prescription for Disaster,* Moore says that "initial drug testing is essential but incomplete."[46] Our "flawed monitoring system" gives people an "illusion of safety" when, in fact, serious drug problems "tend to be slow, insidious, and difficult to see."[47]

A final reason why it can take so long for dangerous effects to come to public attention is that as problems do emerge, pharmaceutical companies and drug proponents typically adopt the strategy of defending the drug to the last. This has been the repeated pattern in the 150 years since potent synthetic drugs targeting the brain were first invented. And we are already seeing this happen in the case of serotonin boosters.

While systematic studies have shown that 60% of patients on serotonin boosters suffer often severe sexual side effects, Eli Lilly's official figure is just 2–5%.[48] The manufacturers of Zoloft, Paxil, and Luvox also provide misleadingly low figures in their official information on the medications.

When people try to withdraw from serotonin boosters—especially Zoloft, Paxil, and Luvox—they may experience debilitating withdrawal syndromes. Mistaking withdrawal for a return of their original symptoms, many patients restart the medication, needlessly prolonging their exposure to the drug. Pharmaceutical companies are so concerned about withdrawal syndromes that Eli Lilly recently funded a panel of drug advocates, prominent academic psychiatrists, who wrote a series of professional papers suggesting the euphemism "antidepressant discontinuation syndrome" as an alternative to "withdrawal," avoiding the latter's negative connotations.[49]

In the case of suicidality and violence, Eli Lilly has adamantly denied this side effect. But new information has come to light that the pharmaceutical giant has paid millions of dollars to victims and survivors of Prozac-related suicides and murders. The test case was the sensational mass murder–suicide of Joseph Wesbecker. In 1989, one month after starting Prozac, Wesbecker opened fire with an AK-47 semi-automatic assault rifle in Louisville, Kentucky, killing eight people and wounding twelve others before taking his own life in the shooting spree. In 1994, Lilly appeared to win a jury verdict in the Wesbecker trial, which they aggressively publicized as "vindicating" their drug.[50]

But the truth is that the pharmaceutical company secretly paid what Cecil Blye, an attorney for one of the victims, Andrew Pointer, later acknowledged was a "tremendous amount of money. It boggles the mind."[51] Pointer was forced to reveal the settlement in his divorce, but the exact amount is still unknown, protected in documents related to the divorce which have been sealed because Lilly has insisted on secrecy. Lilly's lawyers struck the bargain with Wesbecker's victims before the trial was over, making the verdict a sham. In an article entitled "Lilly's Phantom Verdict" in the September 1995 issue of *The American Lawyer,* Nicholas Varchaver describes the verdict as "nothing more than a public relations vehicle, especially when it hardly represents the ringing vindication that Lilly has been proclaiming."[52] The highly unusual, secret deal is "unprecedented in any Western court," in the words of British journalist John Cornwell, who covered the trial for the London *Sunday Times Magazine.*[53]

Eventually the judge in the Wesbecker trial, Judge John Potter of the Jefferson Circuit Court in Louisville, Kentucky, moved to re-examine the trial.[54] Lilly's lawyers fought Judge Potter to the Kentucky Supreme Court until, in 1996, he finally won permission to have the Attorney General's Office conduct an investigation.[55] During the investigation, the lawyers for Lilly and the victims finally acknowledged the deal, although the "mind-boggling" sum has still not been disclosed.[56] Finally, in 1997, three years after its public relations coup in the trial, Lilly agreed to the verdict's being quietly "corrected" to "dismissed . . . as settled."[57] It is difficult to find out exactly how many such cases have been settled, but during the Attorney General's investigation, Lilly acknowledged settling other cases as well, which has kept the issue quiet.[58]

In spite of such efforts at spin control, in the most recent edition of the *Diagnostic and Statistical Manual (DSM IV)*, the American Psychiatric Association added a specific diagnostic category recognizing the neurological side effects being seen with Prozac-type medications, including the untreatable tics that first alerted me to the downside of these drugs.[59]

Having talked with hundreds of patients in my private practice and at the Harvard University Health Services, I know the biggest concern of people on these drugs is the possibility of long-term consequences. Many patients ask, "Will I eventually get some kind of brain damage after years of being on Paxil?" "Will my liver be injured after metabolizing so much Zoloft?" "Will the memory problems I'm having go away when I stop Prozac?"

Numerous authors who have written of their experience with serotonin boosters echo these concerns. Writing in the *Boston Phoenix* in April 1998 about her dependence on prescription antidepressants, in an article entitled "Hooked," Deborah Abramson worries that "research five or ten years down the road might reveal that one of the drugs I take greatly increases the likelihood of some kind of cancer."[60]

In her best-selling memoir *Prozac Nation*, Elizabeth Wurtzel writes, "I can't help feeling that anything that works so effectively, that's so transformative, has got to be hurting me at another end, maybe sometime down the road. . . . I don't know if there are any statistics on this, but how long is a person who is on psychotropic drugs supposed to live? How long before your brain, not to mention the rest of you, will begin to mush and deteriorate?"[61] Expressing her concerns to her psychiatrist, Wurtzel says, "Come on, level with me, anything that works this well has got to have some unknown downside. . . . He says a bunch of reassuring things, explains over and over again how carefully he is monitoring me—all the while admitting that psychopharmacology is more art than science, that he and his colleagues are all basically shooting in the dark. And he acts as if a million doc-tors didn't say the same things to women about DES, about the IUD, about silicon breast implants, as if they didn't once claim that Valium was a non-addictive tranquilizer and that Halcion was a miracle sleeping pill."[62]

Four potent serotonin boosters—Prozac, Zoloft, Paxil, and Luvox—are the focus of the first half of this book. Also called the Prozac group, these four drugs are officially treated as a class because of their similarities. Many patients on Zoloft, Paxil, and Luvox are unaware that these are close rela-tives of Prozac, sharing the same primary mode of action and many side ef-fects. A fifth drug, Celexa, has recently been marketed as the newest addition to this group. I have less to say about Celexa only because it is so new. Four related drugs have also entered the market in the last decade: Wellbutrin, Effexor, Serzone, and Remeron. Many of these also boost sero-tonin and cause some similar side effects. Details on these drugs are pro-vided wherever relevant.

As the more dangerous side effects of the Prozac group come into view, perhaps we will be able to see not only the dark side of these latest miracle cures but also the liability of any potent, synthetic drug targeting the brain. Future generations may well look back on the last 150 years of these drugs as a frightening human experiment. If this happens, either they will be banned altogether because they do more harm than good or their use will be strictly limited to only the most severe cases.

The Good News

Although dangerous side effects are emerging in association with serotonin boosters, the good news is that there are many alternatives. The second half of this book examines clinical experience and research on psychotherapy, cognitive-behavioral treatment, herbal remedies, diet, exercise, couples and family therapy, group therapy, and twelve-step programs. Nowadays, pa-tients looking for alternatives to drugs are often surprised by the array of possibilities, because they have been so poorly informed about them by their HMOs.

I explain what depression is from a psychological point of view and how to distinguish between mild, moderate, and severe cases. Extensive clinical research is reviewed, documenting how psychological interventions are as effective as drugs for mild to moderate depression. Traditional psycho-therapy, cognitive therapy, and behavioral approaches are compared. An approach is outlined for deciding when drugs are indicated and when they are not.

Clinical research has also shown the increasingly popular herbal remedy St. John's wort is as effective as synthetic drugs for mild to moderate depression.[63] In Germany, St. John's wort is the most commonly used antidepressant.

For more severe depression, there are creative ways of combining short-term drug use with other treatment modalities with the goal of removing the medication after six months to a year. Evaluating when one might be ready to go off medication is an important priority. This should be reassessed at least once a year. I explain the relationship between medications, when they are indicated, and psychotherapy.

Many anxiety syndromes, from panic attacks to obsessive-compulsive disorder, are now commonly treated with Prozac-type medications. I present research and cases showing how older, safer drugs and behavioral treatments like exposure, or systematic desensitization, are preferable.

Prozac, Zoloft, Paxil, and Luvox are also prescribed for alcoholism, drug dependence, sexual addictions, and eating disorders. Better, less risky, alternatives exist for treating these forms of compulsive behavior.

Lifestyle changes ranging from instituting aerobic exercise to regularizing one's sleep-wake cycle can also help alleviate mild anxiety, mild depression, and the dozens of other conditions for which the Prozac group are routinely prescribed in this country. Patients can follow programs that are combinations of these approaches, as alternatives to medications or in conjunction with them, to minimize drug exposure.

The book draws on my extensive experience treating patients in my private practice and at the Harvard University Health Services and affords a thorough review of the research published in psychiatric journals. My aim is to provide readers with the most up-to-date information possible about the strengths and weaknesses of serotonin boosters and the available alternatives, so that they can be better informed about whether or not to go on the drugs and how long to remain on them.

PART I

The Dangers of
Prozac-Type
Antidepressants

1

The Awakened Giant's Wrath
Risking Brain Damage

Maura: A Case of Disfiguring Tics

Late in her therapy, Maura took to lying back in the chair in my office, so relaxed she looked as if she drifted into a peaceful, tranquil state as we spoke. This involved a whole ritual for Maura: taking off her glasses and gently placing them on the small table beside the chair, leaning her head back into the soft headrest, closing her eyes, and relaxing her body, which seemed to melt down into the chair.

I would especially watch Maura's face at these times. A thirty-nine-year-old native of Ireland, Maura had milk-white skin and soft, delicate features framed by ringlets of auburn hair. As she continued to converse, reminiscing about her past, her face was a study in repose.

Unfortunately, this peace, hard won throughout a year of psychotherapy, was shattered by a chance observation on my part as I gazed at Maura's face. Suddenly I began to notice intense twitching all around her eyes. Her closed eyelids pressed more tightly shut. Waves of muscular contractions circled around her eyes. Bursts of this abnormal twitching punctuated periods of relative calm in which the muscles appeared to relax with just faint background activity.

How long had this twitching around Maura's eyes been present? I wondered. Was I just imagining that it was new? But I had been scrutinizing her resting face for months. Surely I would have noticed before. After I had observed the distinctive twitching for a number of weeks, I began to look for it when Maura was sitting upright with her eyes open and glasses on. Sure enough, the twitching was present at this time, too.

The image of Maura lying with her head as though on a pillow with twitches dancing around her eyes like fire came to haunt me because of what it portended. Maura had been in treatment with me for nearly a year. She originally had come for a second opinion about her medication, and had decided to stay on as a psychotherapy patient. The year before, her primary-care doctor had put her on Prozac for mild depression, because of her complaints of feelings of anxiety and tearfulness whenever she drove on highways. In two brief follow-up appointments, her doctor had doubled Maura's dose to 40 milligrams a day and given her a year's prescription for the drug. Primary-care doctors often see patients just once a year for an annual checkup. They frequently write year-long prescriptions for a host of drugs, from blood pressure medications to birth control pills. So when they prescribe serotonin boosters, writing a year's supply fits the routine for primary-care doctors even though this is not really appropriate to psychiatric drugs. At the end of the year, Maura consulted with me.

Maura grew up in war-torn Northern Ireland, in the small town of Ballymena. When she was eleven years old, she and her parents were innocent victims of a car bomb that exploded while they were driving to Belfast. Maura was badly injured, but she survived both the explosion and the trauma of witnessing the brutal death of both her parents. After living with an aunt for several years, Maura first came to the United States while in college. At the time that I met her, she was living in a Boston suburb with her American husband and their two daughters. As we pieced together her long-ignored, painful history, Maura realized that her depression began shortly before her elder daughter's tenth birthday. Like many parents, Maura would occasionally find herself daydreaming about what her life had been like at an age similar to her child's. As we talked, she realized her daughter was approaching the age Maura had been when her parents died. Her sudden sense of sadness and loss was worst while driving on highways, perhaps because it was a reminder of the fateful trip from her town into the city of Belfast. After several difficult months of reliving some of her traumatic memories and gaining a greater understanding of her symptoms, Maura gradually achieved the calm I was seeing when she leaned back in the chair. In anticipation of the well-earned end of therapy, we had decided to take Maura off Prozac and had lowered her dose from 40 to 20 milligrams.

"Have you noticed your eyes twitching lately?" I asked after observing the phenomenon for several weeks.

"No," said Maura, surprised.

I decided to write off the twitching as an anomaly, although now I wish I had made more of it. Not that this would have changed Maura's clinical course. A week later we stopped the Prozac. Prozac is a particularly long-lasting drug, lingering in the body for weeks. Two weeks after her last dose Maura called one day, frantic. "Something dreadful is happening to me," she said. "I need to see a neurologist. My lips are twitching and my tongue keeps darting out of my head." I told Maura that I would make time to see her, and to come to my office immediately. When she came, I was flabbergasted to see Maura's symptoms firsthand. Her lips now displayed twitching similar to that which I had observed around her eyes. But worst of all was the tongue-darting: fly-catcher-type movements in which her curled tongue darted in and out. The tongue-darting together with the twitching was disfiguring.

"Have I had a stroke? Do I have a tumor?" asked Maura, distraught.

"No," I said. "I don't think so. I believe this is a medication side effect."

"A medication side effect?" said Maura, dumbfounded.

"Yes. It looks like a tic disorder called tardive dyskinesia."

"Tar . . . what?"

"Tardive dyskinesia. It's a medication-induced tic disorder."

"But I'm not on any medication. I've just stopped the Prozac."

Could Prozac be causing Maura's tics? I wondered. I hadn't heard of Prozac causing these tics, but I had a lot of experience with them in association with major tranquilizers.

"I don't know why you're having these symptoms," I said, "but with other drugs they often worsen or emerge after patients stop taking them."

"What are you talking about?"

My mouth dry, feeling anxious and confused myself, I explained that tics are a well-known side effect of major tranquilizers.[1] Not only do these earlier drugs cause tics, they can also suppress or mask them, as long as the patient is still on the drug. The tics emerge only after the medication is stopped.

"You're not taking any other medications, right?" I asked Maura.

"Right," she confirmed.

"Have you ever been prescribed any other psychiatric medications?"

"Never."

Since Maura had been on Prozac for two years and had not taken any other psychiatric medication, it seemed that Prozac was probably responsible for the tics.

"How can the drug be causing something when it's gone?" asked Maura.

"No one knows the exact process by which the tics come about," I said. "But we do know that they are caused by long-term exposure to certain drugs. Sometimes the tics become severe enough to overcome the drug suppressing them. But sometimes they only appear after the drug is gone. Removal of the drug brings out the tics."

In fact, with major tranquilizers the tics are a result of brain damage brought on by the medication, but in our initial conversation I avoided using these words with Maura, because she was already terribly upset.

"Will this go away?" asked Maura.

"There's a good chance it will."

"A good chance? What are the chances?"

"I don't know. I've never heard of this with Prozac."

"What are the chances with other kinds of drugs?"

"Major tranquilizers? In about half of those cases, the tics slowly go away."

"And the other half?"

"They stay."

"They're permanent?"

"Sometimes they get a little better."

"But they're permanent?"

"Yes."

"Can they get worse?"

"In some cases."

"Oh, my God. Is there any treatment?"

This is one of the most difficult questions to answer, because patients are so desperate to maintain some hope. In fact, no treatment has proven effective for these tics. Many treatments have been tried, without success. The results with one treatment, vitamin E, have been inconclusive. Some studies show that vitamin E improves the course of the tics while other studies show that it does not. Since the results are not conclusive, I suggested vitamin E to Maura without creating too high an expectation.

After Maura left my office, I was distracted for the rest of the day. I was certainly familiar with the kind of tics she had. In fact, I had seen much graver cases, but only in patients who had been treated with older drugs. Physicians always feel guilty when their treatments cause new, sometimes worse problems. I hadn't started Maura on Prozac but had maintained her on it for a year. Had Prozac really caused the tics? I asked myself.

At the first opportunity, in a break between appointments, I pulled out the *Physician's Desk Reference,* a large volume containing the manufacturers' information on every prescription drug. I turned to the information on Prozac and found the section on side effects occurring in the nervous system. Sure enough, "extrapyramidal syndrome" was listed as a neurological side effect.[2] Extrapyramidal syndrome is the technical term for four closely related neurological side effects, including tics like Maura's.

Even more telling was an entry I found under "Postintroduction Reports." This section describes side effects that did not appear during the testing of a drug but only after its introduction to the market. Here I was taken aback to find what sounded like Maura's side effect. It was listed as a "dyskinesia," meaning abnormal movements, and described as a "buccal-lingual-masticatory syndrome with involuntary tongue protrusion," which took months to clear after the drug was stopped. This certainly sounded like the types of tics I was seeing with Maura. Buccal, lingual, and masticatory are technical terms for cheek, tongue, and chewing, respectively. Abnormal movements of the mouth, jaw, and tongue are the most common form of the tics.

Over the next month, Maura's tics worsened. The tongue-darting became more pronounced and more frequent. In addition, she developed chewing-the-cud type movements, indicating involvement of the jaw. I performed a neurologic screening test called the Abnormal Involuntary Movement Scale (AIMS test), used to assess and monitor the severity of medication-induced tics. For the AIMS test, Maura performed a series of exercises while sitting, standing, and walking. I rated a number of different measures of abnormal movements of the hands, arms, torso, pelvis, legs, gait, and mouth, all of which can become involved in the loss of motor control. So far, Maura had only facial tics, the most common form of this disorder. Other facial movements can include grimacing and snorting. Movements around the mouth are typically lip-smacking, blowing, kissing, or puckering.

By now Maura was avoiding social situations. When she did have to go out, she wore sunglasses and scarves in an attempt to hide the tics. Of course her husband was well aware of them and alarmed. Maura suffered from the strain of trying to hide the tics from her children in order not to frighten them.

During this time I began researching the side effects of serotonin boosters. Side effects such as Maura's can take months or years to develop and therefore are not picked up in the short, six-to-eight-week clinical studies required to win FDA approval for new psychiatric drugs. Since the FDA simply does not have the resources for a systematic program for monitoring late-appearing drug reactions, the agency is forced to rely on random, spontaneous reports from individual doctors. As a result, there is no central clearinghouse that makes thorough information on long-term side effects available, even to doctors. Instead, one has to comb through hundreds of often obscure medical journals tracking down spontaneous case reports.

I spent whole weekend days in the bowels of the Harvard Medical School Library poring through esoteric psychiatric journals. I was amazed to find reports estimating thousands of cases of four different side effects involving loss of motor control. The first is tics like Maura's. The second is neurologically driven agitation ranging from mild leg tapping to severe panic.[3] The third is muscle spasms, which, when they are mild, can cause tension in the neck, shoulder, or jaw, but can lock body parts in bizarre positions when severe.[4] The fourth is drug-induced parkinsonism, with symptoms similar to those seen in Parkinson's disease. In this chapter, I refer to this cluster of four, closely related syndromes—tics, agitation, muscle spasms, and parkinsonism—as the neurological side effects of the drugs. I found reports that they were occurring with all of the serotonin boosters: Prozac, Zoloft, Paxil, and Luvox.[5] These neurological side effects represent abnormalities in the involuntary motor system, which is a large group of nerves found deep in the older part of the brain.[6] Normally, these nerves influence automatic functions like eye-blinking, facial expression, and posture. When the brain attempts to compensate for the effects of a drug, it can lead to disorganized, chaotic activity in the involuntary motor system and loss of motor control—an example of Prozac backlash. In my experience, patients with any one of these side effects are at increased risk to develop the others, including tics.

One of the earliest published cases of tics associated with Prozac appeared in April 1992, in the journal *Neuropsychiatry, Neuropsychology, and Behavioral Neurology.*[7] Dr. David Fishbain was the lead author in a team of five doctors at the University of Miami School of Medicine. The patient was a seventy-seven-year-old woman who was taking Prozac for depression and back pain. Prior to treatment with Prozac, she had no abnormal movements.

Forty milligrams a day of Prozac dramatically improved the patient's depression and pain syndrome. However, she developed severe facial tics—described as "bon-bon" (candy-sucking-like movements) and "fly-catch" involuntary tongue protrusion. The movements "were repeated on a regular basis at a frequency of about 2–4 times per minute." The Prozac was stopped immediately and both the bon-bon and fly-catcher tics improved significantly within four weeks and disappeared over the course of several months.

Less fortunate was a forty-three-year-old depressed woman who developed tics while taking Prozac. This case was reported in the October 1991 issue of the *American Journal of Psychiatry* by Drs. Cathy Budman and Ruth Bruun in New York.[8] The patient's "tongue was observed to dart back and forth across her teeth, and it also rolled and curled laterally. There were sucking and blowing movements of her cheeks and intermittent clenching of her teeth. These movements kept her awake at night." This woman's tics subsided but did not fully clear even after the Prozac was stopped.

In the October 1993 issue of the *Journal of Clinical Psychopharmacology,* Drs. Dinesh Arya and E. Szabadi at the Queens Medical Center in Nottingham, England, reported a thirty-eight-year-old depressed woman who developed tics while taking Luvox.[9] The patient's tics consisted of bouts of dramatic rapid eye-blinking occurring four or five times a minute. Her lips would protrude and twist to the left side in "peculiar, repetitive, involuntary movements." She also developed severe clenching of her teeth, which left the muscles of her gums and jaw in pain.

Another published case is of a twenty-nine-year-old man treated with Prozac for obsessive-compulsive disorder, reported in the February 1996 issue of the *Journal of Clinical Psychiatry* by Dr. Nat Sandler of Lexington, Kentucky.[10] After more than a year on Prozac, the patient developed abnormal facial movements, especially around the mouth, including tongue-darting. The patient was aware of the movements but not incapacitated by them. However, Dr. Sandler reported, "Concern over gross thrusting of the tongue led to discontinuation of Prozac. Within two months . . . the tardive dyskinesia symptoms [tics] began to lessen; after six months, there were no signs of mouth movements." Warned Dr. Sandler, "Clinicians should consider the possibility of tardive dyskinesia [tics] occurring in patients taking Prozac."

Not all cases of tics associated with serotonin boosters have been facial. The large muscles of the trunk and limbs can become involved. Doctors Brian Fallon and Michael Liebowitz at the College of Physicians and Surgeons of Columbia University reported in the April 1991 issue of the *Journal of Clinical Psychopharmacology* on a thirty-eight-year-old woman with mild lupus who was started on 20 milligrams a day of Prozac for depression.[11] On Prozac, the patient developed "truncal dyskinesia [tics]" characterized by "mild involuntary pelvic rocking." Fallon and Liebowitz reported that the "pelvic dyskinesia [tics] . . . persisted without much change until after the Prozac was stopped."

Even more "complex movement disorders" after long-term treatment with Prozac were reported by Drs. Kersi Bharucha and Kapil Sethi at the Medical College of Georgia in 1996 in the journal *Movement Disorders.* One patient was a seventy-two-year-old woman admitted to the hospital because of loss of motor control that emerged after two years of treatment with 20 milligrams a day of Prozac. The patient had "constant" movements of her upper lip and jaw that made it difficult for her to speak. She had muscle contractions in the neck, jaw, floor of the mouth, and shoulders. Irregular, jerking movements occurred in both arms and legs. And the patient had involuntary wiggling of her toes. When the Prozac was discontinued "the involuntary movements ceased completely."[12] While some of the patient's tics, twitches, and jerking resembled what is traditionally seen with major tranquilizers, others did not.[13] Bharucha and Sethi advocated the use of the term "complex movement disorders induced by Prozac" because of the combination of a number of different involuntary movements in this and other patients. Much more research is needed to characterize the different types of tics, twitches, and jerking seen with these drugs.

As I told Maura about these and the many other cases I was finding, she asked, "Why aren't patients told about such severe side effects? Why do most doctors not even know?" In a way, this book is my answer to Maura's question, an attempt to remedy the lack of public information on this phenomenon.

While Maura and I anxiously monitored her tics, waiting to see what would happen, she wanted to review why she was put on Prozac in the first place. Here she was like a trauma victim wanting to go over the scene of the crime, looking for clues to how things might have gone differently. In fact, Maura's original symptoms had been relatively mild. For about a month she felt down with sudden feelings of great sadness and loss. She had episodes of feeling particularly upset while driving on the highway. But she had none of the physical symptoms of moderate and severe depression: difficulty sleeping, change in her appetite, poor concentration, inability to function, or suicidality. I thought Prozac was too powerful a drug for her mild distress. When she first consulted with me, I had said this to Maura. She had been taking Prozac for a year, however, and she felt stable on it and did not want to change. Since I had not been aware of the serious side effects emerging with the drug, at the time I did not push too hard for her to stop it. In retrospect, it was awful to think Maura might not have needed Prozac in the first place, given the disfiguring side effect she was now experiencing.

Psychiatric syndromes have two parts: a psychological core and superficial physical symptoms. As we discovered, the core of Maura's difficulty was her parents' traumatic death during her childhood. Long dormant, this trauma was reawakened by her daughter's approaching the age Maura had been when her parents died. Since Maura was not aware of the true source of her upset, she developed symptoms, becoming distressed and tearful, which were a kind of code or flag raised over her distress. Psychotherapy consists of deciphering the code and bringing the flag, or symptoms, down in the process. By contrast, medications only suppress symptoms. They are like crutches or Band-Aids. By themselves, they are never a cure. As such, they should be used only as adjuncts to the real healing, aids used to buy time and protect the healing process. Since medications entail risks and dangers, they should be used only when truly necessary. The least invasive medication should always be chosen, and even then, medication should be used judiciously.

Unfortunately, primary-care doctors do not have the training or time to evaluate and treat the psychological core of psychiatric syndromes. But under managed care and in HMO settings, they are under pressure to treat the psychiatric conditions of their patients. They are trained to follow simple protocols, or algorithms, which look only at the superficial symptoms. Maura, for instance, was medicated according to a simple "If depressed, then Prozac" model. Primary-care clinicians are not trained to explore questions like How mild or severe are the symptoms? How often are they occurring? Why is it happening at this particular time in the patient's life? This more informed, thorough approach requires a specialist—a psychiatrist, psychologist, or social worker—none of which were available to Maura until a year later, when she sought a second opinion from me on her own initiative.

At the two-month mark, Maura's AIMS test showed her tics had stabilized. They no longer appeared to be worsening.

"They seem to get worse when I'm stressed or anxious. I seem to chew and stick my tongue out more," said Maura, unconvinced they were stabilizing.

"Stress exacerbates these tics, for reasons that are not clear," I explained.

Relating a comment of her husband's, Maura added, "John says my tics disappear when I'm asleep."

"That, too, is characteristic."

By the third and fourth month Maura's tics were gradually improving. At the four-month mark, when I performed the AIMS test, the most dramatic of her tics, the chewing-the-cud and fly-catcher tongue-darting, were gone. By six months Maura's tics had largely cleared. She was left with permanent, subtle twitching around her mouth and eyes, but incorporated into her facial expression, these were not noticeable to the casual observer.

Maura only gradually regained her confidence in social situations. Losing the fear that a tic would suddenly act up in the middle of a conversation took months to achieve. Once she regained most of her former ease and was less self-conscious again, Maura no longer needed to be in treatment. She was finally able to stop therapy a few months after the ordeal of her tics.

Maura's case and my research confirming other, similar cases left me thoroughly sobered about the safety of these new serotonergic drugs, tics such as hers being *the* dread side effect of psychiatric medications because no effective treatment exists. With major tranquilizers, the earlier class of drugs associated with the tics, they develop silently, are often masked by the drugs that cause them, and can be permanent in as many as 50% of cases.[14] In some cases, the tics lead to wide-based, lurching gaits; swinging and flailing of the arms; or twisting and writhing of the hands. Why some patients develop the tics more quickly than others is not fully understood. They may be caused by cumulative damage resulting from exposure to certain drugs, viral infections, central nervous system diseases, and the loss of brain cells that occurs with normal aging. Thus the elderly are more likely to develop tics quickly, as are people with prior exposure to drugs causing similar damage. When the tics began appearing with major tranquilizers, it was thought that only certain vulnerable populations like the elderly or medically ill would develop them. It is now recognized that anyone can develop them, including young, healthy patients. With long-term exposure to the drugs, the emergence of tics steadily increases over time. A study being conducted at the Yale University School of Medicine has estimated that 32% of patients develop persistent tics after 5 years on major tranquilizers, 57% by 15 years, and 68% by 25 years.[15] In addition to patients who develop overt tics, many have tics that are suppressed by the drugs. When patients are taken off major tranquilizers specifically to look for tics previously not present, 34% of patients have tics unmasked by stopping the drugs.[16] With tics associated with serotonin boosters, we do not know how many patients will ultimately develop them or what percentage might be permanent. Serotonin boosters are still relatively new and these side effects have not been studied systematically. But what we know from the side effects with major tranquilizers is cause for serious concern.

The research I had done in response to Maura's case had taught me that serotonin boosters cause not only the tics but three other, closely related neurological side effects. Having witnessed the first of these disorders, I now wondered if I would see the other three. From my earliest days as a doctor, I learned to expect that drugs that cause one of these side effects will often cause the others as well. In addition to tics, the other neurological side effects are muscle spasms, agitation, and drug-induced parkinsonism. Had I seen them already, I wondered, and mistaken them for something else?

Might the "caffeinated" feeling so many people describe when starting serotonin boosters, in fact, be neurologically driven agitation in some instances? Later on, after being on the drugs weeks or months many patients develop "paradoxical fatigue." Most doctors consider this fatigue to result from the nervous system's being in chronic overdrive due to the drugs' stimulating effects. But might it be fatigue caused by drug-induced parkinsonism? How would one differentiate these symptoms from the patient's underlying depression? I was soon to find out.

Leslie's Amotivational Syndrome: A Case of Fatigue and Apathy

Leslie's internist asked me to see her in consultation. She explained that significant changes had occurred in Leslie's life in recent years. Leslie was in her mid-fifties, and all of her children were now grown and had left home. Struggling with the changes in her role, Leslie was having difficulty re-entering the job market. Over the course of three years, her internist had prescribed increasing doses of Prozac for her. Her dose was now at the maximum recommended, 80 milligrams per day. Concerned that her depression was still not better and possibly worsening, the doctor now wanted Leslie to have a psychiatric evaluation.

When I met Leslie in the waiting room, her burdened look did not strike me as unusual for a depressed person. Her handshake was limp. She was slow walking into the office. Was Leslie profoundly depressed? Was she showing me the worst of how she felt, wanting to be sure I got the picture of how bad things were? Were characterologic issues going to be prominent?

Once in the office, however, as we talked I gradually began to question whether Leslie was depressed. She was straightforward about missing her children and the role she played as a busy mother. But she seemed to have made peace with this. As she said, the children left gradually, giving her time to slowly adjust.

Leslie's job situation was more frustrating to her. She did not like interviewing for positions: "I hate trying to 'market my skills' in interviews," said Leslie. Surprisingly, she had specific ideas for a business of her own: "I love books. My friends who are librarians or book dealers tell me it's difficult to find people to restore old books—for example, to put new leather bindings on them. Even some new books have leather bindings in limited editions and, again, it's difficult to find people who can do the work. I'd like to take a course or two and invest in the equipment I'd need to set myself up in business. I'd love to do that kind of quality work. I'd also like to be responsible for my own financial fate and be able to make my own hours."

These were lively statements and ideas, not what one would expect to hear from someone profoundly depressed. "Why don't you just do it?" I asked.

Two things held Leslie back. Her husband had not been particularly supportive. He preferred her to get a more "regular, secure" job. But the bigger problem was her fatigue and indifference: "I'm slowed down. I don't get around like I used to. Although I have things I'd like to do, I feel unmotivated . . . apathetic. I don't know what's wrong."

"Is it your depression?"

"I don't feel depressed now. I might have been a few years ago, when my children started leaving. But I don't think I am now."

By this time, I agreed. But if Leslie was not depressed, what would explain her symptoms? Did she have some neurological condition? Was it a side effect of her medication? Could Leslie's lack of motivation and fatigue be due to parkinsonism, I wondered, sensitized to the possibility by Maura's case. Parkinsonism is a term used for drug-induced side effects that resemble the symptoms of Parkinson's disease in the elderly. Parkinsonism is generally considered reversible when the offending drug is stopped, while Parkinson's disease has an inevitably progressive course.

Parkinson's disease can make people feel profoundly fatigued and apathetic. Their facial expression, speech, walking, reaching motions, and all their movements make them look progressively as if they are in slower and slower motion. In severe cases, people are virtually immobilized, stuck in a frozen state of rigidity. Some patients develop a characteristic pill-rolling tremor in their fingers, which contrasts sharply with their prominent, overall inactivity.

As with Maura, Leslie's eyes provided the first clue to her real problem. In parkinsonism, diminished movement in the facial musculature renders the skin, or surface, of the face relatively flat and immobile. The eyes seem to move independently of facial expression. As I watched Leslie, I thought her eyes looked as though they were peering out from behind a mask, rather than a fully expressive face. Parkinsonism, I thought, would explain the incongruity between her mental agility and her slowed physical state. But I did not know Leslie's baseline as a point of comparison. Was this how she looked before the drug? Or was this a change?

As we continued to talk, I observed Leslie carefully. I noted that her slowness had a particular quality: When Leslie moved her body, she tended to do so en bloc, in a somewhat wooden manner. Again, this was subtle, the kind of observation one makes based on experience from having seen patients who developed parkinsonism on older drugs like major tranquilizers.

Finally, I asked Leslie if she would do a diagnostic test. "I'd like to see if you have any stiffness that might be a side effect of the Prozac," I explained. As we stood up, I asked Leslie to relax her arm. Holding her elbow in one hand and her wrist in the other, I slowly moved her arm about the elbow joint. Sure enough, I could feel the ratchet-like resistance to motion one finds in parkinsonism.

I told Leslie I thought her lack of motivation and fatigue were parkinsonism, a side effect of the Prozac. Leslie was quite shocked. She had an elderly uncle with Parkinson's disease. Any comparison with the ravages of his severe illness frightened her. I explained that her symptoms would probably clear up if we lowered or stopped her medication.

In the ensuing weeks, we gradually brought Leslie's dose down, ultimately stopping the medication altogether, since she did not become depressed again. Slowly, her energy and motivation returned. Her facial expression and general body movements became more fluid. Leslie was enormously relieved by her improvement. After she recovered from the shock that it was the medication that had been making her look depressed, Leslie began to pursue her plan for a business. She stayed in psychotherapy, using it for support in overriding her husband's, as well as her own, hesitations. Once he saw Leslie's energy and determination, her husband was actually quite helpful, working closely with her to find the right bookbinding equipment. While Leslie's venture did involve start-up costs, ultimately it was quite successful. She recently saw me in follow-up and told me she now has five people working for her.

As in Leslie's case, the distinction between worsening depression and parkinsonian side effects is often subtle. Making the correct assessment and intervention depends upon an awareness of the side effect and clinical experience. Unfortunately, her primary-care doctor had been unaware of this side effect occurring with serotonin boosters. Instead, the doctor clung to the idea that Leslie was suffering from the "empty nest" syndrome and thought her depression was worsening.

Numerous cases, small-scale studies, and articles on parkinsonian side effects in patients on serotonin boosters have been published. Writing in the November 1993 issue of *Human Psychopharmacology*, Dr. Michael Berk at the University of Witwatersrand Medical School in Johannesburg, South Africa, reported a twenty-six-year-old man with obsessive-compulsive disorder who developed parkinsonism after three months on Paxil, at a dose of 60 milligrams a day.[17] The patient's parkinsonian symptoms included rigidity and excessive salivation. When his dose was reduced to 40 milligrams a day, the parkinsonian side effects cleared.

Many authors have described cases where serotonin boosters dramatically worsened parkinsonian symptoms in patients with pre-existing Parkinson's disease. Patients with this disease have a particularly high incidence of depression and are therefore often prescribed antidepressants. Writing in the December 1994 issue of *Neurology*, a group of Spanish doctors headed by Dr. F. J. Jiménez-Jiménez at the University Hospital in Madrid described a thirty-five-year-old woman with early-onset Parkinson's disease who was put on 20 milligrams of Paxil.[18] Stated Dr. Jiménez-Jiménez: "One month later, all her symptoms had worsened." The patient had developed flattening of her facial expression, rigidity, "difficulty in performing fine finger movements with both hands, short steps, loss of associated movements, and postural instability." These markedly worsened symptoms took two months to clear after the Paxil was stopped.

Much more needs to be learned about the effects of serotonin boosters on existing or incipient Parkinson's disease in elderly patients. In a piece entitled "Serotonin, Depression, and Parkinson's Disease" in the August 1993 issue of *Neurology,* the Dutch neurologist Jan Hesselink laments, "Unfortunately, methodologically sound studies evaluating the efficacy of serotonergic drugs" in depressed patients with Parkinson's disease "are virtually nonexistent so far."[19]

Equally important may be cases of fatigue or indifference occurring in younger patients, in their twenties, thirties, or forties. Many people on Prozac-type drugs report a peculiar "bone-weary fatigue" in which they feel lethargic but not sleepy and, in fact, cannot fall asleep. They describe a "heaviness" in their bones, as though it is just too much to move. This fatigue can be quite severe and is relieved only by reducing the dose or stopping the drug. Other patients emphasize feeling indifferent on the medications. "All the same problems are present in my life but I just don't care anymore" is a frequent refrain. Some patients welcome this more "mellow" attitude toward life, although they may not be aware of the possibility that it entails serious risks. Other patients regard the change as more disturbing, saying that the drugs make them feel "blunted" or "flat" and not at all like their usual selves.

Because parkinsonism with these drugs has not been adequately studied, most doctors do not think of it as a possible cause of fatigue or indifference. But *Principles of Neurology,* the authoritative textbook by Adams and Victor, notes that fatigue and malaise are often the earliest symptoms of parkinsonism: "The fatigue of Parkinson's disease may precede the recognition of [more obvious] neurological signs by months or even years. It is probably a reaction to the subjective awareness of increasing disability occasioned by the akinesia [a disinclination to move]."[20] Since fatigue or indifference are common with Prozac-type antidepressants, they may be particularly worrisome indications of how many people are suffering from mild parkinsonian side effects and therefore are vulnerable in the long term to developing tics.

With major tranquilizers, research has shown the development of parkinsonism, in particular, predicts the later emergence of tics. Psychopharmacologist Guy Chouinard of the Royal Victoria Hospital in Montreal followed ninety-eight patients on the drugs for ten years. He found that the presence of parkinsonism increased the risk of later developing tics.[21] Chouinard presented this important study looking at risk factors for tics at the American Psychiatric Association's annual meeting in May 1990.

Ming and Cora: Cases of Muscle Spasms

Ming is a thirty-eight-year-old Chinese woman who lives in Singapore. Five months after starting Luvox, she developed severe tightening of the muscles in her jaw, resulting in involuntary clenching of her teeth. Ming's lockjaw became so severe that she had great difficulty chewing her food. Obviously, such a dramatic situation would be frightening. Ming's lockjaw improved when the Luvox was reduced from 100 to 50 milligrams but did not fully clear until the drug was stopped. Ming's case was reported by her psychiatrist, Siow Ann Chong, in the September 1995 issue of the *Canadian Journal of Psychiatry.*[22]

Ming's clenched jaw was caused by muscle spasms, another of the four closely related, neurological side effects. Muscle spasms are prolonged contractions of muscles that lock body parts in abnormal positions lasting for minutes to hours. This is in contrast to tics, which are short bursts of repetitive activity.

Cora was a twenty-two-year-old college student in Gainesville, Florida, when she sought treatment for depression. Because she had only a partial response to Prozac, her dose was increased to 80 milligrams over the course of three months. Ten days after reaching the 80-milligram dose, Cora developed severe lockjaw and spasms of the muscles in her neck and tongue.

The spasms were so frightening that Cora went to a hospital emergency room. There she was given Benadryl, which relaxed the muscles. Cora was sent home, but the spasms returned five hours later. She went back to the emergency room and was given a second dose of Benadryl.

Cora's psychiatrist stopped the Prozac, but three weeks later she was feeling depressed and asked to try the drug again. One week after being on just 20 milligrams of Prozac, Cora again developed severe lockjaw, neck tension, and tongue thickening. She again went to the hospital emergency room. This time, even though the Prozac was stopped, the spasms took three days to clear.

Cora's case was reported in the November 1990 issue of the *Journal of Clinical Psychiatry* by three doctors in Gainesville, Florida: Lawrence Reccoppa, Wendy Welch, and Michael Ware.[23] Her case illustrates another important point: Even though a side effect may clear, the nervous system can be left more vulnerable in the future. One sees this dramatically if the patient is re-exposed to the drug and proves more sensitive to developing motor abnormalities. When Cora was re-exposed to Prozac, her reaction was more severe, with the muscle spasms occurring after only one week on 20 milligrams, whereas the first time she was on the drug for three months and up to a dose of 80 milligrams before developing spasms. Say Reccoppa, Welch, and Ware at the conclusion of Cora's case, "Clinicians should be aware of this serious . . . side effect, especially in light of the current widespread use of Prozac."

Some cases of muscle spasms can be even more dramatic and frightening. Spasms affecting the arms, legs, or torso can lock the body in bizarre, twisted postures. In the January 1994 issue of the *American Journal of Psychiatry,* Dr. Mahendra Dave, of Syracuse, New York, reported on a fifty-four-year-old woman who developed acute spasms in her legs and back a month after starting 20 milligrams of Prozac a day.[24] The spasms caused bizarre posturing in which she tilted backward and to the right. When she tried to walk, the spasms caused her to drag her left foot. In addition to the bizarre posturing and foot-dragging, the patient developed a tremor in her lip called "rabbit syndrome" and spasms of the left eyelid that clamped her eye shut.

Instead of stopping Prozac, another medication (Cogentin) was added to suppress the side effects. On the drug combination, the spasms subsided over the course of three weeks. The use of additional drugs like Cogentin or Benadryl to treat muscle spasms is well known to doctors from their experience with the side effects in patients on major tranquilizers. Although many doctors suppress medication-induced movement disorders in this way, I worry that ongoing exposure to the offending drug will cause damage eventually leading to tics. My preference is always to take patients off the offending agent, whenever possible.

Much more common than these dramatic, published cases are milder instances in which patients complain of muscle tension in their shoulders, neck, or jaw. Often, patients have to be asked specifically about these side effects, because it does not occur to them that the muscle tension is related to the drug. The connection may become clear only when the drug is stopped and the pain disappears.

Mild to moderate spasms may affect as many as 10% of patients. This estimate comes from a clinical study of Luvox by the Italian psychiatrists V. Porro and S. Fiorenzoni. Of forty-one patients treated with Luvox, four complained of mild to moderate muscle spasms during the first week of treatment. Muscle spasms were the fifth most common side effect reported in the study published in the April 1988 issue of *Current Therapeutic Research*.[25]

Ironically, one of the first patients ever put on Prozac in the earliest stages of testing the drug developed acute muscle spasms. Writing in the *Journal of Neural Transmission* in 1979, Herbert Meltzer, a psychiatrist at the University of Chicago, described the twenty-five-year-old depressed patient as having neck spasms so severe that they twisted his neck and rotated his head into an abnormal position.[26] He also developed spasms in the muscles of his jaw. Eli Lilly had given Meltzer a grant to study the effects of Prozac and supplied the drug, which was not yet available to doctors. This was a decade before the pharmaceutical company began marketing Prozac for the general public. One wishes this patient had been an early warning sign to Lilly of the potential for serotonin boosters to cause not only muscle spasms but all four of these closely related neurological side effects.

Ron: A Case of Neurologically Driven Agitation

"I feel like I have coffee running into my veins," said Ron, as he crisscrossed the office, pacing compulsively. Ron was a forty-seven-year-old engineer, whom I had started on Paxil because of his severe depression. Since Ron had a large family to support and was concerned that his depression was threatening his job, using Paxil to jump-start him seemed reasonable. Whereas previously Ron had not been able to get out of bed because he was so depressed, now he could not sit still.

"I'm not feeling better," said Ron. "In fact, I'm feeling worse. I'm exhausted, but when I try to fall asleep I lie there tossing and turning with my legs kicking all night." In addition to the physical restlessness, he described the accompanying inner state: "My bones feel like tuning forks humming up and down my body." Ron paced ceaselessly, and looked as if he was going to crash into a table or a wall. "Believe me, I don't do any illegal drugs," he said. "I'm not withdrawing from anything. I don't know what's happening to me."

I asked Ron to sit in a chair so I could examine him.

"I can't sit down," Ron protested impatiently.

"I need you to try," I responded. "It's a test to see what's going on. I want you to sit as still as possible."

Ron had to hold himself down, his white-knuckled hands pulling against the arms of the chair. As he did, his feet displayed a telltale sign, tapping and dancing around the floor uncontrollably. This is a cardinal feature separating medication-induced agitation from psychologically driven anxiety. While patients who are anxious for psychological reasons may move around, they do not experience the same compulsive, relentless activity. Asked to sit still in a chair, an anxious patient might curl up in a ball, petrified but motionless. Ron could not do this. In medication-induced agitation, the patient cannot escape the urge to move, particularly to move the legs.

"Am I going crazy?" Ron asked desperately.

"Not at all," I reassured him. "This is a side effect of the medication."

Had I not known that Paxil can cause agitation, the fourth of the neurological side effects, I might have missed the correct diagnosis and instead thought Ron had developed an agitated depression. The distinction is crucial, because the appropriate intervention is the opposite. If Ron's depression was worsening, one would go up more quickly on the medication. But this would have made the agitation worse. Instead, knowing the agitation was medication-induced, I stopped the drug. Within days, his agitation cleared.

Ron was so "spooked" by the severe side effect that he refused to try another medication. While psychotherapy alone took a while longer to pull him out of the worst of his depression, he did fine without an antidepressant.

When severe, neurologically driven agitation can be quite dangerous, especially if the patient has not been warned about the side effect and confuses it with deterioration of his own emotional state. Some patients describe feeling as if their heads are "going to explode." Others compare the profoundly disturbing inner state to the feeling of fingernails scratching relentlessly up and down a blackboard. Some develop an "abject terror," which can precipitate psychosis and suicidality.[27]

Agitation was the first of the neurological side effects associated with Prozac-type medications to come to the attention of professionals. In 1989 a team of four Harvard Medical School psychopharmacologists at McLean Hospital, led by Dr. Joseph Lipinski, published an article entitled "Prozac-Induced Akathisia [Agitation]: Clinical and Theoretical Implications" in the *Journal of Clinical Psychiatry*.[28] Lipinski and his colleagues described five vivid cases. Within days of starting Prozac, one patient "reported severe anxiety and restlessness. She paced the floor throughout the day, found sleep at night difficult because of the restlessness, and constantly shifted her legs when seated." Two days after starting Prozac, another patient reported, "I couldn't keep my legs still. . . . I would find myself bicycling in bed or just turning around and around. I was embarrassed because I kept my roommate awake."

In this early article, appearing within two years of Prozac's release, Lipinski said the agitation was "clinically indistinguishable" from that caused by major tranquilizers, well known to cause these neurological side effects. Declaring neurologically driven agitation a "common side effect of Prozac," he estimated it occurs in 10–25% of patients. Similar reports of agitation with Zoloft, Paxil, and Luvox appeared after these drugs were introduced.

In mild cases, patients may only experience foot-tapping and a vague sense of needing to keep busy. "I cleaned my house for days when I first went on Zoloft," said one patient. Said another, "I had a desk and six bookcases that I wanted to refinish for some time. Right after I went on Prozac I spent weeks compulsively sanding and finishing the furniture. At the time, I thought it was because my depression had lifted. Now I realize it was because I couldn't sit still."

Lipinski may be right that this agitation is a very common side effect of the serotonin antidepressants. Many patients describe feeling "caffeinated" in the early weeks on the drug. When Prozac was introduced, Eli Lilly researchers coined the euphemism "activating" for the stimulating effects of the drug.[29] How often is this caffeinated effect in fact neurologically driven agitation?

Lipinski's early report might have served as more of a warning. Appearing in 1989, not long after Prozac was introduced, the report on Prozac-induced agitation might have raised concern that all four of the closely related neurological side effects would eventually appear. Unfortunately, this possibility was not adequately considered in the rush to prescribe the popular new medications.

While these four neurological side effects—parkinsonism, agitation, muscle spasms, and tics—are often discussed as separate, distinct side effects, patients can have more than one at a time. Indeed, the four may not be so distinct after all; they may just be different manifestations of the effects of certain drugs, toxins, or viral infections. Patients with Parkinson's disease caused by viral infections also evidence agitation, muscle spasms, and tics like those seen with the drugs. In his book *Awakenings,* neurologist Oliver Sacks vividly describes these postinfectious Parkinson's disease patients.[30] Thus, certain viruses, toxins, and drugs may induce a syndrome of which parkinsonism, agitation, muscle spasms, and tics are just different manifestations.

The Serotonin-Dopamine Connection

These dangerous neurological side effects—parkinsonism, agitation, muscle spasms, and tics—are known to originate in a particular region deep in the brain, the involuntary motor system. We do not know exactly how serotonin boosters induce them, but they appear to represent Prozac backlash, the brain's reaction to intruding chemicals. When a drug boosts serotonin in the brain, the brain's chemical balance is upset. The result is artificially induced fluctuations not only of serotonin but also of the many other chemicals that act in concert with it.

Prozac backlash is the brain's attempt to reverse the effects of drugs in this class. Whenever the drugs step on the chemical gas pedal, the brain tries to slam on the brakes. The result is jerking, stop-and-go oscillations in brain activity that can go out of control. Writing about these kinds of medication-induced side effects, neurologist Oliver Sacks describes them as "sudden and catastrophic oscillations," random, erratic instabilities, which he says are best explained by chaos theory.[31] Although Sacks was writing about the drug levodopa in patients with Parkinson's disease, he compared its side effects with those of major tranquilizers.

There are a number of scientific hypotheses for why this chaos comes about when serotonin is unnaturally boosted in the brain. The leading hypothesis is that boosting serotonin levels has repercussions on the levels of dopamine. Dopamine is a close chemical partner of serotonin. A large body of research over decades has implicated dopamine, not serotonin, in these disorders, regardless of whether they are caused by medications such as major tranquilizers or by diseases such as Parkinson's and Huntington's. As reports of these side effects occurring with the Prozac group have mounted, researchers have been puzzled by the question of how drugs that boost serotonin could cause side effects usually linked to dopamine. Scientists point to research showing a strong link between serotonin and dopamine in the involuntary motor system.[32] Dutch psychiatrist Jan Hesselink wrote in the August 1993 issue of *Neurology,* "From preclinical studies already a decade old, we learned that the relation between the serotonergic and dopaminergic systems is an intimate one."[33] Said Dr. Dinesh Arya in the December 1994 issue of the *British Journal of Psychiatry,* "Serotonin seems to modulate dopamine function."[34] Thus, fluctuations in serotonin levels lead to fluctuations in dopamine levels, which in turn result in loss of motor control.

In particular, elevated serotonin levels trigger a compensatory drop in dopamine. The relationship between serotonin and dopamine can be visualized as a seesaw: When serotonin goes up, dopamine goes down. And it is dopamine suppression that has long been associated with this loss of motor control.

In a particularly relevant study published in the July 1988 issue of *Biological Psychiatry,* Dr. Marc Laruelle used one of the serotonin boosters (Paxil) with a radioactive tag on it to study what locations in the human brain are especially targeted by the drug.[35] Laruelle found some of the highest concentrations of the drug's target cells in the involuntary motor system. Indeed, the highest concentration was found in the specific location (called the substantia nigra) known to be involved in Parkinson's disease.

Because of growing concern about these side effects, in recent years the serotonin-dopamine connection has become an area of active research. Neuroscientists have specifically designed experiments to test whether or not serotonin boosters are associated with a dopamine drop in the involuntary motor system. Dr. Junji Ichikawa at Case Western Reserve University School of Medicine measured dopamine levels in rats before and after administration of Prozac. In the August 1995 issue of the *European Journal of Pharmacology,* Ichikawa reported Prozac produced a 57% drop in dopamine in the involuntary motor system.[36] By contrast, older antidepressants did not produce a drop in dopamine.

A team of neuroscientists headed by Dr. Stephen Dewey at the Brookhaven National Laboratory tested the newest serotonin booster, Celexa. Dewey used not only biochemical measurements but also brain scans to measure dopamine activity in rats and baboons. Writing in the January 1995 issue of the *Journal of Neuroscience*, Dewey reported that Celexa produced a 50% drop in dopamine, again demonstrating that while the drugs put serotonin up, they simultaneously put dopamine down.[37]

Dr. A. DiRocco at the Mount Sinai Medical Center in New York found a dopamine drop in response to Zoloft. Writing in the February 1998 issue of the *Journal of Neural Transmission*, Di Rocco said that "motor activity is highly dependent on a balanced dopaminergic system" and that serotonin boosters appear to "specifically affect dopamine" levels in the involuntary motor system.[38]

Thus, the Prozac group's much-touted "selectivity" for serotonin may, in fact, be a liability: Boosted beyond ordinary levels, elevated serotonin could trigger a dangerous backlash, a compensatory drop in dopamine, resulting in the drugs' most severe neurological side effects. This is like squeezing one end of a balloon only to have it pop out elsewhere. Of course, this kind of secondary, indirect effect on other neurotransmitters renders the drugs not "selective" at all. Indeed, we now know the Prozac group has effects on other neurotransmitters in addition to serotonin and dopamine.[39]

One of the world's leading authorities on serotonin is Efrain Azmitia at New York University. Writing in the December 1991 issue of the *Journal of Clinical Psychiatry*, Dr. Azmitia called the serotonin system a "giant" neuronal system because of its far-reaching effects in the brain.[40] Dr. Azmitia described drugs that externally manipulate the system as "awakening the sleeping giant." The backlash triggered in the brain, reactions like a compensatory drop in dopamine, can be thought of as the awakened giant's wrath.

Working out the full details of the serotonin-dopamine connection may take decades or more. Meanwhile, we are left with the clinical reality of these serious side effects, which in some cases are devastating. The unfortunate irony is that drugs heavily promoted as correcting unproven biochemical imbalances may, in fact, be causing imbalances and brain damage.

To a layperson it may seem surprising that despite reports estimating thousands of cases of such serious side effects, more patients are not advised of them. But only by searching through academic and professional journals one by one does a researcher find the information reported here. In our computer age, a more centralized source of information on side effects would benefit doctors and patients alike. At this time, because we lack a systematic program for monitoring long-term side effects and alerting doctors, many clinicians who prescribe serotonin boosters have not been made aware of the dangers.

The Story of Major Tranquilizers

Of all the earlier mood-altering drugs to have been approved and later heavily controlled or withdrawn from the market, the most pertinent here are major tranquilizers, because they induce the cluster of neurological side effects now emerging with serotonin boosters. The first of these drugs, Thorazine, was introduced in the early 1950s by Smith Kline French. Eventually, there were more than a dozen drugs in this class of agents. Major tranquilizers suppress dopamine directly, whereas the Prozac group are thought to do so indirectly, via their effect on serotonin.

In the 1950s, 1960s, and 1970s, major tranquilizers were immensely popular as treatments for the same everyday conditions for which serotonin boosters are now so popular, including mild depression, anxiety, nervousness, and insomnia.[41] By 1965, Thorazine alone had been prescribed to 50 million patients in the United States.[42] Eventually, an estimated 250 million people worldwide were exposed to major tranquilizers.[43]

By the early 1960s, roughly ten years after Thorazine's introduction, numerous reports of tics, acute muscle spasms, parkinsonism, and agitation resulting from these drugs had been reported in medical journals. Since muscle spasms, agitation, and parkinsonism could all be relieved to some extent with additional drugs, the tics, for which no treatment worked, slowly emerged as the most serious in the cluster of closely related side effects.

By the twenty-year mark in 1973, 2,000 cases of the tics had been reported.[44] Only at this point did some doctors begin sounding the alarm among professionals. They were vigorously opposed by drug proponents, however, who insisted the tics were rare, since there were only 2,000 cases out of the millions on the drug. Drug advocates alleged that only certain "vulnerable" populations like the elderly or those with pre-existing brain damage would get tics. Those concerned about the side effects countered that the reported cases represented only random, spontaneous ones and systematic studies might well show a much higher percentage of patients affected.

In a good, if unfortunate, example of the clash between opposing sides, at the twenty-year mark in 1973, psychiatrist George Crane published a rousing article in the journal *Science* in which he raised the alarm about the neurological side effects of major tranquilizers, especially permanent tics.[45] Twenty years after Thorazine had been introduced, Crane lamented, "Many physicians are still unaware of this problem or seem to be completely unconcerned about it." Crane estimated that tics occurred in "at least 5% of patients exposed to drugs for several years. . . ." He criticized the "indiscriminate and excessive use of potentially dangerous drugs" and called for more thoughtful treatment programs balancing drugs with psychological interventions.

In the same year, in the *Archives of General Psychiatry,* Daniel X. Freedman, a strong proponent of the increasing reliance on medication in psychiatry, blasted back at "uninformed alarmists" trying to raise concerns about the dangerous side effects of the drugs.[46] Freedman excoriated psychiatrists like Crane, calling them "extremists among the consumer advocates."

Eventually, the drug proponents were proven profoundly wrong in their vitriol for patient advocates. By 1980, repeated systematic studies using neurological screening tests to look carefully for early, mild tics found them in an astounding 40% of patients treated with major tranquilizers, many of whom had been on the drugs for less than two years.[47] In addition, landmark malpractice cases awarded patients huge settlements if they had not been adequately warned of the tics. Finally, the medical profession began to take these neurological side effects seriously, severely limiting the use of major tranquilizers to only the most serious conditions, such as schizophrenia. Only in 1985, because of intense pressure resulting from media coverage of the side effects, did the FDA finally require manufacturers to add a warning to the drugs' labels, alerting doctors and patients to these serious side effects.[48] This was more than thirty years after the introduction of Thorazine and decades of indiscriminate use of the popular drugs. Originally, when they were prescribed to the general population, these drugs were simply called tranquilizers. As they fell from favor, however, they were renamed "major" tranquilizers to distinguish them from the Valium-type sedatives, which were called "minor" tranquilizers. As the original tranquilizers became discredited, Valium-type agents replaced them for conditions like anxiety and insomnia in the general population. Valium-type drugs do not cause the same neurological side effects as major tranquilizers, although they have other problems. Eventually, major tranquilizers were renamed again: Today they are officially called "antipsychotics" in an effort to distance the name "tranquilizer" from any association with these dread neurological side effects. But this kind of renaming confuses people, by veiling the history of a discredited class of drugs. Many doctors practicing today are unaware how popular and widely prescribed these drugs were in the 1950s, 1960s, and 1970s. I adhere to the name "major tranquilizers" because it is still used interchangeably with the name "antipsychotics" and serves as a reminder that these drugs were the Prozac of their day.

Experts now acknowledge that all patients on major tranquilizers—

even young, healthy patients—can eventually develop tics. Most psychiatrists consider a key factor to be total, cumulative exposure to the drugs. Being on a low dose for a long enough time can eventually cause the same cumulative damage as being on a high dose for a short period of time. The June 1990 issue of *Clinical Psychiatry News* reported on psychiatrist Guy Chouinard's research on tics induced by major tranquilizers: "It appears that drug exposure of 15 years or more would lead to almost certain risk for tardive dyskinesia [tics]."[49]

Now some of the world's best-informed psychopharmacologists are comparing serotonin boosters to major tranquilizers because of the similarities in their clinical uses and side effects. Ronald Pies, who is on the faculty of both Harvard and Tufts medical schools and the author of a textbook of psychopharmacology, wrote a special editorial in the December 1997 issue of the *Journal of Clinical Psychopharmacology*, entitled "Must We Now Consider SSRIs [Serotonin Boosters] Neuroleptics [Major Tranquilizers]?"[50] In the editorial, Pies discussed the worrisome emergence of neurological side effects with serotonin boosters at some length. Although he concluded that Prozac-type drugs are not exactly like major tranquilizers, he cited research showing that they can be used to treat conditions formerly treated with major tranquilizers, indicating that they may, indeed, have "properties" of these earlier drugs.

Similarly, in a keynote address at an October 1998 Harvard Medical School conference on psychopharmacology, Ross Baldessarini, professor of psychiatry and neuroscience at Harvard, said, "The traditional view of drugs and particular classes as being simply antipsychotic [major tranquilizer], simply antidepressant . . . those boundaries are breaking down. . . . You have to be thinking in a different way of how to categorize these" drugs.[51]

In his 1997 book *The Antidepressant Era*, David Healy also comments on our emerging understanding of the overlap between serotonin boosters and major tranquilizers. Healy is a psychiatrist at the University of Wales College of Medicine and one of Europe's leading authorities on psychiatric drugs. Healy wrote that the effects of serotonin boosters "lie midway between the effects of classical antidepressants and classicial neuroleptics [major tranquilizers]."[52]

Regarding tics associated with serotonin boosters, some doctors point to published cases in which the abnormal movements cleared when the drug was stopped and express the hope that this will be true for the majority of cases. Unfortunately, similar hopes and reassurances were once made on behalf of major tranquilizers. Even drug advocates acknowledge that the published cases reflect a fraction of the true incidence of any side effect. We simply have no idea of the frequency of tics with serotonin boosters or their likely time course. The largest databases on side effects are kept by pharmaceutical companies themselves. Most of the information the FDA has on side effects is forwarded to them by drug manufacturers. Eli Lilly acknowledged in a letter to one doctor who reported Prozac-induced tics that the "true incidence is difficult to determine. . . . It is possible for an event [side effect] to be coded [i.e., recorded in Lilly's databases] as one of several related terms." In other words, a side effect may be logged in databases under a variety of different labels. But experts argue this can obscure the true frequency of side effects. The problems with the labyrinthine databases used by pharmaceutical companies to monitor side effects are discussed in detail in Chapter 4.

Do we this time want to ignore the early warning signs of these effects with serotonin boosters? Should the same pro-drug, authoritarian approach prevail for another decade or two, as it did with tranquilizers? Surely we know too much about these side effects to again take the cavalier attitude "let's see before alerting the public." Even if disfiguring tic disorders turn out to be infrequent, with tens of millions of people having been on serotonin boosters, hundreds of thousands could be affected. If they occur with anywhere near the frequency seen with major tranquilizers, millions would be affected.

Sharon, Jonathan, and Carl: Cases of Memory Problems

Sharon was a hairdresser in her mid-forties who owned her own busy salon with a dozen people working for her. Acutely aware of appearances and hygiene because of the business she was in, Sharon had always been embarrassed by her habit of biting her nails. Most of the women who worked for her and many of her clients had beautifully manicured nails, which Sharon was never able to achieve.

When Sharon complained about her nail-biting to her primary-care doctor, he suggested Zoloft for the "obsessive" habit. Although surprised by the recommendation, Sharon was game to try. Indeed, she was quite surprised when the drug stopped her nail-biting within a few weeks, by which time her dose had been raised to 100 milligrams a day.

Sharon's enthusiasm for the drug changed abruptly when she developed serious memory problems: "I just suddenly forget all kinds of things. One night my husband and I were going to a party at the home of our best friends. I had picked him up after work and was driving. It was dark out and raining heavily, so I was concentrating on the road, hyperfocused on the immediate traffic around me. Suddenly, my mind went blank while I was stopped at an intersection. I couldn't remember where we were going! When my husband told me, I had to ask him for directions! I didn't know where our friends lived, even though I'd been there hundreds of times. Both my husband and I were so unnerved, I pulled over to the side of the road and he took over driving."

When the memory lapses began happening "constantly," Sharon went back to her primary-care doctor. Concerned about the severity of the problem, he referred her to a neurologist. Sharon had a complete neurological workup, which found nothing to explain the dramatic memory lapses. The neurologist concluded the problem must be Zoloft. When her doctor lowered Sharon's Zoloft dose to 50 milligrams, her memory problems improved significantly but did not go away completely. At that point, she consulted me for a second opinion.

Like a great many clinicians, I felt nail-biting was too trivial a reason to be on such a powerful drug, and I advised Sharon to stop altogether. When she went off Zoloft, her memory lapses cleared.

Most patients who complain of memory problems have much more subtle difficulties. Jonathan was in his late twenties and a medical student when I started him on Prozac because he was severely depressed. He responded well to the drug and within a month was no longer depressed.

A short while later, however, Jonathan developed subtle but distinct memory problems. "I have trouble finding the word for something, like a person's name," he said. "I know that I know the name, but I can't retrieve it. I can't bring it up from my memory. Or someone's phone number. A close friend whose phone number I have always known, yet suddenly I can't recall it. This is definitely new. I never had these kinds of problems before. People have always commented that my memory was like a steel trap. It's just not the same anymore."

Yet another difficulty was that Jonathan would forget the "context" in which he learned something: "I've always remembered things in a lot of detail. Now I remember some things without any context. I might remember that a good friend and his wife have separated and are getting a divorce. But I can't remember when I learned it, who told me, where we were at the time, and what else we were talking about. I might have learned it just a few days before, but for the life of me, I can't recall the context."

Being a student whose performance depended on his memory, Jonathan was disturbed by this side effect. He talked to a friend who experienced the same problem on Prozac. Said Jonathan, "If someone told me, 'You've lost five miles an hour on your fast ball,' I'd say: 'Well, it doesn't matter. I don't pitch anymore.' But I feel like I've lost five miles an hour of my mind, and that's a serious problem."

His memory problems motivated Jonathan to get off Prozac even faster than we originally planned. Within a month of stopping the drug, his memory was back to normal.

Some patients have memory problems because of their depression. But Sharon was on Zoloft because of nail-biting, and Jonathan's difficulties started after he was no longer feeling depressed on Prozac.

Memory problems can be more dramatic in the elderly. Carl was a seventy-three-year-old man whom I put on 20 milligrams a day of Prozac for depression. Carl was in excellent physical health. Indeed, he still worked three days a week in the family business, a jewelry manufacturing company, which two of his sons now ran. He worked in the customer service office, overseeing the processing of orders.

Three weeks after starting Prozac, Carl reported, "I'm feeling less depressed but I'm having severe trouble with my memory." When I asked Carl to describe an example, he responded, "At work last week I couldn't close out the new orders. It's a procedure I've done weekly for years. You have to know how to categorize and break down the different types of orders so all the totals come out accurately. I just stared at the blank pages and didn't know what to do. I was so embarrassed I actually considered fudging the report, hoping someone would catch the problem and fix it. But I realized that if it wasn't picked up, it could lead to much worse difficulties. So I went quietly to one of my sons and explained I couldn't remember how to do this task. We were both worried I'd had a stroke or something until we thought of the drug." When he went off Prozac, Carl's memory problems cleared.

In still another example, Lauren Slater, a teacher of creative writing and a practicing psychologist in Boston, says in her 1998 memoir *Prozac Diary*, "I am fearful of the as-yet-undiscovered side effects. . . . Lately I have become especially concerned about Prozac and memory. I used to be able to read a paragraph and recite back its phrases in near-perfect order. I never before needed an appointment book. . . . I am not so old [in her mid-thirties] that I should frequently forget the names of towns I've lived in, streets I've roamed, dishes I have always savored. People I have loved. Gaps in my cognition are appearing, places where the denim is worn so thin the skin shows through."[53]

Major tranquilizers have long been suspected of causing cognitive deficits and impairment in intellectual functioning.[54] These concerns surfaced only after the drugs had been on the market for decades and their use had become limited to schizophrenics. Unfortunately, the concerns have not been adequately investigated and we are not equipped to recognize the signs of these drug effects.

Silent Brain Damage

A final, serious concern with these neurological side effects is silent brain damage occurring in patients who do not develop overt symptoms. We still do not fully understand how tics reflecting permanent brain damage develop with major tranquilizers. But when one looks at the symptoms, the best model to explain them is that the appearance of noticeable tics is merely the final stage in a process of slow, progressive damage. Even in patients who do not develop tics, significant damage may have occurred. One sees this dramatically in patients restarted on a drug who quickly develop tics or other side effects not present during the previous course of the medication. Prior exposure left them with significant injury, which then predisposes them to rapid development of the side effects with just a little additional damage from the re-exposure.

As we age, everyone is vulnerable to developing a variety of neurological conditions such as Parkinson's disease, senile tics, gait abnormalities, stooped posture, and loss of cognitive functioning. These arise from a lifetime of cumulative damage to the brain from many causes: drugs, environmental toxins, viruses, and the loss of brain tissue that accompanies the normal aging process. Will silent damage caused by a serotonin booster accelerate the aging process and make some people more prone to develop neurological symptoms later in life? In some instances, Parkinson's disease is caused by viral infections. In one form of postinfectious Parkinson's disease seen after World War I, some patients did not develop symptoms until twenty-five years after the original exposure to the viral toxin.[55] Their symptoms are thought to have developed because of a variety of factors, including the cumulative effect of the original damage plus the loss of nerve cells and additional damage that accompany aging.

In the case of Parkinson's disease, we know the group of cells in the brain that are destroyed. The cells are believed to be weak links in neural circuitry particularly vulnerable to damage. Autopsy studies have shown that by age sixty individuals who do not have Parkinson's disease have lost about 40% of cells in this region as a result of normal aging.[56] By contrast, patients with Parkinson's disease have lost 80% or more of the cells in this region. If normal aging claims 40% of the cells and patients with Parkinson's disease have lost 80%, this normally leaves a comfortable reserve of 40% offering protection against the disease.

We know a great deal about Parkinson's disease because this is such a well-studied entity, but this model of a comfortable reserve that can be eroded may well apply to other areas of the brain and symptoms that are less well understood. What if being on a serotonin booster for a decade damages a quarter or a third of the cells in a particular region of the brain? This might not be sufficient to produce symptoms in a young patient, but would dangerously narrow the margin of safety later in life. Will someone who has been on a serotonin booster for a decade in her twenties be prone to prematurely develop neurological conditions—senile tics, gait disturbances, memory loss, personality changes, or dementia—because of silent damage sustained years earlier while on the drug?

The best-known diseases of the involuntary motor system, Parkinson's and Huntington's disease, can cause dramatic personality changes and severe dementia as they progress. We now know that the involuntary motor system is crucial not only to motor behavior but to motivation and information processing of all kinds as well, because it is in constant communication with the cerebral cortex, the site of higher cognitive functioning. This is why damage to these deep brain structures can eventually destroy personality, intellect, cognition, and memory.[57] Indeed, some experts believe there is considerable overlap between the dementia seen in diseases of the involuntary motor system and the dementia seen in Alzheimer's disease.

Recently a physician colleague of mine had to travel to California to put his mother in a nursing home because severe memory loss made it impossible for her to continue living independently. In addition to disabling memory deficits, his mother's personality had changed profoundly in the years immediately preceding the move to the nursing home. Whereas all her life she had been a strong-willed, independent woman who ran her own business, now she was a timid, docile shadow of her former self. "For all intents and purposes my mother is gone," said the colleague. "She's semi-living. What's left is not the woman I knew." The changes were all the more tragic because otherwise his mother was in good physical health.

During the trip, my colleague and his wife visited his mother's neurologist, who showed them a CAT scan of her brain. The scan showed significant loss of brain cells, thinning of the tissue, and resulting expansion of the fluid-filled cavities in the brain. While the scan explained his mother's symptoms, what puzzled the doctors was that the tissue loss was so advanced for someone her age. Her brain scan looked like that of someone ten to fifteen years older.

As they left the hospital, my colleague's wife asked, "What could have caused this to happen? Your mother wasn't an alcoholic. She hasn't had any strokes. She didn't smoke. What can it be?"

"The only thing I can think of," he responded, "is that for the past thirty years she's taken every popular psychiatric drug to come along." The majority of them were major tranquilizers and antidepressants, most recently Prozac and Zoloft. The colleague related the story to me because he had seen patients with dramatic memory loss on serotonin boosters. As a physician, he is concerned that psychiatric drugs can cause silent injury to the brain over many years in ways we do not yet understand.

Patients Have a Right to Know

Many patients looking for information on these side effects have to turn to chat rooms on the Internet, support groups in cyberspace for people on the drugs, because so little official information is available. In this Internet correspondence, people post notices or questions to which others can then respond. A number of patients have brought me representative printouts from chat rooms with names like alt.support.depression, alt.support.anxiety-panic, and alt.support.ocd at Web sites with names like www.dejanews.com. Reading the Internet correspondence, I was struck by the similarities between what people are reporting on the Web and what I have seen in my office.

Asked one person, "Anyone on SSRIs [serotonin boosters] get real bad, i.e., terminal leg twitching? Anyone know anything about this?"

Responded another, "There is some research (I've seen it posted here a couple of times) that SSRIs lead to a dopamine drop, which is the current theory for how they cause these side effects."

"In the past, I've occasionally experienced an eyelid twitch or tic, but it seems that the condition has increased considerably since taking the Luvox," said a third correspondent. "Has anybody else experienced this?"

"I find I get a 'flutter' or 'twitch' under my eyelid. I used to get this occasionally if I was tired, but since taking Zoloft, I find I am getting this much more often, even after what seems like a good night's sleep. It's not a blink, just a twitching feeling around the eyelids (sometimes top, sometimes bottom). It seems to happen quite randomly during the day and I'm not sure if it is visible to others. So the proverbial question, 'Am I nuts' or has anyone else had this side effect with Zoloft?"

"Oh, my goodness, yes! I had that happen to me all the time on Zoloft and thought maybe it was my imagination! It's weird, hey? I often wondered if other people could tell, but I don't think they can. So no you aren't nuts, unless I am too."

"I'm curious about the muscle twitches I've had on Paxil. Actually, I'd call them spasms. My stomach muscles will twitch so badly that it'll wake me up at night. Has anybody else experienced these spasms?"

"Yup. Sounds familiar, and otherwise normal, for SSRIs."

"When I was on Effexor, I got this weird side effect: While I was falling asleep or when my body was relaxed, like when I was lying down watching TV, I would get twitching in my legs and head/neck, like involuntary movements. Now that I've decreased my dose from 225 milligrams per day to 150, it doesn't happen nearly as often but does happen on occasion. Am I the only one who's had this weird effect?"

"I started Paxil a couple weeks ago. I've been getting occasional muscle twitches, usually in my legs. Actually, I don't know if 'twitches' really defines it very well. What happens is a muscle will all of a sudden tighten up with a jerk, causing an involuntary movement. Is this muscle-twitch stuff a big deal? Or is it just one of those miscellaneous 'perks' that comes from using antidepressants? If it's relevant I'm on Buspar as well. But this stuff started with the Paxil so I think that's what's causing it."

Reading this entry, I thought, Combinations of Buspar and a serotonin booster may be worrisome, since both have been implicated in involuntary movement disorders.[58] Also worrisome are combinations of serotonin boosters and major tranquilizers. And increasingly, patients are prescribed two serotonergic drugs simultaneously in what psychopharmacologists call "drug cocktails," again, compounding the risks.

Still another person responded to the above entry:

"I've never eaten Paxil but I got lots of twitches from Zoloft and from Wellbutrin. My doctor was a little surprised at my twitches, but not completely. I spoke to a couple of doctors about it including a Parkinson's disease researcher. I just had to get off those drugs because the twitches eventually caused me too much anxiety."

Patients should not have to turn to the Internet in hopes of finding information that ought to be readily available from their doctors. Unfortunately, the history of delayed reaction to these side effects with major tranquilizers appears to be repeating itself with serotonin boosters. In spite of reports estimating thousands of cases of neurological side effects, the reaction is again slow, marked by hesitancy to inform the public. The spontaneous reports by clinicians are considered to represent a small fraction of the total number of cases, which only more systematic monitoring would expose. In recent years some psychiatrists have tried to call professional attention to the problem. In the February 1995 *Canadian Journal of Psychiatry,* Dr. Paul Hoaken wrote an "alert" on involuntary motor disorders with serotonin antidepressants.[59] In the October 1996 *Journal of Clinical Psychiatry,* Dr. Raphael Leo wrote a review article called "Movement Disorders Associated with the Serotonin Selective Reuptake Inhibitors" [SSRIs, i.e., serotonin boosters], in which he said, "This article addresses a previously underrecognized but clinically significant consequence of SSRI use, namely, the development of movement disorders. These disorders can be uncomfortable for patients, influence compliance, and contribute to significant psychosocial and occupational impairments."[60] In the January 1997 *Psychiatric Times,* psychopharmacologist Frank Ayd said of the published reports of antidepressant-induced tics, "In most instances, TD [tardive dyskinesia]-like symptoms [tics] did not improve with Prozac discontinuation."[61]

Concerns have been raised over whether any one or two of the serotonin boosters are more likely to cause these side effects than the others. In February 1993, the British Committee on the Safety of Medicines, the equivalent of our Food and Drug Administration, raised concerns in their newsletter, *Current Problems in Pharmacovigilance,* that some neurological side effects seemed to occur "more frequently with Paxil" than with other serotonin boosters.[62] In test tubes, Paxil is one of the most potent of the serotonin boosters.[63] The following month, however, Vivien Choo in the British medical journal *Lancet* examined the database of the Drug Safety Research Unit in Southampton, England, and concluded that this was not the case. Reported Choo in the *Lancet,* "Comparison with PEM [prescription event monitoring—i.e., side-effect monitoring] data on two other SSRIs, Luvox and Prozac, show that the reactions are not commoner with Paxil than with these two drugs. . . ."[64] Choo concluded that "the reactions seem to be a class effect," meaning they occur with all the drugs in the Prozac group.

Significantly, there is beginning to be some official recognition of the problem: In the most recent edition of the American Psychiatric Association's *Diagnostic and Statistical Manual of Mental Disorders (DSM IV),* the mental health professional's diagnostic bible, a specific category was added recognizing these antidepressant-induced movement disorders.[65] Most recently, psychopharmacologist Ronald Pies (cited earlier for his comparing serotonin boosters to major tranquilizers) published an article in the January 1999 issue of the *Psychiatric Times* in which he advocated that patients on serotonin boosters should be informed of these potentially dangerous side effects and evaluated for whether or not they are experiencing any of them.[66] But not all physicians agree with the approach of Dr. Pies. Shortly after his article was published, I attended a Harvard conference at which another leading psychopharmacologist gave a talk on serotonin boosters. This psychopharmacologist said Pies was "crazy" to suggest informing patients. He protested, "You can't tell patients whom you're giving something that's supposed to help them that it may poison them." He insisted, "We have to put the best face on our treatments."

A colleague in the next seat commented under his breath, "Would he have said the same about Thalidomide [the psychiatric drug that later proved to cause severe birth defects], morphine, and amphetamines when these were popular prescription drugs in their day?" Should doctors not have voiced their concerns to patients taking these drugs as serious side effects began to emerge? Or should they have remained silent and ridden the enthusiasm for the popular medications for as long as it lasted?

While doctors debate what people should be told, many patients with early, mild cases of the neurological side effects of serotonin boosters may go undetected. Instead of diagnosing them early, patients will continue to be exposed to the drugs when this could have been prevented, just as happened with major tranquilizers. Especially in managed care settings, little or no effort is made to periodically reassess whether a patient's dosage can be reduced or the drug stopped. Instead, the drugs are thoughtlessly prescribed year after year. Often the dose needed to maintain the effects of these drugs once they are working is much lower than the dose required for start-up. In my experience consulting to patients who have been treated with these drugs, about 75% are able to dramatically reduce their dose or eliminate the drug altogether.

In light of these neurological side effects, we should especially question how freely these drugs are being prescribed to children. When major tranquilizers were in vogue, they were readily prescribed to children for mild anxiety, insomnia, or hyperactivity. The drugs are no longer used in this way on children because they cause tics. Current estimates are that serotonin boosters are being prescribed to over half a million children in this country, with pediatric use of the drugs one of the fastest-growing "markets."[67] This in spite of repeated studies showing antidepressants are no more effective in children and adolescents than placebos.[68] Should we not be protecting children, with their developing nervous systems, from drugs with potentially serious side effects?

With reports estimating thousands of cases of these serious side effects occurring with serotonin boosters and research documenting the drugs' effects on dopamine as the likely cause, we have strong evidence the drugs are doing something worrisome in the involuntary motor system deep in the brain. How many people on a serotonin booster are silently developing tic disorders? How many others are incurring silent brain damage that could accelerate the aging process, even if they do not develop overt symptoms? Drug advocates and advertisements that portray serotonin boosters as having only trivial, transient side effects are terribly misleading. We need more systematic, long-term monitoring of patients who have developed these side effects and more thorough research on how the drugs cause them. But while we are waiting for definitive answers that could take years, even decades, patients should know about these conditions sooner rather than later in order to make informed choices.

2

Held Hostage

Withdrawal, Dependence, and Wearing Off

Tanya: A Case of Withdrawal

Wearing her bathing suit, a towel draped over her shoulder, Tanya emerged from the locker room of her health club and walked up the flight of stairs to the pool. She was delighted to find only a few people in the pool. Indeed, the lane reserved for swimming laps was empty, so she would have it to herself. Dropping the towel on a bench, she dove into the cool, refreshing water.

On her second lap, Tanya was just beginning to hit her stride when suddenly, like a bolt of lightning, she was struck by what felt like electrical currents coursing through her body. Terrified, she flailed in the water, overcome by the shocks and unable to regain her balance. As the jolting sensations pulsed in her head, she thought a short circuit must have electrified the water in the pool and she was going to die.

Screaming, Tanya was pulled from the water by a fellow swimmer who saw she was in distress. As she gasped for breath, Tanya blurted out, "What's happening? The shocks, do you feel the electric shocks?"

"No." Her rescuer looked at her, perplexed. Another shock reverberated through Tanya. Feeling dizzy and tremulous, she lay back on the cold tile along the pool's edge. Within minutes several people were surrounding her. One particularly warm, gentle woman knelt down beside her and began drying Tanya and wrapping her in towels. Eventually, Tanya sat up on a poolside bench and began to take stock of her situation.

Throughout this time the electric shock–like sensations continued. They were jolting, "zapping" sensations in her brain and traveled down her shoulders and arms. She felt nauseous and dizzy, as if the room were spinning, with a strange "buzzing" in her ears. Something was wrong with her vision. She was seeing shooting-star-like flashes of light. Moreover, her vision kept "jumping," moving back and forth staccato-fashion, jumping a few inches to the left and then to the right.

In spite of the dramatic symptoms, Tanya was fully conscious and alert. The health club manager suggested calling an ambulance to take her to the hospital, but she declined. She had already decided she wanted to talk to me. Just two days before, Tanya had stopped taking 20 milligrams a day of Paxil. She feared the symptoms she was experiencing might be a return of the panic attacks, for which she was originally put on the medication.

Saying she wanted to call her doctor, Tanya made her way back to the locker room with the assistance of the kind woman who had first started to towel her. On her feet, Tanya found herself unsteady and had to hold on to the wall because she had trouble walking in a straight line. She was able to dress herself, although she found the movement caused a worsening of the electric shock sensations and other symptoms.

Fortunately, Tanya was able to reach me. I urged her to take a taxi to the office right away. Half an hour later Tanya, led in by the woman who had helped her at the poolside, was sitting in my office very visibly shaken. She described what had happened vividly: "In the pool I thought I was being electrocuted. What's going on? My panic attacks last summer weren't like this."

"These are not symptoms of panic attacks," I explained. "They may be withdrawal symptoms from having stopped Paxil two days ago."

"Withdrawal symptoms?" Tanya said, shocked.

"I've read about this condition in psychiatric journals, but this is the first time I've seen it with a patient. The only unique circumstance in your case is that the electric shock sensations, dizziness, and visual hallucinations struck when you were in a pool. But the symptoms themselves have been reported before. Though frightening, they are treatable. You'll be all right. Do you by any chance have the bottle of Paxil with you?"

Tanya found the Paxil in her bag.

"I want you to take a pill and rest in one of the empty offices here. I'll check in with you between patients. If the symptoms do not improve, then you'll need to go to the hospital."

When Tanya was back on Paxil, the symptoms she had been experiencing cleared. She checked in with me daily for several days and had no recurrence of the bizarre side effects once she was back on the medication.

Their timing, appearing two days after the Paxil was stopped and disappearing as soon as it was reinstated, clearly indicated they were a withdrawal syndrome.

For weeks Tanya was shaken by her experience in the pool. She found it frightening that withdrawal from the drug had caused such severe side effects when she was in so vulnerable a position. I told her of additional published cases I was now discovering of people who had lost control of the wheel of their car or fallen over furniture because of similar electric shock sensations, dizziness, and visual hallucinations caused by withdrawal from Prozac-type drugs.[1]

"The drugs must be awfully powerful to cause those side effects when they're stopped," said Tanya. I had to agree.

Tanya stayed on the Paxil while we decided what to do next. I explained that the best way to avoid withdrawal symptoms with any drug is to taper off it slowly. I suggested that instead of stopping the medication altogether, we lower the dose from 20 to 10 milligrams a day. Tanya agreed, but she said she wanted to wait a while to "regain her equilibrium" and "prepare" herself for another try at weaning off the medication.

I had been seeing Tanya for only a month when she experienced the dramatic withdrawal symptoms while she was swimming in the pool. She had been started on Paxil five months earlier by a doctor in Seattle. A Harvard Medical School student, Tanya had spent the summer in Seattle working in a hospital laboratory. She had lived in the city for several years before medical school and went back for the summer to see her friends. Near the end of the summer Tanya awoke in the middle of the night having a panic attack. She went to the local emergency room, where her panic responded well to Valium.

Having never had a panic attack before, Tanya was startled to think her mind could have such an effect on her body. A week later, another panic attack landed her in the hospital emergency room again. This time, in addition to giving her Valium, the emergency room doctor told Tanya she needed to go on Paxil to "manage" her anxiety, two emergency room visits in a week being too much. Unbeknownst to Tanya at the time, her managed care insurer, which the hospital called to approve each of the emergency room visits, had urged the doctor to start Paxil.

Not wanting to fall victim to another of these attacks, Tanya readily agreed. The doctor put her on 20 milligrams a day of Paxil and gave her a six-month supply of the medication. Tanya had no follow-up visit with the doctor. She did not receive a psychological evaluation. She tolerated the Paxil well and did not have any more panic attacks.

Five months later, back in Boston, Tanya made an appointment with her primary-care doctor at school to renew her prescription. Her doctor declined, however, saying she wanted Tanya to have a psychiatric evaluation and referring her to me.

When I first met Tanya I was struck by her appearance: She was a tall, thin Eurasian woman, her features a striking combination of her French and Japanese heritage. Tanya was dressed stylishly in black from head to toe. Topping this off, she wore four earrings in each ear, not the look of a conventional medical student.

Hearing Tanya's story, I agreed with her primary-care doctor's concern that the emergency room doctor in Seattle had acted too quickly in putting Tanya on daily Paxil after just two panic attacks, the causes of which were never explored psychologically. Concerned about long-term side effects, I suggested she go off the drug to see whether or not it was really necessary, instead of just automatically renewing it. I explained that had she come to see me originally, I would have used a short course of a Valium-type medication to manage her anxiety while exploring its root causes. In the unlikely event that Tanya had found herself needing daily, high doses of Valium, then switching to Paxil would have been justified.

The most baffling aspect of Tanya's case had been that she had no idea why she was anxious in the first place. "Things have been great for me the past year, really great," she said. "I got into medical school and I like it. In addition, I got into a new relationship with Richard, he's another medical student. I feel lucky." Here Tanya grinned as if still amazed to have found herself in the relationship. "You don't know me, but honestly I didn't expect to fall in love and ever be planning my life with someone else. Never! The relationship with Richard has been wonderful but so unexpected."

Tanya and Richard had met the first week at Harvard and fallen madly in love. They were both older students in their early thirties. Prior to medical school, Tanya had been a painter in Seattle, living a rather bohemian life. Richard had been a researcher at a think tank specializing in health care policy. Both were returning to school with some trepidation, and they gravitated to each other. It was a perfect time in life to have met and the relationship quickly blossomed. With everything going so well, Tanya couldn't imagine any reason for the panic attacks. She was interested in exploring the psychological causes for her anxiety further. We agreed to meet in weekly psychotherapy. In the meantime, she would stop the Paxil. Now her dramatic withdrawal symptoms had put us back to square one.

After several weeks recuperating from the episode in the pool, Tanya was ready to try going down on the dose. Two days after reducing her dose from 20 to 10 milligrams, Tanya developed the same withdrawal symptoms again: zapping electric shock–like sensations, flashing lights, staccato shifting of her vision, dizziness, nausea, nervousness, irritability, and flu-like joint pains. The symptoms brought back fearful memories of what had happened in the pool. She found the one thing that brought some relief from the symptoms was to lie still in bed with her eyes closed. Moving or even looking around the room intensified them. Each day she took to bed for several hours to gain some relief. In spite of "feeling a wreck," Tanya persevered on the lower dose "because at least this time I know what it is and, hopefully, it'll pass."

After several terrible days, Tanya felt somewhat better, although the symptoms persisted sporadically for several weeks. Indeed, at the three-week mark she had several days of prominent symptoms again, including the electric shock sensations and visual hallucinations.

"Why am I still having these symptoms three weeks after reducing the Paxil?" asked Tanya, quite distressed.

The answer was that even though the level of the drug had been reduced for weeks, the brain was still adjusting: "The nerves are in distress because they had become accustomed to the higher level of Paxil and now they're adjusting to there being less of it."

"You mean nerve cells are firing abnormally because the dose has been lowered?"

"They're slowly healing, adjusting to living with less of the drug."

"So it's like I've been feeding them this drug for months and now they're stressed because they're getting less of it? When I have the electric shocks it's like I can feel the nerves going off randomly."

Tanya was so distressed by these events that she was too "scared" to go down on the dose again right away. Instead she wanted to wait a month or so to "recover" from this episode. Throughout this period, most of our attention went to managing Tanya's withdrawal. We made little headway with the question of why she became anxious in the first place over the summer. Apart from the difficulty of getting off Paxil, she continued to feel her life was going really well.

In the midst of all this I arrived in my office one day to meet a new patient who was consulting with me because of insomnia. In his early thirties, he was an older medical school student. He had a somewhat staid, portly look, but his lively eyes betrayed an intense curiosity.

The patient said he had developed difficulty falling asleep only in recent months and was surprised because his life was going well. He was going through significant life changes but felt good about all of them. He had been a specialist in health care policy, which led him to switch fields and come to medical school. He had slight apprehensions about such a big career change but felt he had made the right decision. Eventually, he thought, he would like to combine his interest in health policy with practicing medicine.

The other big change in his life was that he had just gotten engaged. He felt wonderful about this, although it was obviously a big step. His fiancée was another medical student. Indeed at this point he told me his fiancée was Tanya. Only then did I realize he was Richard, whom I had been hearing about from her. When he was telling me about his former career, I thought his story sounded vaguely familiar.

"So the two of you've gotten engaged?" I said, surprised and delighted with this turn of events.

"Yes. On Saturday. It was Tanya's birthday and I surprised her."

"Congratulations," I said, trying to take in this flood of information, meeting Richard unexpectedly and finding out the couple had decided to get married.

"We're still getting used to the idea," Richard added. "Our parents are thrilled. Our friends will be surprised. Most of them don't know yet."

What a curious couple, I thought. Tanya was so offbeat-looking and unconventional. What a curious match with someone as solid and grounded as Richard. Still, perhaps this was what she needed to settle down in life. Richard was quite likable and warm.

Richard said the relationship had taken him by surprise too. "It's been such a wonderful thing for both of us. I was leading the monastic life of a researcher in a think tank. Tanya was leading the life of a hippie painter in Seattle. Medical school felt like a big adjustment. Who would have ever guessed this would happen too?"

As we talked, I began putting two and two together. "Look," I finally said to Richard, "I know you both think your lives are going great, but surely all this change is a little unsettling. You've both become symptomatic, Tanya with her panic attacks in the summer and you with your insomnia. Might the relationship, wonderful as it is, be a little overwhelming?"

"Could something we feel so good about make us anxious?" asked Richard, surprised.

"Sure. It's exhilarating, but a little breathless."

"We never thought of that. But it's true. It's a huge change for both of us."

On the basis of our discussion, Richard decided to forgo prescription medication for his insomnia. Now that he understood it a little better, he was hopeful it would improve without drugs. I suggested he and Tanya talk further about the ideas he and I had begun discussing. I would be seeing her later in the week for our regular appointment.

In fact, Richard and Tanya both came to the appointment. As they arrived, Tanya was beaming somewhat sheepishly. Seeing them together, I was again struck by their contrast. Tall and willowy, Tanya as always looked offbeat and was sporting nearly a dozen earrings. Next to Tanya, the monastic-looking Richard seemed so much more laid-back. As we talked, I could see how comfortable they were with each other, how complementary.

Tanya explained that she had come to a number of realizations about the relationship. Focusing on her bohemian Seattle friends, she said that throughout the previous year she had had a vague apprehension about whether or not they would "accept" Richard: "They had a hard enough time with my switching to something as mainstream as medicine. I wondered how they would deal with my being in a serious relationship. Most of my friends have mohawks and green hair. I didn't know how they would get along with Richard."

Indeed, it turned out that for most of the previous summer Tanya had been on her own in Seattle, working at a hospital and spending her spare time with her friends. Richard had stayed in Boston, working as a research assistant for a professor. He had only just joined her a few days before Tanya had her first panic attack. She now realized she had been anxious over his meeting her friends. In fact, her apprehension had been unfounded: Her friends got along well with Richard for the same reasons she did.

Over the next few weeks I gently shifted Tanya's focus from her friends to herself. Why was she so concerned about their opinion of her relationship? Did this reflect some apprehension on her own part? Gradually, Tanya acknowledged her own concern that between medical school and her relationship with Richard, life was "becoming totally bourgeois." On reflection, she realized these were intellectual concerns. In reality she was really content with the turn of events in her life. Nevertheless, the unarticulated concerns had made her anxious and had culminated in the two panic attacks.

Tanya felt greatly relieved to be getting a better handle on why she had been anxious, but we still had to get her off the Paxil. She was now ready to go down again on the dose from 10 to 5 milligrams. Since there is no 5 milligram pill, this meant cutting the 10-milligram pills in half and trying to collect the right proportion of the fragments.

A day after going down to 5 milligrams, Tanya had a recurrence of her withdrawal symptoms: severe dizziness, nausea, flashing lights, and electric shock sensations. She again felt the need to take to her bed because of her symptoms and feeling unsteady on her feet. Tanya was so "wigged out" by the recurrence of the symptoms that she put her dose up to 7.5 milligrams. Even with this tiny reduction from 10 milligrams, she continued to have withdrawal symptoms, although not as severe. Just as had happened before, the symptoms were worst in the first few days, subsided some, and peaked again several weeks after the dose reduction.

Tanya again wanted to wait a couple of weeks to recover from this dose reduction before attempting another. During this time, one morning she forgot to take her Paxil. In the middle of the afternoon she was suddenly seized with withdrawal symptoms. Leaving school in a cab, she rushed home to take some Paxil, which relieved her of the symptoms.

"I feel hostage to this drug," Tanya said angrily the next time I saw her. "I'm petrified of not taking a dose because of the withdrawal symptoms. I had that terrifying experience in the pool. I probably never needed this medication and now I'm on it because I can't get off it. Why didn't the doctor tell me when he put me on the drug that I could have this much trouble stopping it?" Regrettably, in the current climate many people are put on these drugs indefinitely. Often, getting off them is not even a consideration. This is why patients are often not told about withdrawal effects: The doctor is not even thinking in terms of stopping the drugs.

Tanya and I resigned ourselves to an extremely slow taper off the Paxil. With each 2.5-milligram drop in the dose, Tanya would have withdrawal symptoms for several weeks and take another two to three weeks to "recover" before going down again. Eventually, after months, she was able to get off Paxil.

Many patients like Tanya consult doctors about psychiatric symptoms that they cannot explain. Not only empathy and understanding but a great deal of patience is required to wait for the relevant information to appear. Had Tanya somehow intuited that encouraging Richard to see me about his insomnia would lead to our discovering the important clue relative to her panic attacks? To treat psychiatric patients, doctors need time to build a relationship with them and to learn about the details of their lives as well as the larger picture. Only then can we help solve the mysteries patients come to us about.

After just two panic attacks, Tanya had been put on Paxil by an emergency room doctor who never saw her again. Emergency room doctors are trained to fix acute problems. They should not be forced to consign patients to months or years on potent antidepressants. Tanya needlessly took Paxil for almost a year, had the terrifying experience in the pool, and suffered debilitating withdrawal symptoms, which made her feel trapped, held "hostage," to the drug's adverse effects. That an emergency room doctor might practice in this way instead of referring Tanya to a specialist for a more in-depth evaluation is part of the madness that has overtaken the attitude toward prescribing these drugs in the past decade.

There are now scores of reports of withdrawal syndromes like Tanya's occurring in association with the Prozac group. In an October 1996 article in the *Journal of Clinical Psychopharmacology*, a team of British and Canadian doctors led by Dr. Nick Coupland noted that the most common withdrawal side effect is dizziness, which is "variously described as having a 'swimming,' 'spaced out,' 'drunken,' or 'buzzing' quality."[2] As in Tanya's case, Coupland's group noted that the dizziness is "exacerbated by movement" even "slight head movements or eye movements." The next most common symptom is prominent sensory abnormalities such as staccato or blurred vision, burning sensations, tingling, or electric shock–like sensations.

Writing in the *Journal of Clinical Psychiatry* in 1997, a group of experts headed by Dr. Alan Schatzberg, chairman of the department of psychiatry at the Stanford University School of Medicine, sought to define the characteristic withdrawal effects, both psychological and physical, seen with Prozac-type medications.[3] They defined the core psychological effects as "anxiety-agitation, crying spells, and irritability." The Schatzberg group noted that in many patients "crying spells, in particular, are dramatic and disappear quickly" if the drug is restarted. The group defined the core physical effects as:

1. disequilibrium (e.g., dizziness, spinning sensations, swaying, or difficulty walking)
2. gastrointestinal symptoms (e.g., nausea, vomiting)
3. flu-like symptoms (e.g., fatigue, lethargy, muscle pain, chills)
4. sensory disturbances (e.g., tingling, electric shock sensations)
5. sleep disturbances (e.g., insomnia, vivid dreams)

Many patients experience even worse withdrawal symptoms than Tanya's. Writing in the *American Journal of Psychiatry*, Dr. Lloyd Frost of Toronto, Canada, described one patient who lost control of his car's steering wheel because of electric shock sensations after stopping Zoloft.[4] The patient's withdrawal symptoms lasted thirteen weeks. Other patients have become disoriented, confused, and had memory problems. Writing in the

Journal of the Medical Association of Thailand, Dr. Duangjai Kasantikul reported a woman who "experienced acute episodes of reversible delirium after discontinuation of long-term Prozac therapy."[5] The delirium was "reversible" because it cleared when the drug was reinstated. Dr. William Giakas of Rockford, Illinois, reported a case of "intractable withdrawal" from Effexor in the *Psychiatric Annals.*[6] Many reports describe patients being temporarily "incapacitated"[7] and missing several days of work because of debilitating withdrawal symptoms.[8]

Reviewing a number of studies, Dr. Michel Lejoyeux of the Bichat-Claude Bernard Hospital in Paris, France, says that "children and adolescents who are taking antidepressants could be at higher risk than adults" for withdrawal syndromes.[9] Doctors John Zajecka and Katherine Tracy of Rush Presbyterian St. Luke's Medical Center in Chicago report that in children and adolescents who are withdrawing from serotonergic antidepressants, "marked, uncharacteristic irritability and argumentativeness have been observed."[10] And Dr. L. S. W. Kent of the Queen Elizabeth Psychiatric Hospital in Birmingham, England, reported in the *British Journal of Psychiatry* on a mother who stopped taking Zoloft while breast feeding a three-week-old infant.[11] Within one day the baby developed a withdrawal syndrome of "agitation, restlessness, poor feeding, constant crying, insomnia and an enhanced startle reaction," which lasted several days.

Studies have shown that people who have been taking serotonin boosters for as little as two months develop withdrawal effects when they stop the drug.[12] As discussed in the previous chapter, we are learning that the brain is not passive in the face of drugs that upset its chemical balances. Over the course of months, the nervous system makes numerous adaptations to being bathed in the drug twenty-four hours a day. These adaptations represent Prozac backlash, the brain's attempts to neutralize the effects of a drug. Over time, the nerves have to learn how to cope, how to function, in the constant presence of the drug.

When one stops a Prozac-type medication, suddenly the brain's milieu is altered again. Brain cells that had to adapt to living with the drug now have to readapt to living without it. In effect, they have to dismantle their previous adjustments. The faster the drug washes out, the more abrupt the change and the more distressing for the brain. Since the original adjustments took months to put in place, they take weeks or more to undo. This is why Tanya still had bursts of withdrawal side effects, abnormal brain cell firing, three weeks after stopping Paxil. The bursts of abnormal activity represent the nervous system still distressed, still trying to undo former adjustments to the medication long after the drug is gone. The brain undergoes a similar adjustment when withdrawing from long-term use of other central nervous system drugs, such as alcohol, nicotine, cocaine, barbiturates, or speed (amphetamines).

When Prozac was first introduced, it was thought that this class of drugs would not cause withdrawal. Withdrawal syndromes are unusual with Prozac and have only come to the attention of professionals since Zoloft, Paxil, and Luvox were introduced. We now know Prozac itself rarely causes disruptive withdrawal effects because it is so long-lasting, only slowly washing out of the body over a number of weeks. This provides a slow, built-in taper, which protects most patients from noticing serious withdrawal effects. By contrast, the other Prozac-type drugs are much shorter-acting. Drugs like Paxil and Luvox wash out of the body precipitously in just a couple of days. Zoloft falls in the middle of the spectrum.

How short-acting a drug is relates directly to the frequency of its withdrawal side effects. Withdrawal symptoms are most common with Luvox, estimated to occur in 86% of patients,[13] and Paxil, in as many as 50% of patients.[14] At the other end of the spectrum, few patients stopping Prozac notice withdrawal effects. Their nervous systems are presumably going through the same adjustments, but the withdrawal effects are masked by the drug's built-in taper. In the few reported cases of withdrawal from Prozac, patients experience the same symptoms seen with Zoloft, Paxil, and Luvox but they persist for a much longer period of time, one to two months.[15]

As with other serious, long-term side effects of these drugs, the frequency of withdrawal phenomena cited by pharmaceutical companies is much lower than what one sees in clinical practice and has now been demonstrated in the studies that are available. Indeed, at the end of clinical trials testing new antidepressants for approval, pharmaceutical companies typically do not monitor withdrawal effects. The studies are simply designed to prove the drug's efficacy and end when the patients stop the drug. As a result, the official product information for the drugs merely contains a disclaimer such as: Withdrawal symptoms "were not systematically evaluated in controlled clinical trials."[16]

Many doctors are still unaware of the existence of withdrawal syndromes in association with Prozac-type medications. Doctors A. H. Young and A. Currie of the Newcastle General Hospital in England conducted a survey of over one hundred psychiatrists and primary-care doctors in the northeast of England.[17] Only 30% of primary-care doctors and 72% of psychiatrists were aware that patients can experience withdrawal symptoms. Even fewer, only 20% of psychiatrists and 17% of primary-care doctors, said they warn patients of withdrawal syndromes.

In some instances doctors mistake the symptoms for a serious medical illness and subject patients to medical tests that may involve risks and certainly are costly. Writing in the August 1995 issue of the *American Journal of Psychiatry*, Dr. Eli Einbinder reported a patient who stopped Prozac and developed "extreme dizziness."[18] Because initially the physician did not connect the dizziness with Prozac withdrawal, the patient was evaluated by a neurologist and another specialist in inner ear problems. The patient had a brain scan and also underwent testing for Lyme tick disease. Only when all the tests came back negative was the connection made between stopping Prozac and the dizziness. When the drug was reinstated, the symptoms cleared.

Effexor is another of the popular new antidepressants of the last decade with severe withdrawal effects.[19] Effexor is even shorter-acting than any of the Prozac group. One of my patients on Effexor was rushed to the hospital in an ambulance after she became dizzy, lightheaded, and faint while at work. The emergency room doctors could find nothing wrong with her. Eventually, they concluded she must be anxious. Only when the same symptoms recurred a month later did the patient realize the common feature was that on both days she had forgotten to take her morning dose of Effexor. The severe withdrawal symptoms had emerged within hours. Since then, she has been extra-vigilant never to forget to take the Effexor on time.

A common and serious complication of withdrawal symptoms is for patients and doctors to mistake them for a return of the symptoms the drug was originally used to treat, especially anxiety or depression. As a result, the drug is restarted. Of course this ameliorates the symptoms but in fact it is merely chasing one's tail, medicating withdrawal, and needlessly prolonging the patient's exposure to the drug, often for years. In fact, if a patient is going to suffer a relapse of their psychiatric condition, this typically does not occur until weeks or months after the drug is stopped. To avoid unnecessarily remedicating the patient, both the doctor and patient need to know that new symptoms appearing within days of stopping a drug are almost always withdrawal effects.

The best strategy for avoiding withdrawal effects is to taper the drug slowly. Even then, there are numerous reports of severe symptoms with extremely slow tapers, as in Tanya's case. Patience and perseverance are then required. There are reports of patients who could not get off their antidepressants because the withdrawal effects were so severe they were intolerable.[20]

Yet another strategy that some psychiatrists advocate is switching patients at the end of treatment from Paxil, Luvox, or Effexor to Prozac.[21] Because these drugs all have similar mechanisms of action, the brain has what is called cross-tolerance, which allows one to switch from one drug to the other without discomfort. Switching to Prozac and then stopping the drug gives the patient the benefit of Prozac's built-in slow taper, which masks the dismantling of the brain's adaptations and usually protects the patient from noticing withdrawal.

This strategy is very like using Valium-type drugs to withdraw patients from alcohol. Valium-type drugs and alcohol have similar effects on receptors in the brain, so the brain of an alcoholic has cross-tolerance to Valium. In detoxification centers, alcoholics are switched from alcohol to Valium, which protects them from dangerous withdrawal symptoms. The Valium is then slowly tapered to avoid the withdrawal syndrome that would occur if the patient simply stopped drinking cold turkey. This slow-taper treatment with a Valium-type drug is referred to as "detoxifying" the patient from alcohol. By analogy, some psychiatrists advocate detoxifying patients from Effexor, Paxil, or Luvox by means of the slow built-in taper of Prozac.

Pharmaceutical companies are concerned about the increasing reports of withdrawal syndromes with the new antidepressants. In December 1996, Eli Lilly sponsored a "closed symposium" of a panel of experts in Phoenix, Arizona, to discuss the growing problem.[22] Many of the experts were drug advocates with close ties to Lilly and other pharmaceutical companies.

One of the main outcomes of the meeting was that these phenomena should be renamed "antidepressant discontinuation syndrome," a euphemism avoiding the negative connotations of "withdrawal." In the following year, the group of experts, many of them prominent academic psychopharmacologists, published eight papers on the "antidepressant discontinuation syndrome," thereby helping to establish this new term, free of negative associations.[23] In addition to paying for the private conference in Arizona, Eli Lilly provided assistance for publishing the follow-up papers. The sanitized term "antidepressant discontinuation syndrome" is the kind of well-funded obfuscation doctors and patients frequently face when trying to get honest, reliable information on these powerful drugs.

Paradoxical Weight Gain and Rebound Irritability

Because withdrawal symptoms can last so long, patients often ask if permanent damage can result from effects as powerful as visual hallucinations and electric shock sensations. We do not yet know the answer to this important question. Two late-appearing withdrawal effects are particularly disturbing: paradoxical weight gain and angry, irritable outbursts.

The Prozac group are powerful appetite suppressants for many patients.[24] When starting the drugs, patients report a dramatic loss of interest in food. Some say they lose their sense of flavor as well; food has an unappealing, metallic taste. Many lose weight on the drugs. In some instances the weight loss can be precipitous. I have had a few patients who needed to go off the medication because of dangerous weight loss.

For most people, weight loss is an appealing side effect. Indeed, many go on the drugs expressly for this purpose. Prozac has been prescribed as a diet pill at weight loss centers across the country.[25] Loss of interest in food is also the reason why the Prozac group are commonly prescribed to women with bulimia or compulsive overeating.[26]

Although the medications are appetite suppressants, I have had several patients who, in the initial weeks and months after they went off the drugs, reported a dramatic *increase* in their appetite and "ballooning" of their weight by twenty pounds or more. The patients had always been quite slim and never had a weight problem prior to the drug; all of them lost weight while on the medication. But after the drug was stopped, they found themselves overweight for the first time in their lives. They reported the additional pounds were extremely difficult to take off, even with dieting and exercise. Patients with this kind of paradoxical weight gain have been quite upset. Since the problem only emerged after stopping the medication, they worried the drug did permanent damage to the appetite center in their brains.

Other patients report a paradoxical rebound in their appetite and significant weight gain while still on a Prozac-type drug. This occurs after being on a drug long-term, typically for more than a year. Women are especially distressed by this late-appearing reversal of earlier weight loss on the medication. Bombarded by the media with images equating thinness with beauty, many women are exquisitely sensitive to fluctuations in their weight. In an article in the May 1998 issue of *Clinical Psychiatry News*, Dr. Norman Sussman, director of psychopharmacology research at Bellevue Hospital in New York, was quoted as saying that paradoxical weight gain is one of the most common, long-term side effects of the Prozac group now prompting patients to insist on going off the drugs.[27]

Rebound irritability is another, sometimes quite serious, withdrawal effect of the Prozac group. The drugs have long been recognized to have profound effects on the modulation of anger, leading some doctors to say they would more aptly be called "anger pills." Studies have shown they make people less irritable and more socially cooperative.[28]

In the initial weeks or months after stopping a Prozac-type drug, some patients report a dramatic, rebound irritability. This is not mild irritability. Patients describe angry outbursts in which they lose their temper with family and friends, smash things, or punch walls. In an article on withdrawal syndromes with the Prozac group in the July 1997 *Journal of Clinical Psychiatry*, Dr. John Zajecka reported that the agitation and irritability can cause "aggressiveness and suicidal impulsivity."[29] In the British medical journal *Lancet,* Dr. Miki Bloch of the National Institute of Mental Health reported on patients who became suicidal and homicidal after stopping Paxil, including one man who was distraught over thoughts of harming "his own children."[30]

Unfortunately, many patients with rebound irritability insist they need to go back on the drug, which quickly subdues their angry outbursts. In one such case, published in the *Annals of Pharmacotherapy,* Dr. Andrea Lazowick described a thirty-year-old woman on 100 milligrams a day of Luvox who tried to stop taking the drug after she became pregnant but who "experienced feelings of severe aggression whenever the drug was discontinued" and therefore "continued taking the medication throughout the pregnancy."[31]

Patients with rebound irritability show a remarkable resemblance to people who are trying to stop smoking cigarettes. Nicotine is one of the most commonly used nonprescription stimulating drugs. People who try to stop smoking often feel extremely irritable and describe similar urges to throw objects or punch walls. As with Prozac-type drugs, some people insist they have to resume smoking to control their angry outbursts.

Joanna and Zoe: Cases of Dependence

Increasing numbers of patients report feeling dependent on the Prozac group. Joanna first became concerned about dependence when she started a new, demanding job as a computer programmer and found herself turning to extra doses of Zoloft to get her through difficult, stressful days:

"As the middle of the afternoon approaches I find myself watching the clock, thinking of all the work I have to do, and tensing up. If I have a deadline to meet, I can get so tense I can't think straight. I need to be thinking clearly and able to really concentrate. If I'm stressed or bored and need to crank out work, I've found myself taking an extra Zoloft to get through the afternoon."

"You take an extra Zoloft?" I inquired on hearing these classic symptoms of drug dependence. Joanna was on 100 milligrams a day of the drug.

"I take an extra 50 milligrams."

"And that makes it possible for you to function for the rest of the afternoon?"

"Oh yeah. Within half an hour of taking it I feel much better. My thinking is clearer. I feel more relaxed. I can concentrate much better."

"But you're worried about it?"

"Well, I've been doing it two or three days a week for a month now. I don't like feeling addicted to Zoloft."

In his book *Listening to Prozac*, psychiatrist Peter Kramer describes a patient who took extra doses of Prozac to work more effectively as having "chipped" small amounts of the medication.[32] Chipping is a street drug term dating to the 1960s. It refers to taking extra shavings ("chips") of the crystalline form of a street drug.

"Using the drug for a pick-me-up like that in the afternoon," said Joanna, "I'm afraid I'm becoming dependent on it."

I concurred, and I encouraged Joanna not to use the drug this way.

Joanna was started on Zoloft during her senior year in college. The drug was prescribed by an eating disorders specialist she consulted with because of periodic binge eating. Even though she was not bulimic (bingeing and purging) or anorexic, the psychiatrist diagnosed Joanna as having an eating disorder. Her weight had always been normal, although it had fluctuated by as much as five to ten pounds depending on her eating habits. The specialist saw Joanna only once and prescribed Zoloft. Shortly thereafter, she began psychotherapy with me. Because she had a dependent personality she was already quite attached to the drug, which I continued to prescribe.

Joanna reported an intense, enmeshed relationship with her mother who had always picked out her clothes, told her what to wear, and was "obsessed" with buying her makeup, facial creams, and other cosmetics. "I don't think she sees me as a separate person," said Joanna. "It's as though she's dressing and making herself up when she attends to me." As evidence of the intensity of this mother-daughter bond, Joanna described coming home from college on vacation after having gained almost ten pounds. In horror on seeing Joanna, her mother said, "What have you done to me?"

In a year's psychotherapy, Joanna made considerable progress extricating herself from the suffocating relationship with her mother. She also got into her first serious relationship with a young man, a classmate from college. The relationship provoked a great deal of jealousy in her mother, who was quite possessive of Joanna. As she tried to become more independent of her mother, Joanna received considerable support not only in her therapy but also from her boyfriend.

About six months after telling me about chipping Zoloft at work, Joanna's concerns about being dependent on the drug escalated sharply when she was on a trip out of town and found herself running out of medication. She was visiting her boyfriend's parents for the first time, which was already a stressful occasion. Three days into a ten-day visit, Joanna realized she was running out of medication and would have to ration the drug, cutting the dose in half in order to have a little to take each day.

"I should have asked you for a new prescription and filled it before I left," she said on her return. "After a couple of days on the lower dose, I started to be incredibly anxious. My head got cloudy and I literally couldn't think straight. That really scared me, because I've always depended so much on my intellectual abilities in work and school. I also felt incredibly dizzy and bumped into furniture a couple of times."

I explained that these were withdrawal symptoms occurring because the dose of the drug had been reduced.

"There were times when we were sitting with John's parents over dinner, when I'd become convinced I couldn't make it without more Zoloft, and I'd think of calling you from out of town. I was in such turmoil, because I felt like a drug addict. Sometimes I imagined getting up and saying to John's parents, 'Excuse me, I'm sorry, but I'm a junkie. I need to go call my source.'"

Joanna was truly rattled by this bad experience of feeling "totally dependent" on her antidepressant, a "basket case" without it. I, too, was afraid she was overly dependent on Zoloft and urged her to have a trial off the medication. She had made considerable progress in therapy and her relationship was flourishing. Basing my judgment on experience, I believed she would be fine without the medication if she could extricate herself from it. After weeks of discussion, Joanna was concerned enough that she agreed to a slow taper of the Zoloft, reducing the dose by just 25 milligrams every one to two months. By now she had already forced herself to stop taking extra doses at work.

Joanna took six months to slowly taper off Zoloft. In order to reduce the dose in small increments, she had to buy a pill cutter, which she described as a guillotine. She reported it gave her "great satisfaction" to chop the pills in half in order to take less of them. She described this as a wonderful outlet for her frustration and anger with the pills, and a symbol of her gaining mastery over them. For the last month of her taper, Joanna guillotined a dozen of the 50-milligram Zoloft pills into thirds, producing over 30 fragments of roughly 16.5 milligrams each. Since the crudely cut fragments varied in size, she lined them up from big to small and took one a day beginning with the largest. When Joanna told me this I could just picture the column of fragments on her desk, the perfect visual representation of her waning dependence on the drug.

With the support of myself and her boyfriend, Joanna did fine without the drug. In retrospect, she became quite angry with the eating disorders specialist who had started her on Zoloft: "She never told me I could become dependent on it. I was quite reluctant, but she really sold me on the drug. She told me stories of her patients whose lives it had transformed. Now I don't believe her, because it didn't do that for me. She had a whole drawer full of samples. 'Which one do you want?' she asked, pulling out trays of Prozac, Zoloft, and Paxil. She really hooked me. If she'd just given me a prescription, I might have resisted filling it."

One of the problems in describing the need many people come to feel for their prescription medication is sorting out an array of confusing terminology, words like "dependence," "drug abuse," "addiction," and "craving." A classic paper by psychiatrist Ian Oswald of the University of Edinburgh is helpful in this regard. Writing in the *British Medical Journal*, Oswald and his colleagues describe antidepressants as "drugs of dependence though not of abuse."[33] People rarely take Prozac-type drugs to get high, the way one thinks of in drug abuse. Nevertheless, they can come to feel dependent on them for their well-being, and even begin "chipping" extra doses to cope or function.

Another patient who eventually felt dependent on Prozac was Zoe. When I first saw Zoe she was depressed. Although not on Prozac at the time, she had been on it twice in the past, each time for a year. Like many patients in the 1990s, Zoe had cycled on and off Prozac. She came to me feeling in need of the drug again. In her late twenties, Zoe cited her job as the most significant stress in her life. Zoe was the secretary to the CEO of a growing high-tech company. As she talked about her work, her boss sounded like a driven, self-absorbed man who made excessive demands on Zoe's time and energy. While at times she was exhilarated by working closely with the dynamic president of a young company, at other times Zoe felt near exhaustion and despaired of ever having a personal life. In the months before she first saw me, the company had entered into a complicated merger with one of their competitors. Through intense political jockeying, her boss had emerged the triumphant head of the new company, but only at the expense of grueling hours and ever greater demands on his assistant Zoe.

Zoe was mildly depressed. In fact, she would be better described as exhausted and frustrated over her work. However, she insisted she needed

Prozac to "prop" her up, to prevent sliding into worse depression. At the same time, Zoe worried aloud that she now "reached for Prozac every time something went wrong" in her life. I expressed concern that she was using the drug to cope with being exploited by her boss, when actually she might do better not to just cope, but instead to insist on certain changes at work, or else leave.

Back on Prozac, Zoe felt less frustrated, had more energy, and indeed coped better with the demands at work. Unfortunately, she was quite skeptical of psychotherapy and preferred to rely on medication alone to see her through a difficult period. As a result, nothing had really changed with her job situation after another year on Prozac. At the end of a year, the "crisis" caused by her company's merger had subsided and Zoe felt ready to go off Prozac. Although her stress level was still high, it was now back to her baseline.

I did not hear from Zoe for over a year. Then, a year and a half after I had last seen her, Zoe returned, concerned that she was becoming depressed again. This time, Zoe came to see me before she actually felt depressed, hoping to avert another episode of being unable to cope—and also to avoid taking Prozac for what would be the fourth time. At the time, St. John's wort, the herbal antidepressant, was just beginning to receive considerable press, and Zoe wanted to try this as a natural alternative to Prozac. I recommended a local health food store where she could get the herbal preparation and more information. Zoe told me that in recent months she had begun drinking more, although not heavily. Still, she was concerned about it. I urged her to stop drinking altogether, since alcohol is a powerful central nervous system depressant that worsens depression. We also discussed Zoe's starting a diet and exercise regimen to help ward off depression.

Unfortunately, in retrospect, I now know Zoe's efforts to try alternatives to Prozac were only halfhearted. As with so many patients who cycle on and off these drugs, part of her truly did not want to go back on Prozac but another part of her was inevitably drawn to it. While she cut down on her drinking, she did not fully stop. She did go on St. John's wort, but I learned later that she had only taken one instead of the recommended three doses a day. Although she went to the gym for an evaluation with a fitness trainer, she did not follow up.

For two months I watched Zoe hope that these irresolute attempts would work. During this time she talked endlessly about whether or not to "resort" to Prozac again. Gradually, she sensed herself becoming more and more "a wreck," in her words, over whether or not to start the drug. By the time she finally "succumbed" to the drug (her words again), Zoe looked more like an addict than a depressed person: nervous, jittery, slightly disheveled, and obsessed with the drug.

Finally, Zoe reported during a session that she had resumed taking Prozac, using a supply she had left over from before. When I asked what had happened during the week that tipped the scales in favor of taking the drug, she said she had begun to have trouble sleeping:

"I couldn't fall asleep at night. I just lay in bed running endless lists in my head of everything I needed to do at work. When I start losing sleep, that's when things really start to snowball and I get depressed. I just couldn't let that happen."

"Had anything unusual happened at work? Were the pressures any different from usual?"

"No. They were the same."

At the time, I accepted Zoe's answer. However, several weeks later, I learned in a chance reference she made that the picture was much more complicated than Zoe had thought to mention. It turned out that for months, Zoe had been trying to take a half day per week off from work in order to devote time to considering her next career move. She wanted to meet with career counselors and schedule some job interviews to see what options were available to her. She was even considering moving out of state, back to her home in Virginia.

While, in principle, Zoe's boss was supportive of her taking some time off, it never happened. It was never possible for her to leave in the middle of a busy, hectic day. To research other career options, she had scheduled a week off without pay, months in advance. Again, her boss supported the idea, but as the week approached, it became "impossible" for her to leave because there were so many pressing things for her to assist him with. So Zoe found herself working through a week she was not even being paid for and, once again, forgoing her own personal priorities. It turned out this was the week Zoe restarted the Prozac after lying awake in bed in a panic over everything she had to do. When I heard the more detailed story of what was going on, I became more angry on Zoe's behalf: "When you tell me all this, I'm not so happy about you going on Prozac to sleep," I said. "I think you *should* be losing sleep when you have to work a week you're not even being paid for and had scheduled to take off to devote to your own priorities."

At times I have serious misgivings about writing prescriptions for patients like Zoe. Am I a "source" for a drug they have become excessively dependent on? Should I decline? My concerns were echoed in the title of a front page article in the *New York Times* that read: "With Millions Taking Prozac, A Legal Drug Culture Arises."[34] In fact, according to the terms of their medical license, doctors are expected to practice according to the "professional standards of the day." One can debate the merits of such a mandate, which can easily have a leveling effect, but the fact is that prescribing Prozac has become the standard and is much more easily defended than refusing to prescribe it. I have refused to prescribe the Prozac group for patients without symptoms, who want to feel "better than well," despite the fact that some psychiatrists do not discourage this and the patient can probably get a prescription elsewhere. In a case like Zoe's, however, in which the patient is clearly symptomatic, I do not think the patient will benefit from psychiatrists at either extreme: either rabidly pro-drug or ardently anti-drug. I felt marginally comfortable writing prescriptions for Zoe because I knew in my office she would at least hear messages counterbalancing the drug's seductive affect: that she was overly dependent on the drug, that she ought to pursue more self-awareness and change her work situation, which was at the bottom of her problems, that the drug might wear off, and that its long-term side effects were a serious concern. Patients like Zoe would not keep coming to me if they did not themselves have some of the same feelings, which many of them ultimately heed. Indeed, Zoe said she worried that chronic cycling on and off Prozac weakened her "natural defenses," her innate ability to cope with life's stresses and her will to effect necessary change. Said Zoe, "Once the drug has worked for you, once you've had that experience, it's hard to resist. Knowing what the drug can do for you overshadows the alternatives. Once you've been on it, you can't go back to the state of never having had the drug."

A final concern in Zoe's case was the general effect the drug had on her sense of being. As I got to know her better, Zoe described how Prozac blunted all her emotions, the highs and the lows, making her more compliant and contented in her work, even when it was not healthy to be content. Recent research has confirmed Zoe's description. Funded by the National Institute of Mental Health, a team of researchers led by Dr. Brian Knutson studied the effect of Paxil on the personalities of normal, healthy volunteers with no psychiatric diagnoses. Psychological tests were used to assess changes in the volunteers "personality and social behavior" while on the drug. Writing in the March 1998 issue of the *American Journal of Psychiatry*, Knutson reported that on Paxil people evidenced less "irritability" and were more socially "cooperative."[35] Wrote Knutson: Serotonin boosters "can have significant personality and behavioral effects in normal humans [even] in the absence of baseline depression or other psychopathology."

In a classic psychiatric paper, Doris Mayer labeled this kind of drug effect as the "antidepressed personality." Writing in the *British Journal of*

Medical Psychology, she described how antidepressants "chemically alter, distort and, more especially, stifle feelings."[36] The result is that people lose the "warning sensation" of psychic pain, which might mobilize someone like Zoe to effect change. Mayer feels this "artificial flattening" of emotion alienates people from their feelings and dulls their senses, leaving them "bland" and "tranquilized."

Such sentiments were recently echoed in a moving piece by writer Deborah Abramson that appeared in the April 17, 1998, issue of the *Boston Phoenix.*[37] Writing about her own personal experience, Abramson titled her article "Hooked: Antidepressants Can Take Away as Much of You as They Give Back." Says Abramson of her experience with many different antidepressants: "the medication may have lifted the depression, but instead of allowing me to connect with the world it has surrounded me in another kind of fog. Most of the time, I am simply numb. Everything feels flat, as if I'm living in some uninflected world without substance, depth, or meaning. . . . It's as though a valve inside of me has been turned almost shut, reducing my emotions to a slow trickle, where they once burst forth in a powerful flood."

Abramson describes having "gone through many medications, combinations, and dosages." She is currently on one of the more stimulating new antidepressants, Effexor. At bedtime, she has to take a sedative "to counteract the stimulating effect of the Effexor and help me sleep." Many patients are prescribed such combinations, which psychopharmacologists describe as drug "cocktails." This phenomenon in street drug use is referred to as taking an upper and chasing it with a downer.

The focus of the article, as reflected in the title "Hooked," is Abramson's dependence on antidepressant medication. Because of this dependence, Abramson says, "Lately I've been having a lot of addiction dreams. Heroin, crack, alcohol." In one vivid dream, "I looked down at my arms—there were track marks everywhere, and the skin was tough, impenetrable. . . . I thought to myself, I must be an addict." If she misses a dose, she experiences "a mild form of withdrawal—vertigo and a tingling sensation around my mouth—even after just a couple of hours. The reason I don't panic, as an addict might, when my supply runs out is that I can always get a refill. It's not that I'm any less dependent. This dependence, both psychological and physical, has always made me uncomfortable."

As reflected in Abramson's choice of words, drug dependence is often divided into physical and psychological dependence. Physical dependence refers to a physiological, chemical need for a drug that has been chronically administered. Having been bathed in the drug for a long time, the nervous system comes to rely on its presence as a routine part of its functioning.

Psychological dependence refers to the perceived need for a drug, even if only for a mild or placebo effect. Even dependency that is largely psychological can be powerfully addicting. Of course, physical and psychological dependence are impossible to completely separate. No doubt the dependence patients feel on psychiatric medications is very often a mixture of the two.

Related to dependence is a phenomenon psychiatrists call "supersensitivity," or sensitization of brain cells by psychiatric drugs. In a pair of editorials on "sensitization by antidepressant drugs" published in *Psychotherapy and Psychosomatics* in 1994 and 1995, Italian psychiatrist Giovanni Fava of the University of Bologna questioned whether or not "psychotropic [psychiatric] drugs actually worsen, at least in some cases, the progression of the illness which they are supposed to treat."[38] Fava cited a long-term study of antidepressant use at the University of Pittsburgh in which patients on the drugs more than three years did poorly if taken off them, leading Fava to suggest the results could be explained by "a sensitization to depression leading to the inability to withdraw after three years." In a related piece in the October 1995 issue of the *Journal of Clinical Psychopharmacology*, Fava said the withdrawal effects of the Prozac group in particular raised concern about "sensitization of serotonergic systems . . . leading to *increased vulnerability* to depressive relapse in the long run [italics added]."[39]

Brain cells are known to effect numerous changes in response to antidepressant drugs. Reversal of these changes leads to withdrawal phenomena. But, said Fava, some of the "changes may be irreversible . . . as in tardive dyskinesia," the tics discussed in the previous chapter, which, to date, are our best example of permanent, drug-induced changes in the brain. We tend to think of dependence as something people can overcome with sufficient willpower. But what if long-term use of a serotonin booster sensitizes brain cells such that they cannot function without it? Patients who relapse when they stop medications are often told this is confirmation of the severity of their "underlying condition" and of the need to take drugs indefinitely. In fact, it may be a drug effect. Noting the high relapse rates in patients treated with antidepressants, Fava pointed out that in other branches of medicine similar concerns have been raised that drugs which improve symptoms in the short run may actually worsen the conditions they treat in the long run. The best-known example is the "antibiotic paradox": while treating bacterial infections, antibiotics simultaneously promote the growth of drug-resistant bacteria which come back to haunt us.[40]

Sensitization of brain tissue by psychiatric drugs has been the subject of intense research by leading biological psychiatrists for the past two decades.[41] In spite of this, Fava's articles brought an angry response from prominent drug advocates.[42] However, one of the leading psychopharmacologists in this country, Ross Baldessarini, of Harvard Medical School, came to Fava's defense. In a 1995 article in *Psychotherapy and Psychosomatics,* Baldessarini cited numerous examples of rebound phenomena in people stopping psychiatric medications: Research has shown manic-depressive patients who go off lithium have "a nearly 7-fold shorter time to first recurrence than was found in the shortest cycle before starting lithium."[43] Similarly, patients stopping major tranquilizers have "a gross excess of relapses within the first 12 weeks." Similarly, after long-term use of Valium-type sedatives, patients experience rebound anxiety, especially if the drugs are stopped too quickly. Studies of major tranquilizers, antidepressants, and lithium "suggest that even *partial* abrupt removal of a drug [such as cutting the dose in half] may be sufficient to induce an excess risk of relapse or recurrence of illness." Baldessarini concluded, "It may be timely to reconsider the ethics and scientific interpretation of studies of maintenance treatments broadly, as well as the clinical risks involved."

Exactly what percentage of patients feel dependent on their Prozac-type medication is not known. Certainly many patients are on one of the drugs for a year or two and go off without trouble. But many others share the experience of my patients Joanna, Zoe, and writer Deborah Abramson. Unfortunately this is an area of research that has been sorely neglected. Indeed, pharmaceutical companies and drug advocates have been quite aggressive about insisting the Prozac group do not cause dependence. But it is worth remembering that the same was said of cocaine and amphetamines when they were prescription antidepressants.

In the earlier section of this chapter on withdrawal syndromes, I described a group of experts meeting at an Arizona resort under the auspices of Eli Lilly. In one of their reports, published in 1997 in the *Journal of Clinical Psychiatry,* the group advocated using the euphemism "antidepressant discontinuation syndrome" rather than "withdrawal" because: "Unfortunately, the public often perceives wrongly that antidepressants—like alcohol and barbiturates—are addicting."[44] The group cited a 1996 survey of 2,003 people in England conducted for the "Defeat Depression Campaign" headed by Professor Robert Priest at the Imperial College School of Medicine at St. Mary's in London. The survey, published in the *British Medical Journal,* found 78% of the public felt that "drug treatment for depression was potentially addictive and dulled the symptoms rather than solving the problem."[45] Acting as the "expert" trying to dissuade people from their natural instincts, Priest wrote that the public "may project their prejudices about depression onto the medical profession" and medication. He urged, "Doctors have an important role in *educating the public* about depression and the rationale for antidepressant treatment. In particular, patients should know that *dependence is not a problem with antidepressants* [italics added]." Even more specifically, said Priest, "Patients should be informed clearly when antidepressants are first prescribed that *discontinuing treatment in due course will not be a problem.*"

Writing in the October 1997 issue of the *International Journal of Risk and Safety in Medicine,* Charles Medawar described dependence on serotonin boosters as "the antidepressant web."[46] Medawar is a leading health care consumer advocate in Britain. An authority on dependence on psychiatric drugs, he was influential in bringing dependence on Valium-type sedatives to public and professional attention.[47] Medawar criticized the efforts of Priest and other drug proponents, saying: "Over the past 200 years, doctors have prescribed an almost uninterrupted succession of 'addictive' drugs, always in the belief they would not cause dependence. . . . The public's opinion that antidepressants are drugs of dependence seems much closer to the reality than the exactly opposite orthodox [medical] view."

Eli Lilly's advertisements in the general media for Prozac specifically state: "Like other antidepressants, it isn't habit forming."[48] No wonder so many patients are not informed either about serious withdrawal syndromes or dependence. Obviously such statements by pharmaceutical companies and drug advocates are attempts to "educate" the public out of their healthy concerns about drugs in general, including Prozac-type medications. Although aggressively advanced, such pronouncements are at odds with the clinical reality for many patients on the drugs.

Ron: A Case of Wearing Off

Closely related to withdrawal and dependence is the phenomenon of serotonin boosters wearing off. Ron had been on Zoloft for three years when he moved from Atlanta to Boston for a major job promotion. In Atlanta, Ron had steadily risen through the ranks working at an advertising agency. He moved to Boston to take on an even bigger job managing one of the largest accounts of a major Boston ad agency.

At the time of the move, Ron was on 200 milligrams of Zoloft. In the three years he had been on the drug, every spring he had noticed himself becoming depressed again. In response, his doctor had increased Ron's dose in yearly 50-milligram increments from 50 to 200 milligrams.

Shortly after he arrived in Boston, Ron began having difficulties. At his new company, he found himself in the midst of a political battle between warring factions vying for control of the company's fate. Still worse, the account he was hired to manage turned out to be in serious jeopardy. The account was a Boston-based group of retail lumber stores. Until recently, the stores had thrived as leading home improvement centers, but their business was now being seriously undercut by a national chain that had recently moved into the area. No amount of creative advertising could alter these circumstances, which were beyond Ron's control. Nevertheless, it was easy for him to become the scapegoat in the client's deteriorating situation. For this reason, Ron learned, no one at the agency had been willing to take over the account, which was why he had been recruited from outside. Removed from his network of family and friends back in Atlanta, Ron felt lonely and isolated.

As Ron's mood plummeted, he called his new HMO in Boston. By the time he finally saw a doctor, after waiting a month for an appointment, he was seriously depressed and suicidal. Because of the severity of his condition, the new doctor referred him to a psychopharmacologist.

Ron was shocked when the psychopharmacologist explained that he was on the maximum dose of Zoloft, which had clearly worn off again. When Ron asked what he meant by "again," the psychopharmacologist explained that the yearly increases in his dose had been because the drug had worn off repeatedly. Here again Ron was stunned, because his doctor in Atlanta had never explained the reason for the yearly increments.

Feeling desperate, Ron pleaded with the psychopharmacologist to increase his Zoloft. Many medication doctors are willing to push the dose of Zoloft or another Prozac-type medication beyond the limit set by the Food and Drug Administration and the pharmaceutical company. But even increasing his dose to 300 milligrams of Zoloft was ineffective at halting Ron's slide, and at that point the psychopharmacologist was unwilling to increase the dose further.

In the ensuing months, the psychopharmacologist tried several other antidepressants on Ron, but to no avail. In the meantime, facing increasing job pressures, Ron began drinking heavily. Alcohol is a strong central nervous system depressant, making drinking a deadly combination with depression. One night, after becoming intoxicated, Ron made a serious suicide attempt, ingesting a mixture of potentially lethal pills. Fortunately, a friend from Atlanta called Ron, realized he was slurring his speech and not coherent, and called the police, who rushed him to the hospital.

Ron survived his suicide attempt and spent several weeks in a psychiatric hospital. Just before he was discharged, Ron was informed he had lost his job at the advertising agency. His job termination also left him without health insurance.

I began seeing Ron shortly after he left the hospital. He was devastated by his suicide attempt and losing his job.

"I had no idea the Zoloft had worn off," said Ron angrily. "I thought it was protecting me from a severe depression. This is the worst depression I've ever had."

As part of my evaluation of Ron, I asked what had made him depressed in the first place three years ago when he went on the Zoloft. Ron look at me perplexed. "I have no idea," he said.

Over the years, I have learned not to be surprised by this answer from patients whose treatments have merely consisted of blunting symptoms with medication. "What was going on in your life at the time?" I inquired.

Ron explained that his father had died in the spring of the year in which he first became depressed. As we talked, it emerged that his father was a severe alcoholic who had been physically and emotionally abusive to Ron and his mother. Eventually, during Ron's college years, his mother had mustered the courage to divorce his father. In their bitter divorce, Ron had taken his mother's side. He and his father had not spoken for several years at one point. Ultimately they patched up their relationship superficially, but they had never really talked about the abuse or the difficult years in which they had been estranged. As we talked, Ron began to sob, expressing a mixture of sadness and anger over the abuse, together with guilt that so many things had been left unsaid when his father died. He hoped his father knew that in spite of everything Ron cared for him. He deeply regretted that his father died before he had a chance to express this explicitly.

Here, then, was the answer to my original question of why Ron had gone on Zoloft in the first place: Ron had been medicated to suppress his grief, from which he had been running ever since. Unattended to all these years, the grief was just as fresh and palpable as when his father died. No doubt the yearly recurrences of his depression, which always occurred in the spring, were anniversary reactions to his father's death.

Ron probably never should have been prescribed Zoloft in the first place. He would have benefited much more from a few months of psychotherapy to help him work through his grief. Certainly he had lost valuable years shoring up his mood with Zoloft when he might have more comfortably been working through his grief. Now the medication had worn off and his life was in a shambles.

I was not able to work with Ron for long. Because he had no other supports in Boston, he decided to move back to Atlanta, where he had family and friends. He planned to pursue psychotherapy once he was settled back in Atlanta. Ron's experience is an example of the dire consequences some patients face when their antidepressants wear off and they become severely depressed by the undiluted reality of loss and emotional pain, both past and present.

The wearing off of Prozac, Zoloft, Paxil, and the other serotonin boosters now dominates discussion at many psychiatric meetings. Systematic studies are confirming what has been seen clinically and are finding that the drugs will wear off in at least 30–40% of patients. One such study was conducted by a group of Harvard psychiatrists at the Massachusetts General Hospital led by Dr. Maurizio Fava. The study followed patients who had responded to treatment with 20 milligrams a day of Prozac and were being maintained on the drug long-term. The patients were assessed every two to four weeks for a year for signs that the drug's effect had worn off and their depression had recurred. Published in the February 1995 issue of the *Journal of Clinical Psychiatry*, the study found Prozac wore off in 34% of patients.[49] Most of the patients (83%) responded to an increase in the dose of Prozac to 40 milligrams a day. Within a year, however, the higher dose had worn off in 27% of patients. These patients required an additional increase in their dose or had to be switched to multiple other medications in the search for an antidepressant that might work.

A well-known published case in which medication wore off is that of Elizabeth Wurtzel, the Harvard graduate who wrote the best-selling memoir *Prozac Nation*. In the book, Wurtzel describes her experiences with a host of antidepressants, major tranquilizers, Valium-type antianxiety agents, and sleeping pills. Describing taking "hits" of her prescription medication and feeling "loaded" on the drugs, she characterizes her psychopharmacologist's Manhattan office as the "Fifth Avenue Crack House, because all he really does is write prescriptions and hand out pills. . . . I don't trust him. He's the pusherman."[50]

By the time the book appeared, Wurtzel said in interviews, the Prozac had worn off and she was on Zoloft.[51] Says Wurtzel, "Just as many germs have outsmarted antibiotics such that diseases like tuberculosis, once thought to be under control, have re-emerged in newer, more virulent mutant strains, so depression manages to reconfigure itself" and overcome the medication's diminished effect.[52]

Several examples of antidepressants wearing off are cited in writer Andrew Solomon's personal piece "Anatomy of Melancholy," which appeared in the January 12, 1998, issue of *The New Yorker*.[53] Solomon describes his experiences with "various combinations and doses" of Zoloft, Paxil, Effexor, and Wellbutrin. Says Solomon of being on the drugs, "The real effects, at best, fade with time." He cites a colleague, a young editor named Sarah Gold, who initially responded to Wellbutrin but says "she was one of those people for whom medication is effective for only a limited time." Switched to Effexor, "she got a lift again . . . but that, too, wore off after a year or so." At a depression support group he met a woman named Polly who said, "I took Prozac, and it worked for a year, and then it stopped."

Typically, patients are extremely upset to lose the positive effects of a drug they have depended on, sometimes for years. Patients are often angry they were not warned this could happen. They are particularly angry if a psychopharmacologist or managed care insurer discouraged them from doing psychotherapy. Patients feel they "lost valuable time" when they might have worked through psychological problems in the period of relative calm the drug offered.

In her 1998 memoir, *Prozac Diary,* Lauren Slater describes initially feeling "high," "blissed-out," "delightfully drugged," like a "junkie" on Prozac. She may have felt so good because she was on a high dose, 60 milligrams a day. One year after she started Prozac, the drug wore off. Analogizing Prozac to a lover, she says, "When you fall so deeply in love . . . you don't expect to be betrayed. But then you are."[54]

At the time, Slater was a graduate student in psychology at Harvard. She had gone to Kentucky for the summer to do research on her thesis. A young Jewish woman boarding with a devout Christian family, oppressed by the sweltering Kentucky heat, and separated from her boyfriend and friends, a short while into the three-month trip Slater suddenly awoke one morning depressed: "The Prozac had simply stopped working." Indeed, she felt more depressed than ever: "As fast as Prozac had once, like a sexy firefighter, doused the flames of pain, the flames now flared up, angrier than ever, and my potent pill could do nothing to quell the conflagration."

Feeling desperate, Slater telephoned her psychopharmacologist in Boston. He was on vacation and did not return her call for two weeks, by which time she felt "sick as a dog, my whole mind warped" with depression.

"What is this stuff you gave me?" Slater asked frantically as soon as she heard her doctor on the phone. "It was working perfectly, and now it's not. I've built up a tolerance to it. This stuff is like heroin. What's going on here?"

"It's called Prozac poop-out," he responded, ineloquently.

"Prozac poop-out. You've got to be kidding me." Slater may have been incredulous, but this is a term often used.

"Why didn't you warn me?" pleaded Slater, starting to cry. "You have no idea how shocking this is. I have come . . . to really love, I mean really depend on this stuff, for my functioning."

"It's okay," said her psychopharmacologist, reassuringly. "We can always up your dose. Take eighty milligrams instead of sixty. Let's see what happens."

"You tell me," she responded, still angry, "what happens when we have the little poop-out problem at eighty milligrams [the maximum dose approved by the FDA]. Then what do we do? Keep upping my dose till I die?"

Although she felt "rage at the doctor" and "rage at the two-timing pill," Slater went up to the higher dose. "Prozac never again made me as well as it once had," she says wistfully. "The poop-out problem has remained but not completely. . . . Prozac is not my lover any longer but . . . a slightly anemic, well-meaning buddy whose presence can considerably ease pain but cannot erase it." Having tried many times to go off Prozac and been unable, when her memoir appeared in 1998, Slater had been on the drug for ten years.

Like Slater, many patients are unaware their medication has worn off until they encounter new difficulties in life. Many doctors who prescribe the drugs are equally surprised when patients relapse while on them. Recently, I received a frantic phone call from a colleague, a primary-care doctor, when one of his patients who had been stable for years on Paxil was suddenly depressed and suicidal. "How can he be depressed? He's on Paxil!" asked the doctor in a panic.

"The Paxil has probably worn off," I explained.

"Worn off?" he said, amazed.

"It may have worn off a long time ago and he didn't know and neither did you, until he ran into some new problem in life."

Now feeling in over his head, the primary-care doctor was extremely relieved when I agreed to take over the patient's psychiatric care. Unfortunately, the patient did not respond to increasing his dose or switching to other drugs. Embittered, he said he would have preferred "never to have known" Paxil's mood-elevating effect "if it could not be sustained."

In a related scenario, many patients who have cycled on and off a Prozac-type medication suddenly discover when it is restarted that it no longer works. Jan was a young writer who had been on and off Prozac for a year at a time, over and over again. She would typically go on the drug to improve her concentration when she was working feverishly to finish a book or other major writing project and feeling stressed and vaguely depressed. Finally, one time, after being off Prozac for more than a year, Jan went back on it and was dismayed when it did not work, even when the dose was pushed up to the maximum. Since Jan had been off Prozac for more than a year, it had evidently worn off during the previous stint on the drug. In such cases, the drug's no longer working appears to be permanent.

Further Evidence of Prozac Backlash

Withdrawal, dependence, and wearing off are further evidence of Prozac backlash: They are a triad of closely related side effects all resulting from the brain's reaction to drugs that target the central nervous system. The effects of antidepressants used to be explained simply on the basis of their actions at the junctions between brain cells, where the cells communicate with one another. As shown in the illustrations on pages 18 and 19, the Prozac group boost serotonin by inhibiting—or blocking—reuptake of the neurotransmitter back into the cells that release it. This exposes cells to artificially elevated serotonin levels.

We now appreciate that the effects of these drugs are much more profound than this simple model. In reaction to being hyperstimulated by higher levels of the neurotransmitter, brain cells attempt to compensate by reducing their sensitivity to serotonin and by other long-term adaptations. This backlash involves complex changes in the cells' internal workings. Indeed, recent research on serotonin antidepressants has shown the adaptations of brain cells involve changes in the instructions given by the DNA of the cells—the master code regulating cellular function.[55] Writing in the February 1996 issue of the *American Journal of Psychiatry,* Dr. Steven Hyman, director of the National Institute of Mental Health, describes it this way: "chronic [drug] administration drives the production of adaptations . . . including regulation of neural gene [brain cell DNA] expression."[56] Changes involving DNA expression are complicated, which is part of the reason why the adaptations may take months to fully occur. In some instances, as with patients where the drugs wear off indefinitely, the changes are apparently permanent. This again raises concern about the long-term effects of these drugs on the brain.

Until recently, the changes wrought in brain cells by central nervous system drugs have been presumed to leave the cells intact and functioning, albeit in an altered way. However, in recent years, a much more ominous possibility has emerged: neurotoxicity, that is, the possibility that some central nervous system drugs are toxic to the brain, damaging or destroying critical parts of brain cells. Because we lack adequate studies of neurotoxicity with the Prozac group, one has to turn to studies of other, related drugs. Evidence of neurotoxicity has now accumulated in association with the once popular prescription antidepressants cocaine and amphetamines; the recently withdrawn diet pill Redux; and the currently popular street drug MDMA, or "Ecstasy."[57] Like the Prozac group, all these drugs boost serotonin. To varying degrees, they also boost other neurotransmitters—that is, adrenaline or dopamine.[58] All of them work primarily by one or both of two mechanisms: "Reuptake inhibitors" like the Prozac group block the reabsorption of neurotransmitters by brain cells. Cocaine resembles the Prozac group in that it is primarily a reuptake inhibitor. Other drugs are primarily "releasers": they boost neurotransmitter levels by causing cells to release more neurotransmitters. Redux is an example of a drug that is both a reuptake inhibitor and a releaser. In fact, the distinction between reuptake inhibitors and releasers is blurred: Most of these drugs, including the Prozac group, have been reported to do both, depending on the dose.[59]

Because it was so recently withdrawn from the market, Redux is a particularly relevant example. Introduced in this country in 1996, Redux rode the wave of popular serotonergic drugs of the 1990s. Like the Prozac group, Redux was heavily promoted as a remarkable new designer drug selective for serotonin. By boosting serotonin levels, Redux was said to reduce carbohydrate cravings in patients who wanted to lose weight.[60] Often prescribed in a drug combination known as "fen-phen," Redux was enormously popular, prescribed not only to those who were obese but also to those with normal weight who wanted to slim down. Redux's parent compound had been available in Europe for decades.[61] But in Europe doctors typically used it short term, for up to three months, with severely obese patients. In this country Redux began to be used "cosmetically" by women who were not obese and for periods of up to a year. By 1997 the drugs had been prescribed for an estimated 60 million people worldwide.[62]

In the fall of 1997, Redux was abruptly withdrawn from the market because of potentially fatal heart valve damage.[63] But scientists were also concerned about potential brain cell damage from neurotoxicity caused by the drug. Numerous studies of laboratory animals indicate Redux and its parent compound (fenfluramine) destroy the elaborately branching tentacles of serotonin neurons as they reach out to communicate with other neurons.[64] In other words, the drugs destroy the terminal branches, called axons, of their target cells. Researchers refer to this type of damage as axonal "pruning."[65] Under the microscope, as they are injured, the axons look "swollen," "irregularly shaped," and "seemingly fragmented."[66] In one study, monkeys treated with the drug for just four days showed evidence of "persistent" and "possibly permanent" damage more than a year later.[67] In fact, in the typical experiment, animals are on the drugs for just days at doses that the researchers say are comparable to those that many humans have taken for up to a year.[68] In some instances, if the damage is not too severe, the neurons sprout new branches in what literally amounts to a rewiring of the brain.[69]

The startling photomicrographs (photographs taken through a microscope) on page 97 illustrate the effects of Redux on the cerebral cortex of monkeys. They show apparent widespread destruction of the terminal branches of serotonin brain cells. The photomicrographs are especially chilling when one thinks of the millions of prescriptions written for the popular diet pill until it was withdrawn in September 1997. Could people sustain such damage and still function? Apparently so. In spite of extensive brain damage, the laboratory animals did not evidence any obvious behavioral or other effects. Indeed, neuroscientists argue that the effects of significant damage might not appear until much later in life, when the brain's reserve capacity has been further eroded by the aging process. Writing in the August 27, 1997, issue of the *Journal of the American Medical Association,* a group of researchers headed by Dr. Una McCann at the National Institute of Mental Health (NIMH) stated that Redux's "brain serotonin neurotoxicity" may become "manifest only with advancing age."[70] Since Redux's neurotoxic effects are "dependent on dose and treatment duration," McCann's group raised concern that "the increased duration of use in humans [i.e., up to a year by comparison with days and weeks in experimental animals] could increase the chance of serotonin neuronal injury" in patients.

The neurotoxicity of Redux is often compared to that of Ecstasy. Ecstasy is a popular "designer" street drug targeting serotonin. Ecstasy users say it gives them a rush of energy, a mild euphoria, and a sense of being more trusting, of feeling closer to those around them. For a time, psychiatrists prescribed Ecstasy to patients before the practice was banned.

Studies of Ecstasy have shown that when damaged neurons sprout new branches, the rewiring of the brain is "highly abnormal," a chaotic jumble that does not follow the original pattern.[71] Most alarming, researchers are concerned that the neurotoxicity could cause "increased risk for developing age-related cognitive impairment." Indeed, they are explicit that the "aberrant reinnervation [abnormal rewiring of brain cells] such as that seen after MDMA [Ecstasy] injury may also occur during the course of neurodegenerative diseases (e.g., Parkinson's disease [and] Alzheimer's disease)." This is especially worrisome because patients with Alzheimer's-type dementia

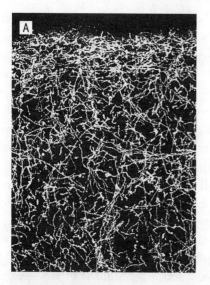 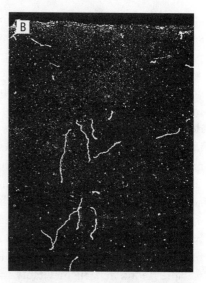

THE NEUROTOXICITY OF REDUX

A. A photograph taken through a microscope (photomicrograph) of the cerebral cortex of a normal monkey, not exposed to Redux. The black background represents brain tissue. The dense white fibers are highly branching serotonin brain cells as they reach out to communicate with other brain cells.

B. A photomicrograph of the cerebral cortex of a monkey exposed to Redux showing apparent widespread destruction of the branches of serotonin brain cells. The monkey was given Redux for just four days. The monkey was sacrificed and the photomicrograph taken 17 months later, indicating that the damage is permanent. The damage has been seen in laboratory animals given the drug for just days at doses that researchers say are comparable to those that many patients have taken for up to a year. Researchers say the effects of the damage may not become apparent until later in life, when the brain's reserve capacity has been further eroded by the aging process.

From U. D. McCann, L. S. Seiden, L. Rubin, and G. Ricaurte, "Brain Serotonin Neurotoxicity and Primary Pulmonary Hypertension from Fenfluramine [Redux's parent compound] and Dexfenfluramine [Redux]," *Journal of the American Medical Association (JAMA)* 278 (1997): 666–72.

"have significant 5-HT [serotonin] deficits in brain regions implicated in learning and memory" as well as deficits in other neurotransmitters.[72] In fact, in recent years, research on neurodegenerative conditions like Parkinson's and Alzheimer's diseases has zeroed in on neurotoxic substances as a likely cause of these debilitating illnesses.[73]

A number of theories of how drugs might be toxic to the brain have been developed. One theory is that high levels of neurotransmitters may result in their being converted into toxins. Writing on the neurotoxicity of amphetamine in the June 1997 issue of the *National Institute on Drug Abuse Research Monograph Series,* a group of biochemists at the University of Oklahoma headed by Dr. Monika Wrona noted that serotonin is "very easily oxidized [converted]" into a "serotonergic neurotoxin."[74] Excess serotonin lingering in the junctions between brain cells is thought to be particularly vulnerable to being converted into toxins.

At the time of the Redux debacle, Dr. McCann at the NIMH was so concerned that neurotoxic brain damage did, in fact, occur in patients taking Redux that she planned retrospectively to study patients for cognitive deficits and emotional disturbances after having received numerous, spontaneous case reports of these effects from doctors and patients.[75] McCann and her group have also speculated that neurotoxicity may explain why serotonergic drugs like Redux wear off in patients: Damage to their target cells renders the drugs ineffective. In their August 1997 article in the *Journal of the American Medical Association,* the group said of Redux's wearing off that "tolerance might be related to the loss of serotonin axons [terminal branches], since these axons are believed to mediate" the drug's effects.[76]

The Redux debacle inevitably raised questions about the Prozac group because of their shared emphasis on serotonin and their overlapping mechanisms of action. Prozac-type drugs are powerful appetite suppressants, prescribed as diet pills.[77] Indeed, when Redux was withdrawn, Prozac replaced it as a prescription diet pill at national weight-loss centers such as Nutri/Systems Diet Centers.[78] The week after Redux was withdrawn from the market, the cover of *Time* reflected the concern about Prozac: "Redux, Fen/phen, Prozac: How Mood Drugs Work . . . and Fail." Inside, the cover article said, "Serotonin drugs treat everything from depression to overeating, but as we learned this week, tinkering with the chemistry of the brain can be risky."[79] *Time* described the neurotoxic effects of Redux as "overdosing neurons and burning them out." Given their similarities with Redux, could the Prozac group be causing nerve cell damage?

There are no published studies of the effects of the Prozac group that include photomicrographic studies such as those shown above for Redux.[80] Meanwhile, many former amphetamine antidepressants, discredited diet pills, and the serotonergic street drug Ecstasy have been tested exhaustively. All of these drugs are neurotoxic in tests of many animal species, including rats, mice, guinea pigs, and monkeys. The research includes experiments in which the drugs were administered in doses believed to be comparable to those used by patients.

Most neurotoxicity studies that produce such photomicrographs also measure a variety of other indicators of nerve cell damage. For example, levels of serotonin drop because the cells are damaged. Also, the levels of receptors normally found on the cells are reduced. These biochemical measures (as opposed to photomicrographic ones) are referred to as "markers" of the cell damage. Studies of these markers are another source of information about the extent of the damage.

There are a few published studies measuring these markers after laboratory animals are given Prozac-type drugs, but the research has not been thorough enough to be conclusive. One critical variable appears to be how long the laboratory animals are treated with Prozac. Studies in which Prozac has been given to animals for twenty-one days show significant reductions of markers (20–50%, depending upon the dose and the region of the brain) when the animals were sacrificed a week after the last dose.[81] But we need experiments in which the animals are sacrificed two weeks, one month, or more after the last dose to see how long the reductions persist as a measure of how long-lasting they may be. Moreover, we need the kind of photomicrographic studies that have been published for the illicit drugs, all of which have been thoroughly researched. In the absence of these studies, the reductions measured so far may or may not indicate lasting damage. Because the additional, needed studies have not been published, we simply do not know. In the absence of thorough research, the few studies we have to date of Prozac are cause for concern. Finally, we need studies in which the Prozac group are administered long-term, as they are to patients, for months or years. Administering the drugs for years would require studying monkeys, since rats do not live long enough.

Some drug advocates have defended serotonin-enhancing medications by suggesting that destroying the terminal branches of brain cells may be part of their therapeutic effect. In a panel discussion on the neurotoxicity of Redux published in the *Annals of the New York Academy of Sciences,* Dr. Mark Molliver of the department of neuroscience and neurology at the Johns Hopkins University School of Medicine said that "it is even possible that pruning serotonin neurons may be therapeutic in some cases. . . . Possibly you have done some psychosurgery [such as lobotomy] on your patients and made them better that way."[82] Another panel member, Dr. John Blundell of the University of Leeds, England, was so shocked by this idea that he said, "I hope this [discussion] isn't being transcribed." But, of course, it was.

I think most patients would be shocked by the idea that a prescription medication could be effecting a chemical lobotomy that might lead to permanent brain damage. At least they would want to be informed if this was a possibility, rather than leaving it up to laboratory scientists to decide whether or not this is a reasonable way to be "therapeutic." Indeed, reading the current literature on neurotoxicity, one finds an unsettling bias. When discussing brain cell damage caused by street drugs such as amphetamines, cocaine, or Ecstasy, researchers speak in the gravest terms, warning of dread effects. Only when referring to prescription drugs do they suggest that pruning nerve cells might be "therapeutic."

Some neurotoxicity researchers argue that cocaine is a better comparison with Prozac than Redux is. This is because cocaine—like the Prozac group—boosts neurotransmitters by blocking their reuptake back into the cells that release them. For years, researchers thought cocaine was not neurotoxic in the way that amphetamines, Redux, and Ecstasy are.[83] This is because cocaine is not toxic to the serotonin and dopamine brain cells commonly tested in neurotoxicity studies. But in recent years, cocaine has been found to be neurotoxic to other, quite unexpected cells. In the early 1990s, a group of researchers at UCLA headed by Dr. Gaylord Ellison reported that cocaine is neurotoxic to specific groups of cells in two other neurotransmitter systems, acetylcholine and gamma-aminobutyric acid.[84] The damaged cells are not cocaine's direct targets. Rather, they are indirectly affected by the drug; that is, they receive messages from cocaine's target cells. Researchers believe the damaged cells are "weak links in neuronal circuitry" particularly vulnerable to neurotoxicity. While not the direct targets of the drug, they are in "pathways overdriven by incessant drug-induced activity [which] may eventually degenerate, leaving the brain in a persistently altered state." This important finding indicates that even though a drug may not be neurotoxic to the brain cells it targets, it may be neurotoxic to other cells that it affects indirectly.

Another finding in the cocaine research is that lower, continuous doses of the drug are neurotoxic, whereas higher, episodic doses are not. Using the same total amount of cocaine administered over five days, researchers have compared giving higher intermittent doses with giving lower, continuous (around-the-clock) doses.[85] Surprisingly, the higher doses did not cause the neurotoxicity. Apparently, even though the doses were higher, the brain was able to recover in the periods when it was free of the drug. But the lower, continuous doses bathed the brain in the drug 24 hours a day, leaving it no time to recover. Reports the Ellison group, "It now appears that, for a number of pharmacological agents [including amphetamines and cocaine], prolonged plasma [blood, and therefore, brain] levels are more crucial in producing neurotoxicity than higher but more transient plasma levels. Apparently neuronal systems [brain cells] have developed more effective ways to cope with sudden and brief insults than with progressive, more prolonged ones."[86] This again raises concerns about the Prozac group, because antidepressants are prescribed daily in order to effect continuous, around-the-clock levels of the drug bathing the brain. The doses used in the cocaine studies are comparable to the higher doses taken by chronic cocaine addicts, not beginners. But as in other neurotoxicity studies, laboratory animals are typically given cocaine for relatively short periods of time, such as five days, by comparison with the years that people are on Prozac-type drugs.

Cocaine is well known to adversely affect the brain by yet another mechanism: Brain-imaging studies have shown cocaine constricts cerebral blood vessels, choking off the blood supply of critical oxygen and nutrients, and thereby injuring brain cells. As a result, both short-term and long-term changes in brain cell function have been reported, even months after cocaine addicts become drug-free. Dr. Nora Volkow at the Brookhaven National Laboratory has been a pioneer of these brain-imaging studies. Writing in the November 1992 issue of the journal *Synapse,* Volkow states that this brain dysfunction is seen in the frontal lobe, which plays an important role in personality, emotions, and cognitive functioning.[87]

There have been few studies of cerebral blood flow and the potential effect on brain cell activity with the Prozac group or other currently popular prescription medications. One rare study using Prozac was conducted by Rudolph Hoehn-Saric at the Johns Hopkins University School of Medicine. In the October 1990 issue of the *Journal of Clinical Psychopharmacology*, Dr. Hoehn-Saric reported patients on Prozac and Luvox whose emotions were so blunted that their "apathy and indifference" resembled that of patients with damage to the frontal lobes.[88] The following year, Hoehn-Saric reported another patient, a twenty-three-year-old man with obsessive-compulsive disorder, who developed a "frontal lobe syndrome" consisting of apathy and cognitive deficits after being on 100 milligrams a day of Prozac for four months. This time, instead of simply relying on a diagnosis based on clinical observation, Hoehn-Saric administered an extensive battery of neuropsychological tests that documented cognitive deficits consistent with "disruption of frontal lobe functioning." Moreover, Hoehn-Saric had used brain-imaging techniques to measure cerebral blood flow in the patient before he was put on Prozac and after developing the frontal lobe symptoms. Writing in the March 1991 issue of the *Journal of Clinical Psychiatry,* Hoehn-Saric reported the imaging study revealed "a decrease in frontal cerebral blood flow" consistent with the "decreased performance on neuropsychological tests sensitive to disruption of frontal lobe functioning."[89]

Reflecting on these disturbing findings, Hoehn-Saric said that "it is conceivable that functional frontal lobe changes of a milder degree are responsible for some of the therapeutic effects of Prozac." Noting that a surgical lobotomy consists of severing the connections "between the frontal lobes and the rest of the brain," Hoehn-Saric speculated that a "similar but reversible and dose-dependent effect of serotonin reuptake-blocking [Prozac-type] medications on frontal lobe functions may be responsible for their effectiveness." Here again, the effects of serotonin-enhancing medications are being compared to a chemical lobotomy. Whereas a decrease in cerebral blood flow and weakening of brain cell functioning with a street drug like cocaine is described by researchers as an adverse consequence of drug use, in the case of serotonin boosters it is described as potentially "therapeutic." Perhaps for patients with severe depression or obsessive-compulsive disorder the risks of a chemical lobotomy may be worth taking. But for the great majority of patients on Prozac-type drugs for whom there are alternatives, I would seriously question the advisability of such a risk. As Hoehn-Saric concludes, "Systematic examination of the effect of serotonin reuptake-blocking drugs [the Prozac group] on cerebral blood flow and metabolism and on mental functions are needed to explore this possibility [of frontal lobe changes]."

Unfortunately, there has been no such systematic investigation. In recent decades, the explosion of published studies about the neurotoxicity of cocaine, amphetamines, discredited diet pills, and street drugs like Ecstasy is impressive. By contrast, there is a striking scarcity of studies on current heavily prescribed drugs like Prozac, Zoloft, Paxil, Luvox, Wellbutrin (also known as Zyban), Effexor, Serzone, and others. Given the enormous amount of research on neurotoxicity, one has to wonder at the large number of studies of illegal drugs and so few on drugs being prescribed to millions of people, most of whom are unaware of the potential risks.

Researchers say one reason for the lack of adequate studies on popularly prescribed medications like the Prozac group is the control pharmaceutical companies exercise over research on drugs as long as they are covered by their patent. For animal research, the pure form of a drug is needed from the manufacturer, as the pill form contains too many additives.[90] But in order to obtain the pure drug, researchers can be required to sign onerous contracts, which, among other things, grant the company the right to veto publication of the results. The careers of scientists depend on publishing their work. Few can invest the time, energy, and money in studies a pharmaceutical company may not allow to be published. All of the serotonin boosters are still covered by their patents. Even when the patent on a drug runs out, obtaining funding for costly animal research can be difficult. Funding for research is typically granted by review boards. Most of the people who sit on review boards are researchers with ties to the pharmaceutical companies that fund at least some of their research. Just one reviewer opposed to a study can easily raise objections that block it.

Is neurotoxicity one of the causes of Prozac backlash? Is it the mechanism by which the Prozac group causes the neurological side effects discussed in the previous chapter, including drug-induced parkinsonism and disfiguring tics? Does neurotoxicity sensitize brain tissue, worsen the long-term progression of psychiatric conditions, and leave people dependent on the drugs? Might neurotoxicity explain the development of tolerance and the drugs wearing off? Is neurotoxicity responsible for memory loss, cognitive deficits, and personality changes on the drugs? Could damage of this type contribute to the development of senile tics, gait disturbances, Alzheimer's disease, Parkinson's disease, or other neurological conditions later in life?

The once popular prescription antidepressants cocaine and amphetamines, diet pills, such as Redux, the street drug Ecstasy, and the currently popular prescription drugs like the Prozac group are all related. These potent drugs are all produced using technology first invented by German scientists only about 150 years ago. All of them target brain cells and boost the levels of neurotransmitters.

When a medication like Redux goes down in a debacle of side effects, drug proponents often point to differences between it and popular drugs like the Prozac group in an effort to protect them from any fallout. Not only are the drugs' differences sometimes exaggerated, often the distinctions do not hold up under scrutiny. At the time of the Redux crisis in the fall of 1997, Prozac's being a "reuptake inhibitor" of serotonin was cited in attempts to distance it from Redux, which was described as a serotonin "releaser." In fact, the distinction may be irrelevant in terms of neurotoxicity; both mechanisms elevate serotonin. For years, researchers thought cocaine was not neurotoxic because it is primarily a reuptake inhibitor. But we now know cocaine is neurotoxic. Moreover, although the Prozac group have been widely promoted for increasing serotonin by inhibiting its reuptake into cells, studies have shown that like Redux they can cause serotonin release as well. The mechanisms of action of Redux, Prozac, and Zoloft were directly compared in a study by a group of Italian scientists in Milan headed by Dr. Silvio Garattini. The study was published in 1992 in the *International Journal of Obesity* in an article entitled "Progress Report on the Anorectic [diet pill] Effects of Redux, Prozac, and Zoloft."[91] Garattini's research showed that in addition to blocking reuptake of serotonin "all three drugs release 5-HT [serotonin] . . . Prozac affected storage of serotonin" as well. Thus, the marketing claims emphasizing a particular mechanism of action of a class of drugs may not be the full story.

Another reassurance that drug proponents often make is that *at prescription doses* currently popular drugs are not toxic. The implication is that drugs targeting the brain are only toxic in the high doses at which street drugs are abused. But animal studies of Redux have been carried out at doses researchers argue are comparable to those taken by patients.[92] Even more important, neurotoxicity research has shown that "toxicity is dependent on both the size of the dose and the length of time over which it is administered."[93] A low dose over a longer period of time may be more dangerous than a high dose over a shorter period of time. Since the drugs are neurotoxic to laboratory animals who take them for days or weeks, what are the implications for people who take them for years, even decades?

Research on Prozac has shown that in humans the drug slowly accumulates in the brain over many months. Writing in the Summer 1993 issue of the *Journal of Neuropsychiatry and Clinical Neurosciences,* a group of researchers at the University of Arkansas for Medical Sciences headed by Dr. Craig Karson reported that Prozac reaches its ultimate concentration in the brain only after six to eight months. After eight months, the level of Prozac in the brain is roughly twenty times the level in the blood.[94] Karson's group said the buildup of Prozac "appeared to depend on duration of treatment and dose," which they called the "cumulative dose" of the drug. While patients often agonize over whether or not to increase their dose by onefold or twofold, the drug is meanwhile being sequestered and concentrated twentyfold in the brain. What might be the long-term effects of these high drug levels on the brain after months of chronic administration?

Still a third reassurance frequently offered is that Prozac is "neuroprotective." That is, when Prozac is combined with known toxins like Redux or amphetamines, the result is less damage than caused by the known toxins alone. But again, this does not hold up to scrutiny. The same argument was made for many years regarding cocaine. When cocaine is given in combination with an amphetamine, it too protects brain cells from some of the amphetamine's neurotoxicity.[95] But recently we have learned that cocaine is neurotoxic to entirely different cells indirectly affected by the drug. Most important, this reassurance is again based on a false premise, because what drugs do in combination is not necessarily any indication of what each one does on its own.

Reviewing the 150-year history of these potent agents, one finds repeated instances of drug advocates providing what turned out to be false reassurances on behalf of popular medications until their dangers were undeniable. Common sense suggests that if all the once popular prescription drugs—including cocaine, amphetamines, and discredited diet pills—

are neurotoxic, then the related, currently popular medications like the Prozac group may be too. Different drugs can be neurotoxic in different parts of the brain depending on the dosage and treatment regimen. Not just one or two experiments but dozens of studies using varying conditions are needed to thoroughly test whether or not a drug is toxic. Truly long-term studies are needed in which animals are given a drug as patients are, for months or years. In addition to the neurotransmitter systems known to be affected by the drug, other neurotransmitter systems, which may be indirectly affected, also need to be investigated.

Are we going to wait decades, until long after these medications have fallen out of favor, for the Prozac group to be thoroughly tested? Surely we already know enough to indicate these drugs should be prescribed far more cautiously than they typically are today.

In the May 20, 1994, issue of *Psychiatric News,* several leading psychopharmacologists were quoted on the controversy over the long-term, potentially damaging effects of prescription antidepressants like the Prozac group. One of the authorities interviewed was Donald Klein, professor of psychiatry at Columbia University and the then president of the American Society of Clinical Psychopharmacologists. Regarding the extraordinary lack of much-needed studies, Dr. Klein said that "the industry is not interested, NIMH is not interested, and the FDA is not interested. Nobody is interested. What balks everybody is that it would be expensive and difficult. *I think the industry is concerned about the possibility of finding long-term risks* [italics added]."[96]

Neurotoxicity studies give one serious cause to wonder whether all drugs targeting specific brain cells and boosting neurotransmitters are potentially toxic over the long term to their target cells. With so many patients being prescribed Prozac-type medications and with so many serious side effects of the earlier drugs now on the horizon, it behooves us to investigate these drugs thoroughly without delay. We do not really need more evidence that cocaine and amphetamines are harmful. What we need urgently are studies of the currently prescribed popular medications.

3

Not Tonight, Dear—
I'm on Prozac
Sexual Dysfunction

Ask any doctor what the side effects of serotonin boosters are and the first ones she will cite are sexual dysfunctions. These are the best-known side effects of the drugs. We now know they occur in 60% of patients.[1] Yet Eli Lilly still lists the seriously misleading figure of 2–5% in their official product information on Prozac.[2] The manufacturers of the other serotonin boosters also give misleadingly low numbers.[3] Why do the official figures not match reality? Because they date to the manufacturers' prerelease testing of the drugs. During most of the short, six-to-eight-week studies, pharmaceutical companies failed to ask patients if they were experiencing sexual difficulties.[4]

The sexual dysfunction induced by serotonin boosters is distinctly different from that seen with earlier antidepressants. Instead, it is remarkably similar to the sexual side effects seen in the 1950s, 1960s, and 1970s in people on major tranquilizers. Of course, these tranquilizers are the class of drugs that, unfortunately, taught us so much about the neurological side effects discussed in Chapter 1. Once the Prozac of their day, they were popularly prescribed for anxiety, insomnia, and mild depression, until their use in the 1980s became strictly limited to only the most severe psychiatric conditions because it was learned that they cause permanent brain damage and disfiguring tics. Unfortunately, this raises the question whether or not the sexual side effects experienced by a high percentage of patients on serotonin boosters are one of the best indications we have so far that many people may be vulnerable, long-term, to the kind of brain damage seen with major tranquilizers.

What Women Report

Inability to Orgasm

"I feel like an adolescent boy with a perpetual hard-on who can't get any action." With this graphic declaration, Sharon told me of her inability to orgasm.

"The worst part is that my appetite for sex isn't dampened, just my ability to really enjoy it. Help!" She grinned ruefully.

"It might be the Prozac, you know," I responded.

"I figured," said Sharon glumly. "It's awful."

Sharon had begun treatment with me just a few months earlier for depression. In her mid-thirties, she was a young mother juggling a marriage, raising two children, and a career. She was a freelance journalist, and had overcommitted to a series of almost-impossible-to-meet deadlines, which were now hard upon her. She wrote in-depth, thoroughly researched articles on environmental issues, several of which had won journalism awards. But the month before consulting with me, Sharon missed a deadline for the first time in her professional career. Missing the deadline scared her, especially with several other big deadlines pending, and made Sharon realize how depressed she was. In addition to threatening her work, the depression had also made her irritable and increasingly distant from her two daughters, aged six and nine. Her husband, Matt, also was concerned about Sharon's depression.

Considering the volume of work on her plate, the tight deadlines, and the concerns about her daughters' suffering from her depressed state, I agreed with Sharon that medication was a reasonable consideration. As with all patients, I explained that antidepressants are never a cure for psychological ills and encouraged her to be in psychotherapy to figure out what she needed to change in her life in order not to require medication. She responded well to 20 milligrams a day of Prozac, which provided the lift in her mood, energy, and concentration that she needed to get her work back on track. But now she was facing significant sexual dysfunction, an inability to orgasm, a difficulty she had never had before.

"In the two months I've been on Prozac," said Sharon, "having an orgasm just became more and more difficult, until now it's impossible. Climaxing took more intense stimulation for longer and longer periods of time: five minutes became ten minutes, became 30 minutes, and eventually I couldn't at all."

The resulting "sexual workout" had spoiled lovemaking for Sharon and Matt, to the point where they were both now "avoiding" sex. Ironically, because she was feeling better on Prozac, Sharon was more rather than less interested in sex, which only heightened her frustration.

"Are you sure you want to stay on a drug?" I asked.

"Yes. I've still got four major articles due in the next six months. I can't afford to get depressed again. The kids are so much happier with me feeling better. I can't go off the medication right now."

Since Sharon was determined to improve her sex life, if at all possible, this meant trying other antidepressants. She actually knew a great deal about the drugs, having researched them thoroughly before she came to see me. She first wanted to try Zoloft, another of the Prozac-type drugs, in the hope that she would get the same benefits but without the sexual side effects. Because Prozac is so long-lasting, lingering in the blood for one to two weeks, switching from Prozac to Zoloft would mean that in the initial weeks on the new drug both would be present, making it difficult to determine which one was causing the orgasmic difficulty if it persisted. We therefore decided to take Sharon off Prozac and wait for the sexual dysfunction to clear before starting Zoloft.

Sharon's ability to orgasm returned within two weeks after stopping the Prozac. "There's no question the drug was the culprit," said Sharon, surprised by how quickly the turnaround occurred. Unfortunately, at the same time Sharon could feel the depression returning. "In the morning, I can't get out of bed to face the day," she said. "After I drop Jenny and Clara off to school, back home I can't face a page, I can't lift a pen to write."

Sharon's depressive symptoms responded to the stimulating effects of Zoloft, just as they had to Prozac. But within a few weeks, her ability to achieve orgasm had again ground to a halt. Frustrated and disappointed, the plucky Sharon was prepared to move on to another drug.

We discussed the possibility of Paxil, but with two of the Prozac-type drugs having had the same effect, we were not optimistic Paxil would be any different. Instead, we decided to move beyond the Prozac group.

In recent years two antidepressants have been heavily promoted as causing fewer sexual side effects than the Prozac-type antidepressants: Serzone and Wellbutrin. After discussing these two possibilities, Sharon wanted to try Serzone first.

Sharon was scheduled to take a four-day vacation with her husband around the time that we were switching from Zoloft to Serzone. She decided to time the period when she would be off medication with the vacation so the couple could enjoy themselves. Nowadays, a surprising number of couples go through these kinds of gyrations trying to buy themselves a few days' relief from antidepressant-induced sexual dysfunction.

Sharon returned from her break having enjoyed herself sexually and all the more determined to be rid of the loathed side effects. We tried Serzone, which unfortunately had the same effect as Prozac and Zoloft, lifting Sharon's mood but ruining her sex life. We were back to square one.

The next drug on the list was Wellbutrin, for which I gave Sharon a prescription. Like many patients, she found Wellbutrin even more energizing and pleasurable than the other antidepressants. "What is this drug?" she asked. "I feel high." What is more, the Wellbutrin did not give her sexual side effects. "Success, at last!" said Sharon, thrilled to have finally found an antidepressant that did not impair her orgasmic capacity, after months of enduring trials of four drugs. One might marvel at Sharon's perseverance in finding a medication without sexual side effects, but in the 1990s her story was not unusual. Many patients have endured such ordeals, undergoing multiple medication trials in the search for a drug that worked for them without causing sexual side effects.

Sharon managed to meet the deadlines for her articles in the ensuing months and continued in psychotherapy, trying to figure out why she had become so depressed in the first place. One day, as she talked about how stressed she felt juggling work and family life, Sharon asked me out of the blue, "Does your wife work?" I was taken aback by the question, wondering why Sharon asked. In fact, over the years, my position on answering this question has changed. I used to answer reflexively, thinking the question mere curiosity, but I learned that no matter what the answer, it quickly became a burden for patients. If my wife worked, then the patient thought this was what I valued. The patient assumed she could only earn my respect if she was a "superwoman," effortlessly juggling raising children with a high-powered career. On the other hand, if my wife didn't work, then the patient assumed my position was the opposite: that I didn't value women working.

Over the years I learned to see the question as a flag for the profound conflict many women, and an increasing number of men, feel trying to achieve a comfortable balance between work and home life. It is not a therapist's job to tell patients what to do, except in dangerous situations. With an issue like balancing work and home life, a therapist is meant to help patients discover what balance works best for them. Therapists themselves are never perfect, and the way they lead their lives is not necessarily right for the next person.

So I declined to answer Sharon's question. Since I don't believe patients benefit from having psychotherapy made mysterious, I explained straightforwardly why I thought it was in her best interest for me not to answer.

Ultimately, like most patients, Sharon appreciated my wanting to leave her free to make her own decisions. But her question opened up an important line of inquiry. As we continued our discussions over months, she realized it was the open-ended demands of freelance work that were making her depressed. When her daughters were young, she had taken up freelance writing thinking it would be the ideal career, giving her complete freedom to schedule working around child-rearing. Now she was feeling overburdened. Since she cared deeply about the pieces she wrote, she could not simply dash them off. As a result, what she thought would be flexible work had instead overrun her life. Even when she was with her children, she was often thinking about the article she was in the midst of writing. Sharon knew she needed the stimulation of work and her family needed her income, but the inflexibility of a job with regular hours had always seemed an obstacle in her mind. Yet, as she struggled with these issues, she began to realize something: "I'm not doing my family any favor being present if I'm so distracted and depressed that I'm short-tempered and distant with them. Nor can I go on indefinitely propping myself up with drugs to do something that's this uncomfortable."

Sharon eventually sought a regular job, turning down several good offers before taking a three-quarter-time position as an editor, which she found genuinely interesting and paid sufficiently. Since nothing is ever perfect, she still fretted over the balance in her life but found the new arrangement much better. Having accomplished this, she was able to go off the Wellbutrin without getting depressed again. In the long term, she expects that once her children are grown and off in college, she will work full-time or go back to freelance writing.

Inhibited Sexual Arousal

Prozac-type antidepressants can wreak havoc on aspects of sexual functioning other than the capacity to achieve orgasm. Christine was an attractive young woman in her mid-twenties who had been put on Zoloft for biting her nails. Her nail-biting improved but she developed difficulty with being sexually aroused on Zoloft. Her libido, her interest in sex, was unaffected by the drug, but Christine was unable to respond physically to sexual stimulation: She could not become lubricated even with intense stimulation by her husband, Eric. Her lack of lubrication made it too painful for Eric to enter her, which had "ruined" their sex life. Because of the combination of feeling highly motivated sexually but unable to respond physically, Christine described herself as being "like a car stuck out of gear. Even with the gas pedal pushed to the floor, the system's straining but going nowhere."

To make matters worse, Eric was taking Christine's lack of responsiveness personally, feeling that she had lost interest in him. Their difficulties as a couple are an example of the profoundly damaging effects that the sexual side effects of these drugs can have on marriages and relationships. I reassured Christine that the problem was probably the drug rather than her feelings for Eric. Because of the distress the couple was experiencing, Christine wanted to stop the Zoloft, which I supported, especially given the relatively trivial symptom for which she had been put on it. When she went off Zoloft, Christine's ability to be sexually responsive quickly returned to normal.

Loss of Libido

Even more basic than the ability to be sexually aroused or to achieve orgasm is one's interest in sex, one's motivation and energy level for pursuing sexual expression or responding to the overtures of another. Ellen was a thirty-four-year-old woman whom I started on Paxil for severe depression. A few weeks after starting the drug, Ellen lost all interest in sex. While irritated with the side effect, Ellen was willing to tolerate it because of the improvement in her energy level provided by the Paxil. At the time, Ellen was not in a relationship and not sexually involved with anyone. Her sex life consisted of masturbating, which she was "willing to sacrifice" to the medication's lifting her out of depression.

Regina was less tolerant of losing even a little bit of her interest in sex. A lesbian, Regina had recently begun her first long-term relationship with a woman and did not want her medication-induced loss of libido to "screw up the relationship." She had been on Luvox for two years for mild depression, but once she stopped the Luvox, buoyed by her relationship and the return of a robust sex drive, she did not relapse into depression.

As Sharon's, Christine's, Ellen's, and Regina's cases demonstrate, the Prozac group can adversely affect all three phases of the sexual arc: sex drive, physical arousal, and the ability to orgasm. Some patients experience more than one sexual side effect, as in Sharon's case, where her inability to orgasm eventually led to diminished interest in sex.

Less Common Sexual Side Effects

In addition to these common sexual side effects, one also finds more unusual ones. Doctors Van King and Ira Horowitz of Baltimore, Maryland, reported in the *American Journal of Psychiatry* on a thirty-seven-year-old woman on Prozac for depression who developed vaginal anesthesia, which they confirmed by physical exam.[5] After just two weeks on 20 milligrams a day of Prozac, the patient developed "convincing, total anesthesia of the vagina and vulva, as determined by needle prick. Urination was unaffected, and sensation was normal on the legs and areas surrounding the vulva." The patient's "genital sensation gradually returned to normal over a four-week period" after the Prozac was stopped. As with many patients, she was fine off the drug, without a return of her depression.

What Men Report

Loss of Libido

On serotonin boosters, men are as vulnerable to sexual dysfunction as women are. Juan's primary-care doctor asked me to see him when his sex drive plummeted on 20 milligrams a day of Paxil. A robust Puerto Rican man in his late thirties, Juan told me his doctor put him on Paxil for symptoms of anxiety. Within weeks, the drug started to dampen his sex drive. Juan was extremely upset that Paxil had "shut down" his libido: "My wife and I used to have sex four or five times a week. Now I feel like a eunuch. I'm not interested in my wife, whom I used to love having sex with. I've never cheated on her, but I've always enjoyed noticing other attractive women. Walking down the street, sitting in a café, or in an office meeting, for me noticing attractive women is part of the electricity, the sexual spark of life. Now everything is dull, gray. I feel like I've been neutered."

When I confirmed that the Paxil was probably responsible for the dramatic change in Juan's interest in sex, he said angrily, "That's it. I'm going off this drug. I don't want to be on medication that can dull my senses to this degree."

When I asked Juan why he had been anxious before going on Paxil he explained it was because of marital tensions. Both Juan and his wife were teachers. Having taught for years in a suburban school system, they both had "tremendous job security" and a good combined income. They owned their own home and had a cottage in Maine where they went for their long summer vacations. Having the summer off was important to him and a big part of why he chose a teaching career. All year long he looked forward to spending more time with his wife and children. In addition, Juan loved to paint the Maine coastline in the summers. "The painting's been ruined, too, by the Paxil," lamented Juan. "With all the color gone from life, who wants to paint?"

The reason he went on the drug, said Juan, was that in recent years his wife had begun pressuring him to take a job during the summer. For several years now, she had been working at a resort not far from their cottage. Recently, she had stepped up the pressure on him to be "earning some income too" during the summer months. The tension in their marriage had made him anxious and irritable. His primary-care doctor recommended Paxil, which alleviated the anxiety and irritability but, Juan commented, "didn't really solve the problem and created a whole new one."

Juan observed that his primary-care doctor seemed "nervous" at the idea of his going off the medication even though, as he said, "Now I'm feeling worse than I did before I went on Paxil. I'm starting to get depressed over what it's done to my love for sex and painting. Because I mentioned feeling depressed, he said perhaps we needed to increase the dose, which is why I think I'm seeing you. But I want to go off Paxil, not take more of it! I don't think he takes my sexual problem, or my generally feeling that life is dulled, seriously enough."

I supported Juan's going off the Paxil and recommended that he and his wife, Jacqueline, do some couples therapy instead. When I met her, Jacqueline proved to be as charming as he was. Interestingly, she had a very different take on the problem of her husband's not working during the summer. From her point of view, the real difficulty was Juan's discomfort with her working: "Juan's much more of an artist and dreamer than I am, so he's quite content to spend the summer on the beach with his easel and palette. I'm a more practical person who needs to keep busy, to be active. When our children were small, they occupied me full-time during the summer. Now they're older and there's not so much for me to do. I need to get out of the house. I enjoy working. We don't need the extra money, although I enjoy having it. It's not that I want Juan to work to earn more money, too. The real problem is that as modern as he is, Juan's still a Latin guy. He's uncomfortable that I'm now earning more than he is and that he's somewhat of a house husband during the summer. I only began suggesting he get a summer job too because he was giving me grief over having one. If he'd stop complaining about my working, I wouldn't care what he does. He's welcome to continue to take the summers off. I'd prefer that. I like the kids having one parent home during the summer, since we both work during the year. This is just a little bit of a blow to his macho ego. That's why he got irritable and anxious."

Over the course of several meetings, Juan and Jacqueline agreed that communication had broken down between them over this problem and that they had lost sight of each other's perspective on the matter. Ultimately, Juan agreed to accept Jacqueline's working and the different family role that would put him in during the summer. In return, Jacqueline assured him that she was quite content for him to take the summers off. The tension between them, together with Juan's irritability and anxiety, cleared. Several months later I received a postcard from Juan from Maine. The front of the card was a scene of the beach at dusk painted by Juan. On the back of the card, he inscribed, "Goodbye, Paxil. Hello, life. Painting, the summer, and you-know-what are all going well!"

Impotence

While Paxil shut down Juan's libido, other men remain interested in sex but have difficulty getting an erection. Within weeks of starting Zoloft, Richard noticed that his ability to achieve an erection "just began to peter out." Said Richard, "The first thing I noticed was that I required more and more intense foreplay to get an erection. Then I realized that my erections weren't lasting very long. If the level of sexual activity dipped for even a minute, my erection just went south. I felt so deflated sexually and otherwise. After two months on the drug, I was completely impotent, unable to get even the weakest hard-on."

Impotence, the inability to perform sexually, is extremely distressing to most men, even when they know it is medication-induced. I had originally put Richard on Zoloft for severe depression and suicidality, as I felt he needed to be on an antidepressant temporarily. I switched him to an older, tricyclic antidepressant, which lifted his energy level and mood without undercutting his ability to perform sexually. After six months of psychotherapy, Richard was no longer depressed and was able to be weaned off medication.

Inability to Ejaculate

Perhaps the most common sexual side effect in men on Prozac-type drugs is delayed ejaculation. With this syndrome, a man's libido is intact, as is his ability to have an erection. Once aroused and erect, however, his ability to ejaculate is delayed, often severely. Dave was a twenty-eight-year-old truck driver taking 40 milligrams a day of Prozac. Dave was prescribed Prozac to help him maintain his alertness, concentration, and energy as a long-distance trucker, often driving through the night. He sought a second opinion with me after the drug made it "impossible" for him to ejaculate.

"At first, it just took me longer to come on the Prozac, which was great," said Dave, a large, down-to-earth, likable man. "I've always been able to last five, maybe ten, minutes during intercourse, which satisfied my wife. Then, on Prozac, it became fifteen to twenty minutes, which we both thought was great. I knew the Prozac was responsible, that I was having difficulty ejaculating. But when it only took fifteen or twenty minutes, it felt good. I felt like I had this indestructible erection. But then it started to take even longer. Karen and I would both become exhausted. After we'd been having intercourse for twenty minutes, I'd withdraw because I was so worn out. Over and over, I'd enter Karen and have to withdraw again because I just couldn't come. She'd get sick of it. She'd want to enjoy the pleasure she had and fall asleep. I can't blame her. I'd feel the same if the tables were turned. Finally, it's gotten to the point where I can't ejaculate. I end up feeling bruised and in pain. On occasion, I've had an erection for two hours or more before finally giving up. Now I'm no longer the big stud. I'm reduced to staring at a swollen erection but unable to get my rocks off."

Because of his prolonged erections and difficulty ejaculating, Dave was "avoiding" sex with Karen, who was upset about his problem as well. "I used to drink coffee to keep me awake when I had to drive through the night," said Dave. "Then a buddy of mine went on Prozac to keep him awake. I tried some of his and it worked, so I asked my doctor to put me on it. Now I'm thinking of going back to the coffee."

I strongly encouraged Dave to do just that. A month later, in follow-up, he told me his sex life had returned to normal. "I was so worried it wouldn't," he confided. "I'd lost confidence in myself sexually. But clearly the problem was due to the Prozac. I'm fine now."

Less Common Sexual Side Effects

As with women, men can experience a host of less common sexual side effects. The first patient I ever started on Prozac, a young man in his early twenties named Jason, complained after a month on the drug that something "bizarre" was happening to him sexually. Jason's interest in sex and his ability to obtain an erection and to orgasm seemed to be fine, unaffected by the drug, but when he ejaculated, no sperm fluid appeared. "Have I stopped making sperm?" he asked anxiously. "Have I become infertile?"

"No," I reassured him, recognizing the side effect but surprised to hear it reported with an antidepressant. In this side effect, called retrograde ejaculation, the patient does, in fact, ejaculate. But because of the presence of the drug, the sperm fluid ends up in the bladder rather than coming out the penis. The result is the impression of having had an orgasm without the appearance of sperm.

I was familiar with this side effect from patients on major tranquilizers.

Indeed, I included a case of retrograde ejaculation, called "The Disappearing Sperm," in my last book, *Sexual Mysteries: Tales of Psychotherapy*.[6] However, I had never seen the side effect before in association with an antidepressant. Of course, when I started Jason on Prozac, it was a brand-new type of antidepressant. Since the side effect occurred in the first patient I put on the drug, I had no idea that it would prove to be a harbinger of things to come. Over time, I saw with Prozac many other side effects previously associated with major tranquilizers, including the neurological side effects discussed in Chapter 1.

While retrograde ejaculation is considered a relatively benign side effect, it is disconcerting to most men. I was not surprised that Jason insisted on going off the Prozac because he was "freaked out" by ejaculating without the appearance of sperm. Off medication, his sexual functioning quickly returned to normal.

Another unusual side effect is penile anesthesia, analogous to vaginal anesthesia occurring in women. Writing in the November 1991 issue of the *American Journal of Psychiatry*, Dr. John Neill of Lexington, Kentucky, described a man in his mid-forties who lost sensation in his penis when his Prozac dose was increased from 40 to 60 milligrams a day.[7] Putting his dose back down to 40 milligrams produced "no improvement of the penile anesthesia." The side effect caused the patient, who normally enjoyed sex with his wife, "a great deal of distress and did not disappear over the ensuing months." Eventually, the patient demanded to go off the medication "against medical advice." When he was off Prozac, sensation in his penis returned to normal.

Paradoxical Sexual Effects

Paradoxically, the sexual side effects of serotonin boosters have been the rationale for some doctors to prescribe them. Under what circumstances might one want to *inflict* sexual dysfunction on a patient? Premature ejaculation and sexual addictions are two of the most common difficulties for which the drugs are prescribed for their sexual side effects.

Premature ejaculation is easily treatable with behavioral techniques pioneered by Masters and Johnson. These behavioral exercises teach ejaculatory control and are effective in virtually all (98%) cases.[8] My last book included a case study of a couple who were able to cure the male partner's long-standing problem with premature ejaculation in just eight weeks using those techniques.[9]

Even though such a simple, behavioral approach exists, nowadays many doctors still advocate the slightly quicker fix of a Prozac-type medication. The drugs are used to impair a man's sexual functioning sufficiently to prolong his erection for the desired length of time. The dose of the drug is adjusted strictly to address the mechanics of sexual functionality, as though it were purely a plumbing matter. Since the drugs are not a cure for the underlying problem but merely mask it, they have to be taken for an indefinite course. Of course, this exposes people to the potential problems caused by the drugs' wearing off, the return of the initial difficulty, and long-term side effects.

Several clinical studies have been published documenting the effectiveness of serotonin boosters for premature ejaculation. Dr. Marcel Waldinger of the Netherlands published a study using Paxil in the *American Journal of Psychiatry* in 1994.[10] Dr. Joseph Mendels of Wynnewood, Pennsylvania, used Zoloft in a study published in the December 1995 issue of the *Journal of Clinical Psychiatry*.[11] Wrote Mendels, "Zoloft produced clinically and statistically significant improvements . . . in time to ejaculation and in the number of successful attempts at intercourse as well as in overall clinical judgments of improvement." Dr. A. Graziottin presented a study utilizing Prozac to the 1995 Annual Meeting of the American Urological Association.[12] And in the Summer 1996 issue of the *Journal of Sex and Marital Therapy*, psychiatrist Richard Balon of the Wayne State University School of Medicine in Detroit, Michigan, wrote a lengthy article reviewing these and other studies in which he said the Prozac group "seem to be a safe treatment option for patients with premature ejaculation."[13]

In my estimation, Prozac, Zoloft, Paxil, and other serotonin boosters should almost never be used in this way. Masters and Johnson–style behavior treatment provides a permanent, natural alternative. Why needlessly expose patients to long-term use of drugs with serious side effects when such a safe, effective alternative exists?

Another problem area for which serotonin boosters have been widely prescribed for their sexual side effects is sexual addictions. A relatively new term introduced only in recent decades, "sexual addictions" refers to sexual obsessions and compulsive sexual behavior. The best treatment for sexual addictions is a combination of psychotherapy and twelve-step programs. The twelve-step programs go by a number of different names, such as Sex and Love Addicts Anonymous, SLAA, or Sexaholics Anonymous, SA. I have used the combination of psychotherapy and twelve-step programs to treat patients with a wide range of sexual addictions, from Don Juans to cross-dressers to people compulsively drawn to sadomasochism. Unfortunately, despite these natural alternatives, many doctors prescribe serotonin boosters to suppress the sex drive of these patients.

The opening case in Peter Kramer's *Listening to Prozac* is a forty-year-old man who compulsively bought pornography and "insisted his wife watch hard-core sex films with him despite her distaste."[14] On Prozac, as his compulsive behavior waned, the patient felt "freed of an addiction."

Among the proponents of using drugs in this way are psychopharmacologists Donald F. Klein at Columbia Medical School and Martin Kafka at Harvard Medical School. Reviewing their publications, one finds serotonin boosters used for "compulsive masturbation," fetishes (such as "fetishism with women smoking"), "obsessions about [the] sinfulness of sexual fantasy and masturbation," "compulsive staring at crotches," "promiscuity," "phone sex," and "voyeurism."[15] With drug treatment, says Kafka, sexual desire, fantasies, urges, and activity can become "surprisingly conventional." Psychiatry ventures into dangerous territory trying to make people "conventional" in this way. This is especially true when the methods used are chemical. Some psychiatrists have even reported that antidepressants can change the sexual orientation of gay patients.[16]

In an astute critique, Stanley Althof, a psychologist specializing in the treatment of sexual disorders at the Case Western Reserve University School of Medicine, describes the use of serotonin boosters for premature ejaculation as "exploiting the medication-induced ejaculatory impairment" to achieve a superficial, quick fix.[17] Says Althof, "The compelling economic argument that the drug should be the first line of treatment is countered by the potential of a psychotherapeutic approach to enable lifelong ejaculatory control." Althof concludes, "I worry that pharmacologic intervention will be recommended indiscriminately by busy physicians unaware" of the complex emotional issues underlying an individual's or couple's sexual difficulties. I could not agree with him more.

While most patients on serotonin boosters report impaired sexual functioning, a few describe paradoxical hypersexuality. I have not seen these rare side effects in my practice, but a number of reports have appeared in medical journals. These range from a woman in her mid-forties put on Prozac for agoraphobia who developed a "newly emergent obsessive preoccupation with sex" to a sixty-nine-year-old man who began having "bursts of sexual excitement," the frequent sensation of becoming erect when he saw a woman, which made him feel "deeply ashamed" because he felt he was "being unfaithful to his wife."[18]

A number of reports have appeared of patients having become spontaneously aroused to the point of orgasm when they exercised or yawned. In the *Journal of Clinical Psychopharmacology,* Dr. Jack Modell reported a young woman who developed "yawning, clitoral engorgement, and orgasm" when her Prozac dose was increased from 20 to 40 milligrams a day.[19] The patient had frequent episodes of yawning and spontaneous orgasms, which "returned each morning following medication ingestion, continued for several hours, and disappeared by mid-afternoon." The patient complained the side effects were "interfering with normal activity" and was so disturbed by them that she went back down on her Prozac dose. The yawning and intrusive orgasms "disappeared within one day of the dosage decrease."

Writing in the *Journal of Clinical Psychiatry,* psychiatrist James Ellison of Burlington, Massachusetts, reported a fifty-year-old woman who developed "unintended exercise-induced orgasms" when her Prozac was increased from 10 to 20 milligrams a day.[20] The spontaneous orgasms occurred during exercise sessions in which she "walked vigorously on a treadmill."

Drugs that rob most patients of the ability to orgasm while causing an overabundance of unwanted orgasms in a few prompted Dr. Thomas Gualtieri of Chapel Hill, North Carolina, to write a piece on the "paradoxical effects" of serotonin boosters in the *Journal of Clinical Psychopharmacology.*[21] Gualtieri cited a number of areas in which the drugs may cause paradoxical reactions. These include "apathy and indifference," overeating, "suicidal rumination," and "compulsive self-injurious behavior." Said Gualtieri, "There are other examples of paradoxical response in neuropsychopharmacology, to be sure. . . . *But there has never been anything quite like this* [italics added]." He attributed the "paradoxical nature of the clinical effects of Prozac . . . to the complexity of the serotonin system itself." The system is so widespread in the brain and so complicated that the drugs can do all kinds of different things in people.

How Common Is Sexual Dysfunction?

As I mentioned earlier, the official and real numbers for the sexual side effects of serotonin boosters do not tally. In Prozac's official product information, Eli Lilly says sexual dysfunction occurs in 2–5% of patients. This figure is based on Lilly's clinical testing of Prozac in the 1980s to win FDA approval for the drug. During most clinical trials—which were remarkably short, typically lasting only six to eight weeks—Lilly did not specifically *ask* patients about sexual side effects. The 2–5% figure represents those patients whose side effects were so severe they *volunteered* them to technicians working in the drug-testing centers.[22] The official rates for the other drugs in the Prozac group are also misleadingly low.[23]

More careful attention to the sexual effects of serotonin boosters began as early as 1989.[24] Throughout the early 1990s, small-scale studies were conducted by individual doctors who inquired about sexual dysfunction in their patients. Reported in medical and psychiatric journals ranging from the *Southern Medical Journal* to the *American Journal of Psychiatry,* these studies revealed rates as high as 75% of patients on these drugs reporting sexual dysfunction. A recurrent theme of these early reports was that especially since these side effects involve such intimate, personal matters, asking patients directly about sexual dysfunction is required to detect the true, much higher rate.

By the mid-1990s, many psychiatrists, therapists, and primary-care doctors realized sexual dysfunction was a serious problem with Prozac and the other serotonin boosters that had begun appearing on the market. The sexual dysfunction seen with serotonin boosters was unlike anything seen with older antidepressants. In 1994 Dr. Michael Gitlin of the UCLA School of Medicine wrote in the *Journal of Clinical Psychiatry* that the severity of sexual dysfunction seen with an antidepressant correlates with how strong an effect it has on serotonin, "with more powerful serotonergic effects being associated with higher rates of dysfunction."[25]

Systematic, large-scale studies involving hundreds of patients were conducted in the mid-1990s. One of the most comprehensive studies was conducted by a group at the University Hospital of Salamanca in Spain. Headed by Dr. Angel Montejo-González, the study followed over 300 patients on Prozac, Zoloft, Paxil, or Luvox. The patients were interviewed before starting medication and thereafter every one to two months for five to eight months. The patients were on the drugs for a range of problems, including eating disorders, obsessions, compulsions, anxiety, depression, and personality problems. In a report published in the Fall 1997 issue of the *Journal of Sex and Marital Therapy,* the Spanish researchers reported that when patients were studied systematically, 58% suffered sexual dysfunction, most commonly decreased libido, loss of the capacity to orgasm, erectile dysfunction, or ejaculatory problems.[26] Montejo-González noted that while only 14% of patients spontaneously reported sexual side effects, 58%, over four times as many, reported them when questioned directly.

The study confirmed that sexual side effects are dose-related: "Patients experienced substantial improvement in sexual function when the dose was diminished or the drug withdrawn." All four of the Prozac-type drugs evidenced a high incidence, ranging from 54–65%. The Montejo-González study is probably the best assessment we have of the incidence of sexual side effects with the Prozac-type antidepressants, because of the large number of patients, the length of time they were followed, and the inclusion of all four drugs in the Prozac group.

Nowadays, most psychiatrists and primary-care doctors are well aware of how common sexual dysfunction is in people on serotonin boosters. Severe sexual problems are one of the most frequent reasons patients ask to go off the drugs. In 1995, two of the country's leading psychiatric experts on sexual dysfunction, the late Dr. Helen Singer Kaplan and Dr. Barbara Bartlik, wrote in the *Journal of Sex and Marital Therapy,* "More than other classes of antidepressants, the SSRIs [serotonin boosters] appear to profoundly affect sexual dysfunction."[27] Indeed, Kaplan and Bartlik described sexual side effects as "almost universal" with the Prozac group.

Obviously, this is a far cry from official figures, such as Eli Lilly's 2–5% of patients in clinical studies where they typically did not ask directly about sexual side effects. Writing in the September 1994 issue of the *Journal of Clinical Psychiatry,* Dr. Michael J. Gitlin of the UCLA School of Medicine, an expert on drug-induced sexual dysfunction, described Lilly's approach as "less than systematic" in light of the high incidence of sexual dysfunction seen in later studies.[28] Dr. Jack Modell of the University of Alabama characterized it more sharply in the April 1997 issue of *Clinical Pharmacology and Therapeutics* as: "if you don't ask, you won't find out."[29]

The Serotonin-Dopamine Connection, Again

The mechanism by which serotonin boosters cause sexual dysfunction is not fully understood. Libido, arousal, and sexual behavior involve complex interactions between a number of neurotransmitters and hormones. A variety of mechanisms involving disruption of normal functioning in both the brain and the genitals are thought to be responsible for the drug-induced sexual dysfunction seen with serotonin boosters. One mechanism is raising the level of serotonin, which has an inhibitory effect on sexuality; another is an indirect effect on adrenaline, which plays an important role in regulating ejaculation.

One of the mechanisms commonly cited as a likely cause of sexual side effects is the compensatory drop in dopamine that results from boosting serotonin. This, once again, implicates Prozac backlash in yet another major group of severe side effects of the drugs. Many researchers have pointed to this serotonin-dopamine connection.

Writing in the *Journal of Steroid Biochemistry and Molecular Biology* in

1990, Dr. Gaetano Frajese reviewed animal and human studies of sexual functioning and concluded, "Dopamine (DA) and serotonin (5-HT) are the neurotransmitters most directly involved in sexual activity. DA [dopamine] plays a stimulatory role while 5-HT [serotonin] has an inhibitory effect. The two monoamine systems [i.e., the serotonin and dopamine systems] modulate the secretion of many hormones . . . involved in sexual functional capacity."[30] Indeed, the hormones cited by Frajese play crucial roles in regulating estrogen, progesterone, and testosterone secretion; the menstrual cycle in women; and sperm production in men. Thus, serotonin and dopamine have widespread effects on sexual functioning mediated via critical sex hormones.

Writing about Prozac-induced inability to orgasm in the June 1992 issue of the *Journal of Clinical Psychiatry*, Dr. Scott Balogh of Omaha, Nebraska, said, "Animal studies suggest that serotonin inhibits while dopamine facilitates ejaculation. These findings complement each other when coupled with the observation that Prozac can indirectly decrease dopamine stores in brain regions that [normally] exhibit increased dopamine release during copulation" in laboratory animals.[31]

Dr. Angel Montejo-González, who headed the most comprehensive study to date of sexual side effects with these drugs, wrote in the *Journal of Sex and Marital Therapy* in 1997: "Serotonin appears to play a very important role in the development of SD [sexual dysfunction] by inhibiting libido, ejaculation, and orgasm. This effect can be explained, especially at the central [brain] level, as there is evidence that serotonin causes a decrease in dopamine levels (a neurotransmitter enhancing sexual function) in the central nervous system of laboratory animals."[32]

A study of the indirect but potentially potent effects of serotonin boosters on dopamine in humans was conducted by Herbert Meltzer at the University of Chicago Pritzker School of Medicine.[33] Dopamine is generally acknowledged to be the critical neurotransmitter controlling release of the sex hormone prolactin. Meltzer measured prolactin levels in a patient before and after starting Prozac. Writing in the *Journal of Neural Transmission*, Meltzer reported the patient's prolactin level tripled "within 24 hours of initiating Prozac treatment." Within a week, the patient's prolactin rose sevenfold. Given dopamine's critical influence on prolactin, Meltzer reasoned that Prozac's dramatic effect on the hormone was via dopamine.

In addition to the elevated prolactin on Prozac, Meltzer's patient suffered a severe case of the neurological side effects described in Chapter 1. Meltzer said the patient had "torticollis [muscle spasms in the neck severe enough to rotate his head], rigidity of his jaw [due to spasms of the jaw muscles], cogwheel rigidity [a sign of drug-induced parkinsonism] and loss of fluid motion in his gait." Said Meltzer, "These symptoms appear *indistinguishable* from those associated with neuroleptic [major tranquilizer] treatment [italics added]." Of course major tranquilizers cause these neurological side effects by directly lowering dopamine activity in the brain. Moreover, these tranquilizers are well known to cause elevated prolactin levels like those Meltzer obtained in his patient on Prozac.

While the sexual dysfunction caused by the Prozac group has mystified researchers because it is unlike what was seen with the old antidepressants, it is remarkably like the sexual side effects of major tranquilizers. These tranquilizers cause loss of libido, impotence, difficulty achieving orgasm, and ejaculatory problems.[34] Studies have shown that major tranquilizers produce these sexual side effects in as many as 60% of patients, the same percentage range seen with serotonin boosters.[35] In another remarkable parallel, major tranquilizers were prescribed in their heyday for sexual problems like premature ejaculation[36] and to control sexual behavior (including "excessive masturbation,"[37] "sexual hyperactivity,"[38] wet dreams,[39] and "sexual preoccupation"[40]) just as serotonin boosters are today. Thus, we come upon a convergence, once again, of the most serious side effects of serotonin boosters and those of major tranquilizers. Whereas major tranquilizers cause both neurological side effects and some of the sexual dysfunction by directly inhibiting dopamine, serotonin boosters are thought to do so indirectly.

Meltzer's report was published in 1979, before Prozac's large-scale clinical testing and its approval, a decade later, by the FDA. Meltzer's research was funded by Eli Lilly, as part of the earliest testing of the drug in small numbers of patients. In fact, Meltzer later described the patient as "one of the first patients [ever] treated with Prozac."[41] Did Meltzer's findings not alert Lilly to the neurological side effects of the drugs, to their potential to cause sexual dysfunction, to the serotonin–dopamine connection, and to Prozac backlash? Why, under these circumstances, would one fail to ask patients in Prozac's clinical studies if they were having sexual side effects and come up with the strangely low figure of 2–5%?

The striking similarities between the sexual and neurological side effects of both major tranquilizers and serotonin boosters raise a disturbing question: Is the high percentage of patients with sexual dysfunction on serotonin boosters one of the best indications we have that many people on the drugs are experiencing dopamine suppression and will therefore be vulnerable long-term to developing the kind of brain damage seen with major tranquilizers? This is an aspect of the sexual side effects of these drugs that has not been adequately addressed and should be an area of active research.

How Doctors and Patients
Cope with Sexual Side Effects

A variety of options are available to doctors trying to help patients who develop intolerable sexual side effects.

Stopping the Drug

Having helped many patients cope with the sexual side effects caused by serotonin boosters, my preference is to try to discontinue the drug whenever possible. Too often patients have been put on these drugs for relatively trivial reasons. Severe side effects can be an important opportunity to reconsider the wisdom of being on the drug at all. Whenever possible, the best practice is to stop the medication and observe the patient to see if his or her symptoms return. All of the issues raised in the previous chapter need to be observed with regard to tapering the medication and distinguishing between withdrawal effects and a true relapse. Many of the patients who consult with me do fine when taken off medication and sometimes they do even better than when they were on the drug. Certainly, for people who can do without a drug, discontinuing it eliminates unnecessary exposure to long-term risks.

Dosage Reduction

Reducing the dose of a drug usually does not result in complete remission of sexual side effects, but it may improve them enough to be tolerable. A patient who cannot orgasm on 40 milligrams a day of Prozac may be able to orgasm, albeit with considerable effort, on 20 milligrams and feel this is a reasonable compromise. Unfortunately, for many patients, even at a lower dose their sexual dysfunction remains severe. Reducing the dose is purely empirical, that is, trial and error. One is always dealing with trade-offs. In some instances the sexual problem may improve only at the cost of losing some of the therapeutic effect of the drug.

Drug Holidays

Anthony Rothschild recommends what he calls "weekend drug holidays" for patients with sexual dysfunction. Writing in the October 1995 issue of the *American Journal of Psychiatry*, Rothschild described having patients discontinue their Zoloft or Paxil "after the Thursday morning dose" and restart it "on Sunday at 12:00 noon. Patients were instructed to have sexual relations between Thursday evening and Monday morning."[42] The point of the drug holiday is to buy patients and their partners a brief reprieve from medication-induced sexual dysfunction. For many patients, however, scheduling sex in this way robs it of its spontaneity and pleasure. What is more, Rothschild concedes that a brief hiatus does not work with a long-lasting medication like Prozac, which takes weeks to wash out of a patient's system. While the sexual side effects of the shorter-acting drugs like Zoloft and Paxil may disappear more quickly, the problem is that after just one or two days off the drugs, patients can experience withdrawal effects.

Rothschild's drug holidays are controversial within the profession because of fears that if patients stop their drugs briefly they may be tempted to stop them altogether. Many drug proponents are concerned with "noncompliance," patients not taking their medication as directed. In the December 1996 issue of the *Journal of Clinical Psychiatry,* Dr. Troy Thompson expressed concern that "drug holidays may be used as an invitation to noncompliance" since "patients may start to taper off medications on their own" once they begin experimenting with not taking them.[43]

Switching to Another Medication

For those patients whose symptoms do warrant being on medication, a number of alternatives to Prozac-type drugs exist. Two new antidepressants—Serzone and Wellbutrin—have been heavily promoted as Prozac alternatives. In my experience and that of my colleagues, Wellbutrin is far more successful than Serzone for treatment of depression without sexual side effects. Indeed, Wellbutrin has enjoyed a surge in popularity as the alternative for patients who develop sexual dysfunction on serotonin boosters. Not only does Wellbutrin produce fewer sexual side effects, many patients report heightened sexual pleasure. In a large study conducted by Dr. Jack Modell at the University of Alabama published in the April 1997 issue of *Clinical Pharmacology and Therapeutics,* 77% of patients on Wellbutrin reported "heightened sexual functioning," increased libido, and more intense, prolonged orgasms.[44]

Wellbutrin is not without problems, however. Just before it was originally introduced, Wellbutrin was withdrawn because it was so stimulating it caused seizures in some patients. The manufacturer, Glaxo Wellcome, persevered, however, and three years later won approval for Wellbutrin with a more gradual dosing schedule to allow the nervous system time to slowly adapt to the drug.[45] But the fact that it is associated with a high rate of seizures if not dosed carefully makes me cautious.

Like Sharon, the first patient described in this chapter, many people report that Wellbutrin is so pleasurable it makes them feel "high." Wellbutrin raises levels of the brain chemical dopamine. Historically, drugs that raise dopamine tend to be more stimulating and more addicting than drugs that only raise adrenaline and/or serotonin.[46] Cocaine, amphetamines (speed), and the amphetamine-like drug Ritalin all raise dopamine levels and all can be addicting.

Like cocaine, amphetamines, and Ritalin, Wellbutrin is short-acting, starts to wear off within hours, and is often taken more than once a day.[47] The rapidly alternating peaks and valleys of such short-acting drugs make them more prone to causing addiction. Patients report being very aware of the "hit" of one dose wearing off and needing to take another.[48] One also hears of Wellbutrin being abused, crushed, and snorted for a faster, greater high.

For all these reasons, many psychiatrists openly refer to Wellbutrin as being a "stimulant-like," or "amphetamine-like," drug. Harvard psychiatrist J. Alexander Bodkin described Wellbutrin as "stimulant like" in an article on antidepressants in the April 1997 issue of the *Journal of Clinical Psychiatry.*[49] Dr. Jack Modell of the University of Alabama, commenting in *The Atlanta Journal* on May 22, 1997, on his study of Wellbutrin's sexual effects, described the drug as a "stimulant," adding, "But nobody in our study was hanging from chandeliers."[50]

Wellbutrin is also being heavily promoted under a different name, Zyban, to help people give up their addiction to smoking.[51] This is reminiscent of how earlier prescription stimulants were used to treat addictions. At the turn of the century, when cocaine was a prescription drug, it was used by many doctors, including Freud, to treat opium and morphine addicts.[52] Later, in the middle of the twentieth century, amphetamines were prescribed for addictions to narcotics, alcoholism, and smoking. In this pattern, popular "cures" for addictions often turn out to be addicting themselves. I worry that psychiatric patients and smokers being encouraged to take Wellbutrin/Zyban may find themselves addicted to this popular new remedy. Indeed, in my experience, Wellbutrin has proved to be one of the most difficult antidepressants from which to wean patients. The most frequent withdrawal effect is severe irritability and anger, which often causes patients to insist on going back on it.

Even the use of Wellbutrin to avoid sexual dysfunction may be shortsighted. Drugs that increase dopamine are well known to be aphrodisiacs, to heighten sexual interest and pleasure, but only in the short run. With long-term use they too can dampen sexual function. A leading authority on sexual dysfunction, the late psychiatrist Helen Singer Kaplan, wrote in her groundbreaking 1974 book *The New Sex Therapy* that when used short-term, dopamine-enhancing drugs have "*transient* aphrodisiac effects [italics added]" on "both erotic interest and sexual performance."[53] However, with chronic use, patients "claim they cannot function [sexually] without it" and "experience a diminution in sexual interest and capability." Indeed, I have now seen a number of patients who lost interest in sex, even developed an aversion to it, after being on Wellbutrin long-term.

Antidotes

Still another strategy advocated by many psychopharmacologists is adding another drug, a so-called "antidote," to a patient's regimen to reverse sexual dysfunction without stopping the Prozac-type medication. Here again, Wellbutrin is advocated for this purpose. Writing in the *Annals of Clinical Psychiatry* in 1994, Drs. L. A. Labbate and M. H. Pollack recommend adding 75 milligrams of Wellbutrin to Prozac to treat drug-induced sexual dysfunction.[54] Of course, this means the patient is on two mood-altering drugs with their combined risks of long-term side effects.

Similarly, Barbara Bartlik, professor of psychiatry at the Cornell University Medical College, advocates the use of dextroamphetamine in the Winter 1995 issue of the *Journal of Sex and Marital Therapy*.[55] Of course, dextroamphetamine is speed. While most forms of speed have been illegal for decades, a few still can be prescribed by doctors. Thus, Dr. Bartlik prescribes 5 to 10 milligrams of speed to patients suffering sexual dysfunction on serotonin boosters. Patients are instructed to take a dose of speed "one hour before sexual activity." Reports Dr. Bartlik, This leads to "a marked increase in desire, sexual fantasy, lubrication, and arousal," which persists "for up to 12 hours." Dr. Bartlik acknowledges speed's "potential for untoward side effects and addiction" but states that "with the use of an increasing number of [Prozac-type] medications that inhibit sexual functioning, there is certainly a need for an antidote to these side effects." Saying that the "use of stimulants in enhancing sexual functioning has been overlooked" because of "a backlash in response to stimulant abuse a generation ago," Bartlik concludes, "Today, the significance of stimulants for a variety of new indications is increasingly recognized."

Other dopamine-enhancing drugs recommended as antidotes include pemoline, amantadine, and Ritalin.[56] Since all of these antidotes increase dopamine, they may work by compensating for dopamine suppression caused by the drug. Advocating the use of Ritalin in the November 1996 issue of the *Journal of Clinical Psychiatry*, Manhattan psychiatrist Carol Roeloffs comments that it "not only can . . . relieve sexual dysfunction caused by SSRI [Prozac-type drug] therapy," but the addition of the stimulant can also "boost the antidepressant action" of the Prozac-type drug.[57]

As with other classes of side effects, my preference is to avoid treating the side effects of one drug with yet another. This is especially true of speed and other stimulants, which can cause their own severe side effects, including addiction. With these drugs and any newer agents resembling them, we should not forget the lessons of the past, especially when there are other, safer ways of dealing with sexual side effects.

One recommended antidote is an herb rather than a prescription drug. Writing in the *Journal of Sex and Marital Therapy* in 1998, Drs. Alan Cohen and Barbara Bartlik describe the use of ginkgo biloba to treat drug-induced sexual dysfunction.[58] Ginkgo biloba is an extract derived from the leaves of the Chinese ginkgo tree. Having been used for centuries in Chinese herbal medicine, ginkgo biloba has become popular in this country as a memory-enhancing agent. In their article in the *Journal of Sex and Marital Therapy*, Cohen and Bartlik report that ginkgo biloba improved libido, erectile functioning, and the ability to orgasm in patients with antidepressant-induced sexual dysfunction. The dosage of ginkgo biloba taken by the patients ranged from 60 to 240 milligrams a day. Although an herb may be safer than a prescription drug as an antidote, it is still covering up potentially serious side effects of Prozac-type antidepressants. If possible, stopping the antidepressant is preferable.

Should Children Be Taking These Drugs?

More than half a million children are on serotonin boosters, with the numbers growing rapidly. Doctors prescribe the drugs to allegedly depressed children as young as six and seven years old, even though the FDA has not approved them for depression in children. Some of the Prozac-type drugs have been approved by the FDA for children with obsessive-compulsive disorder. This has opened the door to much more widespread pediatric use of the drugs.

Should children who have not yet matured be taking drugs with such profound sexual side effects? If the balance between serotonin and dopamine influences the release of testosterone and other important sex hormones, what are the consequences to a child's developing reproductive system?[59] In addition to physical consequences, what are the psychological implications of shutting down sexual interest in pubescent and teenage children, at a time when their sexuality is normally awakening?

Sarah was a fifteen-year-old girl referred by her pediatrician for help in dealing with her parents' bitter, protracted divorce. Throughout the divorce, Sarah had agonized over being caught between her parents and "forced to take sides." Even though it was "not really necessary financially," Sarah's father had forced her mother to sell the family home. Since then her mother had moved with the children to three different apartments. Since the divorce was finalized, a year prior to my consultation with her, Sarah's father had "disappeared," moving to California and having only sporadic telephone contact with his daughter.

At the time of her father's disappearance, a psychopharmacologist put Sarah on Paxil for vague anxiety. When I questioned her, Sarah said that she had been anxious about the possibility of never seeing her father again, an anxiety that thus far was proving legitimate. The anxiety had not been severe; she had not had panic attacks. But Sarah was reluctant to go off the Paxil because she didn't want to disrupt her "routine," given how much had already changed in her life in the last year.

Early in our work, Sarah confided that her reason for seeking psychotherapy was a loss of any interest in dating boys. While her friends were all beginning to date and enjoy their newfound interest in the opposite sex, Sarah had "lost all interest" in the romantic arena. Becoming tearful, she expressed the fear that this might be the "lasting legacy" of her parents' divorce. She had recently broached the subject with her mother, who expressed concern and said she would feel "guilty" if this proved to be true. Sarah volunteered that she had not masturbated in a year. I commented that she went on the Paxil at the same time and explained that the drug could have shut down her sex drive. This amazed Sarah, who had not been told of the medication's sexual side effects.

I suggested a trial off the Paxil, to clarify whether or not the drug was responsible for the change in Sarah. After discussing the matter for several weeks both with me and with her mother, Sarah decided to go off the medication. Within a week she was "stunned" when her sex drive and interest in boys abruptly returned. "One day in school it just hit me like a thunderbolt," said Sarah. "Suddenly the world was alive again." Sarah was upset to think a drug had caused her so much self-doubt. What if she had stayed on the medication throughout her teenage years, such a formative period of sexual and social development? "I would have blamed everything on my parents' divorce, having no idea it was a side effect of the medication!" said Sarah.

Since I am not a child psychiatrist, I have no clinical experience with younger children on these medications. As a parent of school-age children, however, and as one who hears many stories of youngsters in the community being put on the drugs, I have grave concerns. When President Clinton proposed requiring testing of the efficacy and safety of drugs in the pediatric population before allowing widespread prescribing to children, pharmaceutical companies vigorously protested, citing safety concerns.[60] How can safety concerns be allowed to block testing of these drugs, meanwhile allowing doctors to prescribe them to such a vulnerable population? The United States is the only country in the world where potent, synthetic drugs targeting the brain are routinely prescribed to children.

Human sexuality is not merely a matter of plumbing or even just sexual performance. Sexuality colors much of everyday life. Drugs that shut down sex drive can shut down vitality in general. Said one college-age patient, explaining that the loss of her sex drive had broader ramifications, "I don't have strong feelings about anything anymore. I used to write passionate essays in my classes but I've stopped. I don't get upset anymore when my roommates leave the apartment a mess, but that's just because I'm apathetic." What is the overall effect of drugs with such far-reaching consequences on the development of children?

Side Effects and Politics

Eli Lilly's original figure for the incidence of sexual side effects on Prozac was 2–5%, based on their clinical studies of the drug in which they typically refrained from asking patients about sexual difficulties. Remarkably, Lilly still lists the outdated, gross underestimate in Prozac's product information, found in the drug's package insert and in reference books like the *Physicians' Desk Reference (PDR)*. The manufacturers of Zoloft, Paxil, and Luvox list similarly low figures. This poses serious problems for doctors and patients trying to get accurate information. I recently told a patient considering Prozac about the drug's sexual effects, saying they occur in 60% of patients. The next week the patient said she was relieved to find I was wrong, having researched Prozac on the Internet and discovered Lilly's figure of 2–5%. I had to correct Lilly's misinformation by giving her half a dozen published papers documenting the much higher incidence found in later, systematic studies in which patients were asked specifically about sexual dysfunction.

The sexual effects of serotonin boosters are a prime example of the disparity between research performed by pharmaceutical companies on their own drugs and that of outside investigators. Most side effects never receive the kind of thorough investigation that has been done on sexual dysfunction caused by serotonin agents. The reason sexual dysfunction has been so well publicized when other, even more dangerous side effects have not is that funding for these studies came from competing pharmaceutical companies trying to establish market niches. By the mid-1990s, serotonin boosters had become so popular that it was difficult for new antidepressant drugs to compete. As reports of sexual side effects mounted, the manufacturers of Serzone and Wellbutrin, two other new antidepressants, recognized a potential weak spot that might be exploited in an effort to gain market share. Serzone's manufacturer, Bristol-Myers Squibb, funded two studies comparing their drug with Zoloft. One was done by Dr. Alan Feiger at the University of Colorado; the other by Dr. James Ferguson at the University of Utah.[61] In both studies, Zoloft caused sexual dysfunction in about 67% of patients, while Serzone caused sexual difficulties in only 18%. Meanwhile, Burroughs Wellcome funded studies comparing Wellbutrin favorably with serotonergic agents.[62]

Feiger published his Bristol-Myers Squibb–funded study in 1996 in the *Journal of Clinical Psychiatry*.[63] In May 1996, Feiger and Ferguson presented their findings at the annual convention of the American Psychiatric Association in New York City. Following the presentations, Feiger held a press conference to announce the findings to the media.[64]

The result was a spate of publicity on the sexual side effects of serotonin boosters in the popular press. "Wonder drugs to brighten moods can dim libido but there are solutions available to those left sexually bereft," wrote columnist Jane Brody in the Minneapolis *Star Tribune*.[65] Her articles on this subject appeared in papers across the country, including the May 15, 1996, *New York Times*.[66] "Some Antidepressants Put Hex on Sex," read the headline of an article by Sandra Boodman in the *Des Moines Register*.[67] In a related article in the *Washington Post,* she quoted Ferguson as saying sexual dysfunction is the "cruel kicker" of serotonin boosters.[68] "Not tonight dear, I had a Prozac . . . ," read the headline of *Elle* magazine.[69] Feiger and Ferguson were widely quoted, as was Taylor Segraves, professor of psychiatry at Case Western Reserve University, who conducted one of the Wellbutrin studies for Burroughs Wellcome.[70]

The manufacturers of serotonin boosters fired back a series of obfuscating defenses. One standard response is to blame the patient's underlying condition rather than the drug. "Clinical depression is a multifaceted illness and various types of sexual impairment are common symptoms. . . . Patients suffering from depression frequently report a loss of sexual desire or changes in sexual functioning," said Eli Lilly in the *Sunday Times.*[71] But the loss of satisfaction with sex sometimes seen in depression differs sharply from the profound sexual dysfunction brought on by the drugs.

Doctors Eric Nofzinger and Michael Thase at the University of Pittsburgh School of Medicine have conducted detailed studies of the effects of depression. For the studies, they do extensive assessments of patients' sexual functioning during depressive episodes and in the period after recovery. Writing in the January 1993 issue of the *Archives of General Psychiatry,* Nofzinger and Thase reported "contrary to expectation" sexual activity per se is "not reduced during the depressed state."[72] Depressed patients "did *not* show decrements on most . . . measures of sexual function including sex drive, activity, and interest [italics added]." One change that does occur regularly is a "loss of sexual satisfaction that then improves with remission from depression." Thus depression seems to change the emotional valence of sex.

Some depressed patients report that the loss of satisfaction has made them less interested in sex, but when their sexual activity is tracked, the data show that it does not actually decrease. In fact, in many instances, the patients' sexual activity actually increased, in what Nofzinger and Thase interpreted as "a way of coping with ongoing dysphoria [depression] or anxiety."

This is very different from the dramatic physical problems—like impotence, ejaculatory abnormalities, and inability to orgasm—seen with serotonin boosters. The effects of depression versus the side effects of the drugs are distinctly different and should not be confused. Efforts by pharmaceutical companies to blur the difference are attempts to paper over the drugs' ill effects.

In its statement Lilly continued, "Antidepressants can relieve these [sexual] and other symptoms [in those who are depressed], enabling patients to return to normal functioning in all aspects of their lives."[73] By "antidepressants" did Lilly mean drugs like Wellbutrin and dextroamphetamine (speed), which do temporarily enhance sexual performance? If so, this is a very misleading defense of Lilly's drug, Prozac. Or did they mean that by improving mood, serotonin boosters can reverse the loss of sexual satisfaction experienced by some depressed patients? This, too, would be misleading: To suggest that drugs that produce serious sexual impairment in 60% of patients instead improve people's sex lives is spurious.

Another common response is to distract attention from undesirable side effects by scaring people about not taking drugs. "Undue emphasis on this side effect trivializes the serious medical illness of depression. We need to be reminded that depression is a serious medical illness, just like diabetes or cancer," said a Lilly representative in *The Spokesman-Review* of Spokane, Washington.[74] In this response, one senses the paternalistic irritation with patients judged too upset over severe sexual side effects. This echoes the comments of many patients who feel their medication doctor did not take their sexual dysfunction seriously. Again, the statement is misleading on several points: Most people are not on these drugs for serious depression. Instead, they are on them for a plethora of more minor conditions. In most instances, their conditions are not like having diabetes or cancer, which are unfair, needlessly frightening comparisons. Moreover, a drug's therapeutic effects will often have worn off and the patient does not need it anymore. In other instances, the patients' medications have not been re-evaluated in years and they are taking far more of the drugs than they need. Such summary dismissal of people's distress over serious sexual difficulties is not a reasonable or appropriate response. Unfortunately, it happens all too often with these and other side effects.

Still another standard response is to defuse the problem by insisting other drugs cause it too. In a panel discussion on antidepressant-induced sexual dysfunction published in the December 1996 issue of the *Journal of Clinical Psychiatry,* Dr. Troy L. Thompson stated, "The level of sexual dysfunction is no higher now with SSRIs [serotonin boosters] than it was with the older agents."[75] This is simply not true. For some time, clinicians and researchers have recognized that sexual side effects are far more common and severe with serotonin agents than with older antidepressants.[76]

Another typical response is to push more drugs as antidotes to unwanted side effects. In the same panel discussion, called "The Experts Converse," published in the *Journal of Clinical Psychiatry,* Dr. Thomas Wise said, "I generally use Wellbutrin as an adjunct [antidote] on a regular basis ... [at a dose of] 75 mg. daily, sometimes in combination with yohimbine [yet another sexual enhancer] 5.4 mg. given daily. I have also given Ritalin 10 mg. daily on occasion, with beneficial results."[77] Here Wise is recommending not just one but possibly two additional drugs in order to maintain the serotonin booster. So the patient ends up taking three drugs daily—what psychopharmacologists refer to as "drug cocktails"—each with its own side effects and potential long-term risks.

One of the most serious obfuscations occurred in this particular panel discussion, in the dialogue between Drs. Thompson and Wise. Said Dr.

Thompson at one point: "Occasionally, we have the opportunity to turn lemons into lemonade. If a patient develops sexual dysfunction while taking an antidepressant, the physician should encourage the patient to talk with the partner about the problem. This may provide the first opportunity for partners to discuss their sexual desires, likes, and dislikes."[78] Responded Dr. Thomas Wise: "I agree. This may provide a unique building block for a better sexual relationship." So inflicting severe sexual dysfunction is rationalized as improving people's communication around their sex lives. Sounds more like a lemon than lemonade to me.

These strategies—blaming patients' underlying conditions, asserting the drug has the opposite effect, instilling fear of not taking drugs, claiming other drugs are as bad, and pushing antidotes (more drugs)—are the stock-in-trade responses of pharmaceutical companies and drug proponents. Reading dozens of articles on a variety of side effects, one begins to discern the pattern of these predictable responses, poor substitutes for genuinely empathizing with patients' problems and trying to find them the least toxic solutions.

The public debate over the sexual side effects of serotonin boosters has been relatively superficial, focusing on the incidence of the side effects. Many patients missed the publicity, which peaked in 1996. The public debate has not included the many other issues raised in this chapter: the details of the different types of sexual dysfunction, concerns about alternative drugs, possible mechanisms by which the drugs cause the side effects, the potential connection between them and the neurological side effects discussed in Chapter 1, concerns about children on the medications, the regrettable financial ties between drug "experts" and pharmaceutical companies, and the behind-the-scenes spin control and public relations in the debate.

These difficulties notwithstanding, the sexual side effects of serotonin boosters have certainly received more systematic study and publicity than any other side effects. Unfortunately, this kind of aggressive research and publicity only happened because rival pharmaceutical companies were seeking a market share. This state of affairs is regrettable. We need the same kind of aggressive study and public education for phenomena like brain damage, memory loss, drug dependence, withdrawal syndromes, the drugs' wearing off, neurotoxicity, and their association with suicidality and violence. But in these areas there have not been the same vested interests to fund this desperately needed research.

4

Bones Rattling
Like Tuning Forks
Startling New Information
on Suicide and Violence

The Suicide and Violence Scare

In early 1990, two Harvard Medical School psychiatrists, Martin Teicher and Jonathan Cole, reported in the *American Journal of Psychiatry* that Prozac could induce "intense, violent suicidal preoccupation."[1] The two psychopharmacologists at McLean Hospital described a number of patients who became severely anxious, agitated, and obsessed with violence within two to seven weeks of starting Prozac. Occurring in people who were not seriously suicidal when they started the drug, the reactions were sudden and dramatic: One patient reported feeling like "jumping out of her skin." So great was her "anxiety, fear, and turbulence that she felt 'death would be a welcome result.'" Another described "nearly constant suicidal preoccupation, violent self-destructive fantasies," and "resignation to the inevitability of suicide." Another patient felt she "could not fight or control her suicidal impulses." One patient escaped from the hospital but was brought back by hospital security guards. Once in the hospital again, she "became violent, banging her head and mutilating herself, and physical restraint was necessary." Another patient made a suicide attempt with her medication. Two contemplated purchasing guns. Indeed, one woman put a loaded gun to her head.

"None of these patients had ever experienced a similar state during treatment with any other psychotropic drug," said Teicher and Cole. The virulent obsessions subsided when the drug was stopped, disappearing in as little as three days but in some instances lasting as long as three months. "No patient was able to articulate a reason for feeling so suicidal," said the authors. Ironically, even at the height of her suicidality, one patient wished to stay on Prozac, hoping the new drug would work for her as it had for others. Teicher and Cole labeled the suicidal and violent impulses a "paradoxical" reaction to Prozac, estimated it might happen in 3.5% of patients, and warned physicians to prescribe the drug with caution.

Numerous similar reports and discussions of the phenomenon appeared in other medical journals, including the *New England Journal of Medicine*,[2] *Journal of the American Academy of Child and Adolescent Psychiatry*,[3] *Journal of Family Practice*,[4] *American Journal of Psychiatry*,[5] *Archives of General Psychiatry*,[6] *Human Psychopharmacology*,[7] and the British medical journal *Lancet*.[8] Teicher and Cole's report was particularly influential because of their detailed analysis and the stature of the two authors: Both had national reputations as research psychopharmacologists. Cole had conducted research on Prozac for Eli Lilly.[9] Coming from prominent psychopharmacologists with ties to the pharmaceutical industry, the report had a particularly strong impact.

Teicher and Cole's announcement suddenly gave credibility to reports that had been circulating of sensational murder–suicides associated with Prozac. Following publication of their article, in the summer of 1990 the issue exploded in the media. Just a few months earlier, the cover of *Newsweek* had proclaimed: "The Promise of Prozac."[10] Almost overnight, Prozac went from being a "miracle cure" to a "deadly drug."

One of the most lurid stories was that of Joseph Wesbecker, a printing press operator distressed over job pressures at the Standard Gravure printing plant in Louisville, Kentucky.[11] Wesbecker had a long history of psychiatric problems, including two prior suicide attempts, and had been on many psychiatric medications. Just weeks after he started Prozac, however, Wesbecker's distress turned extremely violent and was directed not only at himself but toward others when he went on a shooting spree at Standard Gravure with an AK-47 semi-automatic assault rifle. Wesbecker wounded twelve people and killed eight others. He then committed suicide, shooting himself to death. The mass murder–suicide made national headlines, gripping the country as SWAT teams descended on the building, police and medics searched for bodies, and the fate of several of the wounded hung in the balance. Wesbecker's friends and psychiatrist said he had changed dramatically on Prozac, becoming severely agitated. In their last appointment, just three days before the shootings, his psychiatrist had urged Wesbecker to stop the drug and come into the hospital, but he refused.

Over the next year, scores of patients came forward saying Prozac abruptly made them anxious, agitated, and obsessed with suicide and violence. Many had made near-lethal suicide attempts or mutilated themselves. Families told of suicides and murder-suicides. The widow of Dell Shannon said Prozac was responsible for the rock star's death.[12] Within days of starting the drug, Shannon developed severe restlessness, pacing, agitation, and insomnia. In the midst of a full schedule of performances, he shocked his family and friends by shooting himself to death.

Many told their Prozac nightmares on daytime talk shows hosted by Geraldo Rivera and Phil Donahue. One Donahue show was titled "Prozac—Medication That Makes You Kill."[13] Around the country, networks of Prozac survivor groups sprang up. In what became known as the "Prozac defense," people accused of violence or other crimes attributed their actions to the drug.[14] Multimillion-dollar lawsuits were filed against Eli Lilly, including one brought by the survivors and family members of the victims of Joseph Wesbecker's mass murder–suicide.[15]

Prozac proponents insisted the professional and public attention was a reaction against the glowing publicity the drug had received earlier. To allay doctors' fears, Lilly offered to pay all legal expenses for any physician sued in connection with prescribing Prozac.[16] The pharmaceutical giant vowed Prozac would be vindicated in court.

During this turbulent period, I found the stories of colleagues and patients particularly compelling. One colleague told me that he unequivocally saw Prozac trigger severe suicidality in a young man admitted to the hospital for depression. Ten days after starting Prozac, the patient developed a severe obsession with suicide and stabbed himself multiple times in the chest. He was in intensive care for almost a week because one of his lungs collapsed from deep stab wounds. Although he survived, the patient was left with permanent brain injuries from the period in which he almost bled to death. Such extremely painful, gruesome behavior is not typical of suicidal patients. Even severely suicidal patients typically express concern about not wanting to be in prolonged pain if they were to make a suicide attempt. Typically, they imagine overdosing and falling into a painless sleep from which they will not awaken. Or they imagine shooting or hanging themselves in order to die quickly. How could someone tolerate the horrendous pain of multiple, self-inflicted stab wounds? My colleague was deeply shaken by the incident, because the patient had not been at all suicidal prior to starting the drug. Convinced Prozac was the cause, he wondered what kind of drug-induced state the patient must have been in.

Another colleague reported that shortly after starting Prozac her mother underwent a "marked change," becoming "distant" and "remote," like she "was on the other side of a barrier" where her family "could not reach her." A few weeks later, her mother took a massive overdose which left her unconscious in an intensive care unit for over a week. This period was "terrifying" for my colleague and her family because the doctors were unsure what brain functioning her mother would be left with if she regained consciousness. Fortunately, her mother recovered fully.

Several reliable patients said members of their families had similar reactions. Two weeks after starting Prozac, one patient's mother tried to stab her father to death as he lay sleeping in bed. The father was able to subdue her; then, as he called the police, the mother tried to hang herself. Fortunately they both survived, but my patient was reeling from this "unfathomable behavior" in a woman she had known all her life.

Another patient's father tried to kill himself by carbon monoxide poisoning. A month after starting Prozac, he closed himself in the garage and sat in his car with the engine running. By chance, he was found unconscious. He was rushed to the hospital and was lucky to survive.

In every instance, the stories are remarkably similar: a dramatic, noticeable change occurred in an individual soon after starting the drug. Phrases like "severely anxious and agitated," "felt like jumping out of her skin," and "couldn't sleep, pacing all night" were recurring themes. The suicide attempts and violence toward others were described as "shocking," "completely out of character."

The anguish that friends and relatives feel in the aftermath of suicides or suicide attempts is profound. Guilt spreads like spores upon the wind, inhaled by anyone even remotely near the scene. "I talked to him on the phone the day before, how could I not have known?" "Why didn't she tell me? Did she think I was too busy or didn't want to hear?" For years, people go over and over the events in minute detail, looking for pieces of evidence, hints that might explain what happened. In these Prozac-related cases, everyone thought the drug was responsible. The argument could be made that Prozac is just an easy target, a scapegoat for people looking for something to blame, and that people who become suicidal or violent on Prozac must have had psychological problems to begin with. But the key elements in these stories appeared to be the "dramatic change" observed in these people after starting Prozac, how "out of character" their behavior was on the drug, and the often extraordinary degree of violence not only toward themselves but toward others.

One of the most compelling stories was that of Anna, who told me Prozac caused her to make a serious suicide attempt while in the care of a previous psychiatrist. As a freshman in college, Anna had been miserably depressed, missing her family and feeling unhappy with her roommates. As the year wore on, she consulted with a psychologist who referred her to a psychiatrist for medication. Anna was started on Prozac but became severely anxious, agitated, and sleepless. She felt "all sped up inside," as if she were "in fast forward while the rest of the world was in slow motion." Having never been suicidal before, two weeks after starting Prozac, Anna went to her HMO because she felt like killing herself. The psychiatrist on call told Anna the Prozac was indeed making her worse and hospitalized her. But her original psychiatrist disagreed, restarted Prozac, although at a lower dose, and added a second, sedating antidepressant (Trazodone), which, however, Anna only took for two days.

After she was discharged from the hospital, Anna felt worse. Sleepless, crying, and at times tremulous, she "walked around like a zombie," devising a plan to overdose. This zombie-like state was a strange depersonalization in which Anna felt she was outside herself, watching herself walking around campus plotting her death with a cold, mechanical detachment.

A few days later, Anna executed the plan. Sitting in her dormitory room, she methodically took dozens of over-the-counter sleeping pills, "horrified" by what she was doing but "unable to stop" herself. By chance, a friend discovered Anna slipping into unconsciousness. When she awoke in an intensive care unit the next day, she was "stunned" by what she had done. She was "humiliated" to find herself tied down in the hospital bed in order to ensure her safety.

Once she was stable, Anna was admitted to McLean Hospital, where she was described as having had a "paradoxical" reaction to Prozac. A nurse told her one of McLean's psychopharmacologists, Dr. Teicher, had written about patients like Anna who became suicidal on Prozac. She was put on a different type of antidepressant, which did not precipitate the same reaction. At the end of the three weeks she was discharged and returned with her parents to their home in Michigan. She was unable to finish the semester and had to take a year off before returning to college.

When she returned to school, I met Anna for the first time. She was an engaging, somewhat anxious young woman. I found her to be excessively polite, cautious, and fearful, as so many depressed people are. Smiling, she tried to put a good face on her history, but she broke down as she told of her suicide attempt the year before, its "devastating" effect on her parents, and the feeling that she might "never live it down." In a gesture one often sees in depressed patients, Anna kept apologizing for crying, as though her display of emotion was somehow unacceptable.

As Anna gradually became more comfortable, she confided her worst fears: How would anyone become her friend? How would anyone date her? How would anyone marry her, if he knew that she had tried to kill herself? As she walked me through the details of her close encounter with death, she repeatedly broke down in tears. Anna said that both she and her parents believed Prozac had caused the strange, "zombie-like" state during which she had nearly died. I hesitated, not wanting to take this explanation away from her, but also not quite prepared to agree. I had not yet seen the reaction myself, firsthand. I told Anna I hoped one day she would accept her suicide attempt as an integral part of her life history regardless of its cause. On this point I feel I did Anna a disservice. Had I known what I know now, I would have readily agreed the Prozac could have precipitated her suicide attempt. But at the time, I had no idea what the truth was.

The FDA's Review of Prozac's Safety

In the early 1990s most doctors did not know what to make of the Prozac scare. Psychiatrists had long recognized that in the early weeks and months on any antidepressant, patients are at increased risk to act on suicidal impulses. Over the course of just a few weeks, antidepressants can jump-start patients, reinvigorating people who have been without energy for some time. Most depressed patients are deeply angry and do not even know it. Abruptly reinvigorating people under these circumstances entails risks. Depression may be nature's way of protecting people from anger they do not yet understand. The newfound energy provided by an antidepressant can suddenly enable a patient to act on suicidal or violent urges. Classic papers dating as far back as the 1930s describe the risk with amphetamine antidepressants.[17] For decades pharmaceutical companies and drug proponents adamantly denied the phenomenon, but by the 1970s, when strict limitations were imposed on prescribing amphetamines, their ability to trigger suicide and violence had been firmly established.

In the 1980s, a similar phenomenon was recognized with tricyclic antidepressants, the class of drugs used between the fall of amphetamine antidepressants in the 1970s and the rise of serotonin boosters in the 1990s.[18] But whereas earlier antidepressants gave people more energy to act on suicidal thoughts, in their report in the *American Journal of Psychiatry*,

Teicher and Cole suggested Prozac did something different. Prozac seemed to *induce* a unique form of agitation and obsessive preoccupation with suicide, which emerged in the early weeks after starting the drug or increasing its dose.[19]

In response to the rising tide of public and professional fear, the FDA appointed a panel of independent experts to look into the matter. In the meantime, the rise in Prozac sales slackened as doctors and patients backed away from the drug. Perhaps the older tricyclic antidepressants were not so bad after all. In fact, their side effects had been exaggerated in the promotion of Prozac.

While the FDA looked into the matter, reports continued to appear in the medical literature. The highly respected British medical journal *Lancet* ran an editorial on Prozac that, while generally favorable to the drug, described one of its more severe side effects as "the promotion of suicidal thoughts and behavior."[20] In the spring of 1991, the Public Citizen Health Research Group, a Ralph Nader–associated consumer advocacy organization, publicly requested the FDA to warn doctors and patients that "a small minority of persons taking Prozac have experienced intense, violent, suicidal thoughts, agitation, and impulsivity after starting treatment with the drug."[21]

Not all psychiatrists supported the inquiry into Prozac's safety. Writing in the *American Journal of Psychiatry*, Dr. Gary Tollefson decried the Prozac controversy, saying that "we should not lose sight of its beneficial addition to our therapeutic armamentarium."[22] Tollefson said that raising the alarm about a drug from which so many people benefited was "potentially counterproductive" and might set a dangerous "medical-legal precedent." Tollefson failed, however, to identify himself as an employee of Eli Lilly.[23]

In the fall of 1991, the FDA committee looking into Prozac's safety exonerated the drug. In an opinion that Eli Lilly later described as "unanimous," the panel found "no credible evidence" that Prozac caused suicidal or violent impulses. Not only would Prozac stay on the market, the FDA rejected any changes in the prescribing guidelines for the drug. No warning would be added to the drug's label.

This was a momentous, highly publicized decision.[24] Naturally, doctors and patients felt reassured. Decisions by the FDA have enormous influence on the medical profession and on the public's perception of drugs. One assumes their positions are thoroughly researched and impartial. In a seemingly bizarre twist, the media reported that a "front" for the Church of Scientology, a group called the Citizens' Commission on Human Rights, had fanned the flames of the Prozac scare by spreading word of the findings of Teicher and Cole in the media. In addition to the FDA's decision, the link between the Church of Scientology and the scare greatly diminished its credibility. One patient brought me copies of a cover article in *Time* magazine detailing the Church of Scientology's purported role.[25] Another showed me a succinct summary of the controversy and the Church of Scientology's alleged role as it appeared in the *Wall Street Journal.*[26]

Reassured, doctors—including myself—again increasingly prescribed Prozac and the other serotonin boosters, which were introduced soon after. Once again, patients began requesting the new medications. Most doctors and patients want to believe in the safety of drugs that seem to make so many distressed people feel better. Sales of the drugs climbed steadily.

But doubts about serotonin boosters causing suicide and violence persisted. Some patients remained skeptical. References to the scare continued to appear in the media and on Internet Web sites. Whenever I told patients about the Church of Scientology connection, they invariably looked at me strangely. So far-fetched was the story, they seemed to wonder if I was making it up. Instead, I began giving people copies of the *Wall Street Journal* article describing the Church of Scientology's role.

The parents of one patient, a Harvard undergraduate, flew from California to meet with me in the spring of 1992 after I recommended Prozac for their daughter. What about suicide and violence, they wanted to know. I told them of the FDA's decision and gave them the articles to read. I reassured them I would be happy to work with their daughter without medication. As with any patient, the decision whether or not to start a drug was ultimately hers. Two months later, the patient requested Prozac because she continued to feel depressed and her final exams were approaching.

While the FDA had cleared the drugs, my colleagues continued to describe some cases in which they appeared to have caused severe reactions—agitation, paranoia, psychosis, suicide, and violence—in a small number of patients. Rumors within psychiatric circles held that the FDA panel of outside experts had been flawed, beset with conflicts of interest and deeply divided on the issue of Prozac's safety, in spite of the impression given to the public. Could it be true that a majority of the panel members had conflicts of interest? Had the vote not been unanimous? Was the panel so divided that one-third of its members pressed for a warning and changes in the guidelines for prescribing antidepressant drugs? What was one to believe?

Joanna and Sunita Become Suicidal on Prozac

For some time, I remained unsure what to think about the Prozac scare. I was cautious about reaching any conclusion, since I had not seen any patients of mine react violently or suicidally to Prozac. In general, I was inclined to believe the FDA's conclusions. That is, until the mid-1990s, when I personally witnessed patients develop acute, suicidal obsessions shortly after starting a serotonin booster.

A week after Joanne began taking Prozac, I received a call from the psychologist who initially evaluated her and referred her to me for medication. The psychologist said Joanne had called to say Prozac was making her suicidal. While I was shocked, the psychologist seemed much less so. "Have you seen this reaction before?" I asked.

"Yes. I've seen it in other clients," she replied. She called because she advised Joanne to stop the Prozac and wanted to be sure I agreed.

"Absolutely," I said. "She should stop it immediately."

"That's what I told her."

"I should see her right away. I'll stay late and see her at the end of the day."

"She's out of town."

"What?"

"She's in Chicago, on a business trip."

"Good grief," I gasped. The idea of a patient becoming suicidal in response to a drug and being away from home, alone in a strange place, beyond our reach, was mind-boggling. "Tell her to please call. Tell her I'll see her the day she gets back."

I wondered if Joanne's reaction would subside once she was off the medication. But when she appeared in my office two days later, she told me she was still acutely suicidal. "I can't stop thinking about ways to kill myself," said Joanne. "I imagine jumping out a window or shooting myself in the head. My brains splatter everywhere. I'm starting to think about where one buys a gun. It's terrible. I can't get the thoughts out of my head."

She was visibly anxious and agitated. She had difficulty sitting still in the chair. Joanne said the agitation and suicidal thoughts had begun at the same time, at the end of her first week on Prozac. She described the same kind of depersonalization that I had heard attributed to the drug before: feeling she was outside herself, observing her own behavior in a detached, "surreal" way. Joanne had not been suicidal before starting Prozac. She was convinced it had triggered the obsession.

"I think you should come into the hospital," was my first impulse.

"No. I don't want to disrupt my life like that."

"But you're not safe."

"I think I am."

"You can control the impulses?"

"So far."

I did not find this very reassuring. However, thinking out loud, I said, "Now that you're off the medication I suppose the urges will subside."

"I'm still taking Prozac."

"I thought your therapist told you to stop," I said, shocked.

"Yes, but I didn't."

"What do you mean?"

"I feel it's working a little."

"How?"

"I have more energy."

"But at the price of feeling suicidal?"

"Won't these thoughts go away?"

I was completely stumped. I told Joanne I had no idea what the answer to her question might be. Since the FDA review cleared the drugs, doctors have no official guidelines to follow. Even if the reaction did go away, what if it returned at a later date? In the absence of reliable information, staying on Prozac hardly seemed worth the risk.

But Joanne persisted. She was "being driven crazy" by the drug but "didn't want to give up hope" in it. There was a desperate quality to her wanting to stay on the medication.

Even as an experienced psychiatrist, I felt utterly unprepared for this moment. I thought it imperative Joanne stop the Prozac. I continued—unsuccessfully—to press her to stop the drug, but being accustomed to supporting people making their own choices, I was truly at a loss. Moreover, I knew Joanne was in the driver's seat. She still had half the prescription I had written for her. What good would it do to force her to pretend to stop Prozac and then not know what I was dealing with? As Joanne insisted on continuing the medication, I reluctantly agreed, on the condition that we meet daily to assess the situation and that she call me in the meantime if the suicidality was worsening.

After Joanne left, I wondered what I had agreed to. What if she killed herself? Should I bring her back into the office? Should I call the police? Should I hospitalize her against her will? I decided none of these actions would be justified. But as I thought about it throughout the evening, I resolved that the next day I would press her again to stop the drug.

At our meeting the next afternoon, even before I spoke, Joanne informed me she was stopping Prozac. She had taken a dose again that morning and was feeling worse; the obsession was getting more intense. She now agreed that the experiment was not worth the risk. I felt enormously relieved.

I continued to check in with Joanne daily. The suicidal preoccupation subsided quickly and was completely gone within a week. Given what had happened, Joanne did not want to try another antidepressant. Once the obsession cleared, she said the whole episode had "jolted" her out of the worst of her depression: "Feeling that terrible for a week put everything in perspective. I wasn't feeling *that* bad before I started Prozac." Indeed, Joanne did fine without medication.

Within months, another patient, Sunita, had an even worse reaction shortly after starting Prozac. Sunita was an extremely isolated, vulnerable student from India, whom I had been seeing in therapy for over a year. She initially came to see me because she was distraught over her mother's death from breast cancer. As she worked through her grief, it emerged that her father was a severe alcoholic who had been psychologically and physically abusive.

During the year, Sunita chose to switch the focus of her studies from history to the premed requirements, with the goal of going to medical school. In the spring of the second year of our work, she became depressed as the anniversary of her mother's death approached. Under increasing pressure in difficult science courses, she asked about going on an antidepressant.

I was reluctant to prescribe one, feeling that Sunita should simply work through the grief she was suffering. But she was fearful of doing poorly in her classes and had read many advertisements and articles promoting the new drugs. I certainly did not want her to fail the semester and become even more depressed.

In her second week on Prozac, Sunita's clinical picture changed dramatically. Trembling because she felt so "panicky," Sunita told me she felt like she was being "brutalized" on campus.

"What do you mean?" I asked, alarmed.

"My body parts are strewn all over the campus."

"Your body parts?"

"My arms, my legs, my torso . . . when I walk around campus I see them strewn through the trees."

"Trees?"

"Yes. They're hanging in trees, all bloodied. I've been dismembered."

Sunita went on to tell me the professor in one of her most difficult premed courses was now forcing her to "fellate" him.

"He is?"

"Yes. Most days when I go to class."

"When does this happen?"

"*In* class. He's been making me perform oral sex on him in front of the whole class!"

"In front of the class?"

"The whole class, one hundred fifty students," Sunita insisted, desperately. "He keeps staring at me, singling me out, talking to me instead of the others, looking at me sexually until I come down and perform oral sex on him in front of everyone, and then he stops bothering me. It's so humiliating."

Obviously, this could not possibly be happening in front of a huge class of students. Sunita was psychotic.

Still worse, she was also preoccupied with killing herself. Disjointedly, she said, "I'm dead anyway. People are killing me. My body parts are strewn all over campus. I can't stop thinking I should just kill myself and get it over with."

Sunita had never been psychotic or suicidal before. Gently, I reminded her that she had felt under a lot of pressure with her classes and the anniversary of her mother's death. I said I thought the Prozac might have tipped her into being so fearful and suicidal. I wanted her to stop the drug and come into the hospital.

Sunita became even more agitated: "Don't put me in the hospital. Please don't do that. If I go in the hospital, I'll never finish the semester. I'd be devastated. Then I'll really kill myself."

"I didn't say I was going to force you into the hospital, but I think we should seriously consider it. Just for a week. Just for observation."

"No. Please. I don't want that."

Sunita also wanted to stay on Prozac: "I know it's making me panicky. But it's going to work, isn't it? The ads—I saw another one this week—it said these medications 'give you back your life.' I want my life back. . . ." Sunita broke down, sobbing.

Once Sunita was composed, I explained: "I've seen this reaction in other people. The obsessive thoughts of violence and suicide only get worse. It's too dangerous."

Gradually, Sunita and I worked out a compromise. She would stop the drug and bring me the bottle of remaining pills. I wanted the pills so I could be sure she stopped taking the Prozac. Sunita agreed to call me in the evening to let me know how she was doing. She also agreed to meet daily to check in with me until her suicidality had cleared. In return, I agreed that she would not have to go into the hospital unless her condition worsened.

Agreeing to Sunita's not going into the hospital was risky, even with these safeguards, but psychiatrists have to deal with these risks all the time. Hospitalization is no guarantee a patient will be safe. Hospitalization can make some patients feel worse, especially if they feel betrayed by a doctor who forces them to go against their will. Angry, embittered patients can find ways to kill themselves in the hospital or soon after leaving.

The single most important protection against patients' killing themselves is a strong alliance with a clinician who they feel understands their situation and whom they trust. Sunita was willing to check in with me daily and to call me if she felt she was actually going to harm herself. Since she was adamantly opposed to hospitalization, I felt following her closely on an outpatient basis would be the best arrangement.

When she went off Prozac, Sunita's suicidality gradually waned, but it did not completely clear for weeks. Unfortunately, even after the suicidality disappeared, she remained psychotic, delusional about the oral sex and body parts for months. She declined antipsychotic medication "after what happened on Prozac." Indeed, she became paranoid of me, feeling I was part of a "conspiracy," with my role being to "drug" her. At this point, Sunita announced she was stopping therapy.

Obviously, this was an extremely rocky period in Sunita's treatment. Given her clinical condition, this was no time for this already extremely isolated student to be without anyone monitoring her. I suggested that instead of stopping, we cut back to what had been our original, once-a-week format. With paranoid, psychotic patients, meeting less frequently is often better. They are exquisitely sensitive to anything they perceive to be intrusive. Now that she was no longer suicidal, I felt cutting back to once a week would be safe.

Sunita stayed in therapy and did quite well. She managed to finish the semester with "respectable grades," in her words, even though her psychosis did not completely clear until three months after the Prozac was stopped.

The Influence of Dose and Setting

After having seen firsthand the reaction Teicher and Cole described in 1990, I no longer had any doubts about what colleagues and patients had told me. But what caused the reaction? I wondered. How were other psychiatrists and therapists coping with it?

To answer these questions, I sought out professional forums—talks, symposia, and continuing medical education conferences—where serotonin boosters and their side effects were discussed. Often, I brought up the subject of agitation and suicidality. Privately, I also talked with colleagues: psychiatrists, psychologists, social workers, and primary-care doctors.

I discovered that while no official guidelines exist for this sort of reaction to Prozac-type drugs, and while none of the drugs' package inserts give any advice or warning of the possibility of their triggering suicide and violence, many psychiatrists were quietly learning to deal with the problem through trial and error. One strategy psychiatrists developed was to start patients at much lower doses of the drugs than officially recommended. Typically, psychoactive drugs are started at low doses, which are gradually increased as the patient's nervous system adjusts. The earliest prescription antidepressants, cocaine elixirs, were liquids that were measured out of a bottle or flask. The liquid form of a drug is the easiest to administer in small, incremental starting doses. With cocaine elixirs it was easy to adjust the dose so a patient remained comfortable. When amphetamine antidepressants were introduced, they came in graduated sizes: 5-, 10-, and 20-milligram pills. Patients could be started on as little as 5 milligrams and slowly increased to 20 milligrams or more. Tricyclic antidepressants, the immediate precursors of Prozac, are similarly started at low doses and gradually increased. The drugs' side effects (such as dry mouth, lightheadedness, and nausea) are monitored as signs of the nervous system's adapting. With each increase in dose, the side effects flare up and then subside. Their subsiding is the sign that the nervous system has adapted and one can go up again. Slowly, one gradually reinvigorates the patient, typically over two months.

When Prozac was introduced, one of the most striking differences between it and its predecessors was that its prescribing guidelines indicated that there was no need to slowly increase the dose and balance this with the drug's side effects. The starting dose, one 20-milligram pill per day, was the maintenance dose for most depressed patients.[27] Similarly, when Zoloft and Paxil were later introduced, the starting dose could also be used as the maintenance dose for depressed patients.[28] Obviously, their one-dose-fits-all-patients was much simpler and a large part of their attraction.

But psychiatrists learned the one-dose-fits-everyone schedule exposes patients to a relatively high starting dose. For most patients this may be all right, but for sensitive individuals, it can be extremely problematic. These patients are jump-started too quickly. Their nervous systems are thrown into overdrive without adequate time to adjust. These are the patients who become anxious, agitated, and sleepless. Still worse, they can be tipped into paranoia or psychosis. Worse yet, they can become acutely suicidal and violent. This is especially true if the dose is rapidly increased above 20 milligrams a day of Prozac. This was a striking feature of Teicher and Cole's cases reported in the *American Journal of Psychiatry*. In one case, the patient's dose reached 60 milligrams a day in less than two weeks. In others, the dose continued to be increased even after the patients became suicidal or violent, until Teicher and Cole began to suspect the drug.

As I researched the phenomenon, I discovered many psychiatrists had quietly changed how they prescribe serotonin boosters, returning to the way they prescribed earlier antidepressants. These doctors start Prozac at 5 or 10 milligrams and slowly increase it to 20, allowing the patient's nervous system to slowly adjust to the drug, resulting in a lower incidence of anxiety, agitation, paranoia, psychosis, and suicidality. Starting patients on a lower dose was particularly difficult when Prozac was first introduced, because it only came in a 20-milligram size and is a capsule rather than a tablet. With their grainy, powdery contents, capsules are difficult to divide.[29] Psychiatrists instructed patients to open the capsule, pour a quarter or a half of the powder into a glass of water, drink the water, and save the rest of the capsule for the next day.

Another strategy was adding a sedative for any patient who became anxious, agitated, or sleepless. The concurrent sedative takes the edge off the side effects, preventing the patient from escalating to suicidal or violent impulses. For anyone who is anxious before starting an antidepressant, a sedative can be added from the start.

Here, too, psychiatrists had been left to their own devices in the absence of official guidelines. Cocaine elixirs were made by mixing cocaine—a stimulant—with red Bordeaux wine, a sedative. Amphetamine antidepressants were routinely prescribed in concert with sedating barbiturates. The tricyclic antidepressants provide a mixture of stimulation and sedation in one pill. This is not unlike mixing stimulants and sedatives socially or recreationally. People often combine smoking cigarettes (containing the stimulant nicotine) with drinking alcohol. Intravenous drug users mix cocaine and heroin in what are called "speedballs." Drug users refer to such practices as "mixing uppers and downers."

When mixed, stimulants and sedatives enhance each other's desired effects, take the edge off each other's side effects, and allow the use of increased doses of both. Nowadays, the sedatives that informed psychiatrists prescribe in concert with serotonin boosters are either a Valium-type sleeping pill (Dalmane, Restoril, Serax, etc.) or an antianxiety agent (Ativan,

Xanax, etc.). Alternatively, they combine a morning dose of a serotonin booster with a bedtime dose of a second antidepressant, one of the older, sedating ones such as trazodone or amitriptyline. The concurrent sedative calms patients while their nervous system adapts to the serotonin booster. Usually, the need for the sedative is temporary. Once the patient's nervous system has adjusted, the sedative can be withdrawn, typically after two months. But by then many people are attached to the sedative and too often remain on both indefinitely.

Practices like adjusting the dosing schedule or adding a sedative have no official precedent, and in order to learn them, doctors must become connected to an underground, word-of-mouth network of critical, clinical information. As I learned these techniques from colleagues, I thought, These suggestions should be in the official prescribing guidelines for the drugs, especially given the risks involved for patient and public safety.

In addition to adjusting the dosing schedule and adding a sedative, the third key variable in a patient's response to a serotonin booster is the setting in which the drug is prescribed. Psychiatrists refer to the setting, or context, as a patient's "holding environment." This is the care and concern evidenced by the clinician, important ingredients in the healing process. A prerequisite is appointments that are frequent enough and long enough for the clinician to convey his or her commitment to the patient and to explore any underlying psychological issues. Another requirement is continuity of care—the presence of a consistent clinician with whom the patient has a good rapport and can develop feelings of safety and trust. The clinician brings experience, intuition, and empathy to the process, helping patients penetrate to the heart of what is bothering them.

This holding environment is the modern equivalent of the settings in which ancient cultures have used naturally occurring psychoactive compounds for centuries. Whether Andean Indians chewing coca leaves, Chinese herbalists prescribing ephedra, or North American Indians ceremonially smoking peyote, these low-potency, naturally occurring agents have always been used in the context of complex rituals and close cultural ties. Today, we use much more dangerous, potent, synthetic drugs to treat individuals who very often are isolated, making the setting all the more important for safety.

What is the setting in which patients have been prescribed serotonin boosters? As I listened to psychiatrists discuss serotonin antidepressants and their side effects, I heard over and over again that patients are more likely to have bad reactions in managed care settings. In managed care–delivery systems (health maintenance organizations and preapproved physician networks), distressed psychiatric patients are given minimal, fragmented treatment emphasizing medication with little or no psychosocial support. Often, the medication dose is rapidly increased to quickly jump-start patients. In these anxiety-amplifying circumstances, patients are much more likely to have bad reactions to the drugs.

In recent years, the context in which psychiatric patients are treated has only worsened. Managed-care administrators see clinicians as interchangeable and often deliberately disrupt continuity of care in the interest of efficiency. Doctor-patient appointments are treated like an assembly line. Doctors are under enormous pressure to see patients for brief, cursory appointments. All that matters is processing the largest number of patients in the shortest period of time possible. Obviously, this is not a holding environment for anyone.

The Serotonin-Dopamine Connection, Yet Again

How do serotonin boosters catalyze suicidal and violent impulses? Does the phenomenon occur because of the drugs' stimulating, re-energizing effects as with previous antidepressants? Or might something different happen with these new drugs, as Teicher and Cole suggested in their original report?

While a psychiatrist at Harvard Medical School, Anthony Rothschild conducted a particularly important study reported in the December 1991 issue of the *Journal of Clinical Psychiatry*.[30] In a risky gamble, Rothschild represcribed Prozac to three patients who had previously become suicidal on the drug to see if they would have the same reaction. The patients chosen were dramatic cases. The first patient was deemed safe to enter the study because she could be easily monitored: She was "confined to a wheelchair" after injuries sustained in a near-lethal suicide attempt the first time she went on Prozac. On that occasion, about two weeks after starting the drug, the patient became extremely agitated and anxious. Seeking relief from the severe discomfort, she leapt from the roof of a building. Although she did not die, the impact of the fall caused hemorrhaging in her brain and multiple fractures of her arms and legs. She spent a month in a general hospital recuperating from these injuries before being transferred to McLean Hospital, where Rothschild restarted her on Prozac.

Eleven days later, after he started the patient on Prozac for the second time, she again developed "severe anxiety, restlessness, and an inability to sit still." Observing the patient closely, Rothschild realized she was suffering from a severe case of neurologically driven agitation, one of the four neurological side effects caused by Prozac backlash as described in Chapter 1. The patient described the panicky agitation as "identical" to what she felt prior to her suicide attempt the first time she was on Prozac. Said the patient, "I tried to kill myself because of these anxiety symptoms. It was not so much the depression." When Prozac was stopped, the patient's agitation and suicidal urges cleared within seventy-two hours.

When the second patient was first put on Prozac, he jumped off a cliff because he felt as though he were jumping out of his skin. In Rothschild's rechallenge study, when this patient was restarted on Prozac, he again developed severe restlessness, pacing, and insomnia. The patient insisted, "This is exactly what happened the last time I was on Prozac, and I feel like jumping off a cliff again."

This time, instead of stopping the Prozac, Rothschild gave the patient an antianxiety agent (propranolol) known to counteract drug-induced agitation. Rothschild wanted to test whether or not this *particular* side effect was responsible for the patient's suicidality. In fact, the addition of the second medication "led to the complete disappearance within 24 hours of the restlessness, the anxiety, and the desire to jump off a cliff."

The third patient had "jumped off the roof of a tall building" the first time she went on Prozac. In Rothschild's rechallenge study, two weeks after restarting the drug, the patient "began complaining that she had to move her legs back and forth and pace constantly to relieve anxiety. On examination, she constantly shifted her legs while seated and would get up from the chair many times to walk around the office. She stated that this restlessness was driving her 'crazy' and that she was feeling like she did during her last suicide attempt." Once again, in this case, addition of an antianxiety agent "led to a complete remission of the restlessness, anxiety, and suicidal feelings."

All three of the patients in Rothschild's study "developed severe akathisia [the technical term for drug-induced agitation] during retreatment with Prozac and stated that the development of the akathisia made them feel suicidal and that it had precipitated their prior suicide attempts." In other words, the patients were *not* simply re-energized on Prozac. Instead, they experienced a virulent form of drug-induced restlessness and anxiety that seemingly drove them to suicide and violence. Of course, neurologically driven agitation is one of the serotonin boosters' side effects, well known to psychiatrists from major tranquilizers. Whereas major tranquilizers directly decrease dopamine in the involuntary motor system, serotonin boosters are thought to cause these side effects via the serotonin–dopamine connection. Thus, this same mechanism has been implicated in many of the drugs' most severe side effects.

One of the world's leading experts on drug-induced agitation until his recent death was Theodore Van Putten, a psychiatrist at UCLA. In the 1970s and 1980s, Van Putten published classic papers on the "behavioral toxicity" of major tranquilizers.[31] Among the toxic effects, Van Putten described vivid cases of severe agitation leading to suicidal and violent impulses. Other psychiatrists published similar cases of suicidality, violence, and deaths due to major tranquilizer-induced agitation that read eerily like those later seen with Prozac.[32]

The classic papers on drug-induced agitation describe it as an "abject terror" that can be "more difficult to endure than any of the symptoms for which they [the patients] had been originally treated."[33] Mild cases are often "difficult to articulate" and can involve subtle, almost "evanescent" feelings of being "all nerved up," "tense," or "impatient."[34] Some patients describe feeling as if their bones are tuning forks rattling inside their bodies. Others say it is like living twenty-four-hours-a-day with the sensation of someone scratching their nails on a blackboard. Even mild cases "can be unbearable."[35] In some instances observable restlessness is minimal but the patient experiences "a subjective state [that] can, nevertheless, be tormenting." In a particularly dangerous scenario, patients who have not been warned of the side effect can misinterpret it as a grave worsening of their condition and become despairing and suicidal.

In July 1992, Van Putten, together with Dr. William Wirshing and four other colleagues at UCLA, published a report in the *Archives of General Psychiatry* comparing Prozac-induced "restlessness, pacing, insomnia, and obsessional suicidality" to that seen with major tranquilizers.[36] As in earlier Prozac cases, one of their patients felt an "obsessive need" to kill herself; another "begged for relief" from her inner turmoil. One patient who had previously become agitated on a major tranquilizer reported that the Prozac-induced syndrome was "one hundred times worse than anything I've experienced before!" Another patient was tipped into psychosis as well as suicidality. Although usually considered an early side effect, in one instance a patient developed agitation and suicidality only after she was on Prozac for four months and no longer depressed.

When Van Putten and Wirshing took their patients off Prozac or lowered their dose sufficiently, the agitation and suicidality cleared. When antianxiety agents were used to temper the agitation, the suicidality also improved. As in Rothschild's study, when one patient was rechallenged with a higher dose of the drug, she experienced a return of the side effects. Van

Putten and Wirshing concluded, "Our cases appear to confirm that certain subjects experience akathisia [agitation] while taking Prozac and that this effect is dose-related in the individual patient. Further . . . the 'Prozac akathisia' can apparently be associated with suicidal ideation, sometimes of ruminative intensity."

In November 1992, Drs. Margaret Hamilton and Lewis Opler published yet another report citing Prozac-induced agitation as the cause of suicidality on the drug in the *Journal of Clinical Psychiatry*.[37] Hamilton and Opler are in the Department of Psychiatry at Columbia University College of Physicians and Surgeons in New York. Together they reviewed the many previously published cases and presented one of their own, a young woman who developed severe agitation and suicidality a month after starting Prozac. The patient had been depressed but not suicidal before going on the drug. Her depression actually improved on Prozac but, they said, "the patient stated that although her mood was good, she was afraid that she would kill herself because of these restless and out-of-control feelings." Hamilton and Opler quoted the patient: "I feel I need to hold on to my chair or else I'll jump out the window." The patient developed the potentially lethal side effect "at a very low dose" of Prozac, just 5 milligrams a day.

Much of Hamilton and Opler's paper on Prozac-induced agitation and suicidality focused on the serotonin–dopamine connection. They cited animal studies in which it is "well documented" that serotonin nerves "project directly" into the involuntary motor system. Numerous studies suggest that "serotonin inhibits dopamine" in this system. Via these pathways, said Hamilton and Opler, serotonin boosters could indirectly produce the same side effect as major tranquilizers, which directly inhibit dopamine. Indeed, they proposed a model for wiring within the involuntary motor system to account for how elevated serotonin levels could cause a drop in dopamine, resulting in this severe side effect.

Hamilton and Opler concluded that suicidality in association with serotonin boosters "is really a reaction to the side effect of akathisia [agitation] and not true suicidal ideation as is typically described by depressed patients experiencing suicidal ideation." They characterized it as an "extreme" version of the "behavioral toxicity" of the drugs.

While all of these later researchers focused on drug-induced agitation and, therefore, the serotonin–dopamine connection, it is important to note that other effects of the drugs may contribute to suicidality and violence. In severe cases, the overstimulated, caffeinated feeling that some patients experience soon after starting a Prozac-type medication is another potential factor. This anxious, panicky state is different from the restlessness of neurologically driven agitation. Insomnia, a common side effect of the drugs, may be another contributing factor. The drugs tip some patients into mania or psychosis, both of which can increase the risk of suicidality and violence. Because this issue still needs more research, at present we have no way of knowing how each of these drug effects may contribute to the problem.

In lawsuits involving Prozac's association with murder-suicide, discussed in detail later in the chapter, surprising evidence has emerged regarding how Eli Lilly handled drug-induced agitation as a side effect during Prozac's clinical studies. After reviewing internal Lilly documents in one case, Dr. David Healy, one of Europe's leading psychiatrists, reported, "There appears to be a pattern that obscures the occurrence of akathisia [agitation] on Prozac. . . . Akathisia was named as a side effect of Prozac in the very early trials. The 31 July 1978 Prozac Project Team Meeting minutes state that 'There have been a fairly large number of adverse reactions. . . . Akathisia and restlessness were reported in some patients.' On 19 December 1979, Lilly canceled the clinical trial being conducted by Dr. Joyce Small. . . . It is interesting that Small is one of the few researchers to list akathisia as one of the side effects she observed in persons on Prozac—and she found it in one out of 11 persons on the drug, a rate of 9%."[38] But, says Healy, "Despite this large early incidence of reported akathisia, in the later trials [clinical studies] the use of the term *unaccountably disappears*. A widely held hypothesis has been that this was done deliberately for fear that the drug would not have been registered with [approved by] the FDA were the extent to which stimulatory effects occurred more salient [italics added]."

Moreover, internal Eli Lilly documents reveal that the pharmaceutical company knew years before Prozac was approved by the FDA and marketed to the public that the drug could affect dopamine and other neurotransmitters indirectly. These documents have become part of the public record in Prozac murder-suicide trials. One of these documents, an early 1983 draft of Prozac's official product information, stated that the drug affected serotonin but "would not be expected to affect noradrenergic [adrenaline] or dopaminergic [dopamine] neurons."[39] But a later, August 24, 1983, memo commenting on the draft says that the wording should be changed to "would not be expected to *directly* affect" adrenaline or dopamine (italics added).[40] The rationale for the change is stated this way: "The key word in this description is directly. Indirect effects on the noradrenergic and dopaminergic neurons may be mediated by Prozac's direct effect on serotonergic neurons." In other words, Lilly knew that Prozac's direct effects on serotonin could have secondary, indirect effects on other neurotransmitter systems linked to it, such as the serotonin–dopamine connection. How could Prozac have been widely promoted as "selective" for serotonin when Lilly knew that it could affect other important neurotransmitters, albeit indirectly?

Later, as doctors struggled to understand Prozac's side effects and began writing about the serotonin–dopamine connection, Lilly was critical of these efforts. After Drs. Margaret Hamilton and Lewis Opler published their paper on Prozac-induced agitation and suicidality, which included proposed wiring for the serotonin–dopamine connection in the involuntary motor system, Charles Beasley, an in-house doctor at Eli Lilly, criticized their observations and model as "premature."[41] Beasley published his critique in the February 1994 issue of the *Journal of Clinical Psychiatry.* This was more than a decade after Lilly's 1983 memo indicating Prozac could have indirect effects on other neurotransmitters, including dopamine. What was "premature" about doctors trying to puzzle out what Lilly apparently knew at least a decade earlier?

While prominent psychiatrists continued to report on Prozac-related suicidality and violence, unfortunately, coming after the FDA panel exonerated the drugs, these later reports, including the rechallenge studies, were largely ignored. Most physicians and the general public were left with the impression that the problem did not exist.

Revisiting the FDA Panel's Investigation

In addition to continuing reports of the grave side effects of suicidality and violence, other disturbing information about the political handling of this information began to emerge in the mid-1990s. For one thing, the FDA committee looking into Prozac's safety had indeed been seriously flawed.

In the early 1990s, when Prozac's dangerous effects surfaced in the media, the FDA asked a special committee to look into the matter of suicidality and violence. On important issues that come to public attention, the FDA often turns to an advisory committee, a panel of "independent"— meaning outside the FDA—"blue ribbon" experts. The panel is asked to render an opinion to aid the FDA in deciding what to do. The panel's findings are nonbinding, but obviously the opinion of an independent, "blue ribbon" committee will influence the FDA in its course of action and weigh heavily on public opinion.

Who were the blue-ribbon, independent experts on the Prozac panel? There were nine doctors, five of whose financial ties to the pharmaceutical industry—including the manufacturers of serotonin boosters—required the FDA to "waive" its own standards regarding conflicts of interest.[42] In addition, six consultants were appointed to advise the panel. Four of the six consultants required conflict-of-interest waivers. Among the committee members receiving waivers was Dr. David Dunner of the Department of Psychiatry and Behavioral Sciences at the University of Washington in Seattle. Dunner had been a lead investigator for Eli Lilly in one of the four Prozac placebo-controlled clinical studies which Lilly submitted to the FDA to win approval to market the drug.[43] Among the consultants receiving waivers was Dr. Stewart Montgomery of the Department of Psychiatry, Saint Mary's Hospital Medical School in London, England. Montgomery, too, had been a principal investigator for Eli Lilly in a study of Prozac.[44]

To investigate the Prozac scare, the panel held a one-day hearing on September 20, 1991. According to an FDA memo summarizing the many conflicts of interest, the waivers were justified on the following grounds: "In accordance with the prepared agenda [for the hearing], *there will be no specific issues dealing with a specific product [drug] or sponsor [pharmaceutical company] presented to the committee for review and evaluation during this meeting.* Therefore, it has been determined that all committee members may fully participate in today's meeting without the risk of any conflict of interest [italics added]."[45] But concerns about Prozac's safety were the reason the committee was meeting. Prozac was what patients, doctors, and the public were concerned about. Indeed, half of the formal presentations on the agenda were made by Eli Lilly. Reading the transcript of the hearing, which runs almost 350 pages, one sees that the vast majority of the discussion is about Prozac.[46] Under these circumstances, how could one justify waivers on the grounds that no specific drug would be evaluated? An advisory panel with conflicts of interest serious enough that the FDA had to waive its own standards for the majority of members hardly seems appropriate for such a serious question of patient and public safety.

The daylong hearing was divided into three parts. In the opening segment, fifty members of the public who had signed up in advance on a first-come-first-served basis were allowed to address the committee for up to five minutes each. Many people told dramatic, moving stories. Some were patients who told of how they had become suicidal and violent on Prozac. Others were family members of people who had committed suicide. Many of the patients and family members had traveled great distances to testify at the hearing. But a different approach was taken by a number of psychiatrists and drug proponents who also testified, warning the committee that any changes in Prozac's prescribing guidelines would undermine the public's confidence in psychiatric drugs.

In the second part of the hearing, the FDA's staff reported on the information in their databases. They explained that there is no systematic program for monitoring the side effects of drugs once they are on the market. The FDA's spontaneous monitoring system, in which doctors or patients take the initiative to report side effects, captures only a "fraction" of the true incidence.[47] Most reports are made to the drug's manufacturer, who processes them and then passes the information on to the FDA. Many reports are "incomplete" and "difficult to interpret." The FDA's system was described as "weak" and having "flaws." Especially with complicated phenomena like suicide and violence, at best the system might provide a preliminary, inconclusive "signal [i.e., suggestion] of something that may need further investigation [in a more rigorous, scientific way] and does not itself constitute evidence of causality."

Finally, four doctors made presentations on behalf of Eli Lilly. With the aid of numerous overhead slides, the Lilly representatives presented the committee with hard numbers that they said scientifically proved Prozac was a safe drug. Lilly's focus was on a retrospective analysis of statistical data from Prozac's large-scale clinical studies, looking at the emergence or intensification of suicidality in patients. These were the studies Lilly had performed to win FDA approval for the drug. According to Lilly, the data showed that patients given Prozac did not have a higher incidence of suicidality than those given a placebo. Just as other side effects of the drug—such as its sexual side effects—have been blamed on the patients' underlying depression, this was the explanation given for suicidality and violence. Summarizing Lilly's presentations, Dr. Robert Zerby insisted "the only scientifically valid approach to the evaluation and treatment of emergent suicidality in depression is through an analysis of appropriately controlled data [such as Lilly's]. Neither anecdotes [the stories told by people in the first part of the hearing and the many published cases] or spontaneous reporting [the FDA's inadequate data]" could compare.[48] Dr. Charles Nemeroff, professor and chairman of the department of psychiatry at Emory University, in Atlanta, concluded his presentation for Lilly by saying that he had "little confidence in these anecdotal [case] reports . . . there is no substitute for controlled prospective double-blind clinical trials [such as Lilly's].[49]

Coming on the heels of the public's "anecdotes" earlier in the day and the FDA's inconclusive data, Lilly's seemingly scientific evidence gave the committee members and consultants considerable comfort. Said one, "The Lilly data are obviously very reassuring." Said another, Lilly's data "provide for me, as a scientist, the frame of reference that I feel most comfortable with. . . ."[50] Announced a third, As a "committee of science advisors . . . I think that the kind of advice you get from a group like us needs to be based on the numbers."

Another theme in the discussion was an academic debate over whether or not Prozac could be *proven* to cause suicidality and violence. Another psychiatrist speaking for Lilly was Dr. Jan Fawcett, professor and chairman of the Department of Psychiatry at Rush Presbyterian Saint Luke's Medical Center in Chicago. Fawcett acknowledged that research has shown anxiety and agitation, not depression per se, correlate with suicide and violence. In fact, he testified his own research "found that anxiety, panic attacks, poor concentration, and insomnia formed a cluster which predicted suicide" in depressed patients.[51] While it was acknowledged that Prozac causes these specific side effects, it was still not *proven* that Prozac caused the suicidality. This was analogous to tobacco companies insisting for decades that no one had *proven* cigarettes caused lung cancer, addiction, and many other health problems.

Also at the hearing was Martin Teicher, the Harvard psychiatrist whose case reports helped bring the issue of suicidality and violence to national attention. Remarkably, although four doctors representing Eli Lilly had been scheduled to make formal presentations to the committee, Dr. Teicher was not. Eventually, toward the end of the day, Dr. Ida Hellander of the Ralph Nader–associated Public Citizen Health Research Group protested, "I am very disappointed [that] . . . we have not heard much from [Dr.] Teicher today. . . . [Dr.] Teicher is here, and I would actually really appreciate it if he would have a few moments to talk, because I am very interested in his views and fully expected them to be more elucidated."[52]

Dr. Teicher briefly summarized the clinical experience with Prozac inducing suicide and violence, proposed several mechanisms by which the drug might do so, and said he had data showing that Prozac is associated with a "threefold" higher incidence of suicidality than other antidepressants. But Dr. Teicher was not able to present the data. Presiding over the hearing was the panel's chairman, Dr. Daniel Casey, a strong drug proponent from Oregon Health Sciences University in Portland. As Teicher spoke, Casey repeatedly cut him off, admonishing him to keep his comments "brief" and "focused." At one point Casey interrupted Teicher to say, "I am soon going to ask for a vote of the committee."[53]

Teicher was in a three-way conversation with Casey and Dr. Paul Leber, director of the FDA's Division of Neuropharmacological Drug Products, which was responsible for originally approving Prozac and for now investigating the issue of suicide and violence. Leber criticized Teicher for not having hard "evidence" from "controlled conditions." The data Lilly had presented were from controlled—meaning placebo-controlled—clinical studies.

Teicher explained that he did have some hard data: A re-evaluation of a published study, which was important because Eli Lilly and drug proponents originally said it showed that Prozac is not associated with a higher incidence of suicidality.[54] Teicher's re-evaluation of the data actually demonstrated that patients on Prozac had a "threefold" higher incidence of newly emerging suicidality than patients on older antidepressants.

Apparently questioning the validity of Teicher's data, Leber asked whether "maybe it would be useful if you would say precisely where these data that show an excess risk for Prozac actually are cited or published."

"I will be happy to show you," answered Teicher. Wanting to present the data to the committee, Teicher asked, "May I show you a couple of slides?"

"I would rather not. . . ," responded Casey.[55]

Teicher made one more appeal to Leber and Casey but did not prevail. Even though Eli Lilly was allowed lengthy presentations by doctors who showed multiple slides, Teicher never got to present his. Instead, Casey announced, "I would like to offer my opinion—everyone else has offered an opinion—and then call the question, form a question for us to vote on. . . . I do not believe there is credible evidence to date to support the idea that antidepressant drugs cause intensification of suicidality."

Shortly thereafter, the committee agreed, voting unanimously that antidepressants do not cause suicide and violence. This was the unanimous, "no credible evidence" vote that was widely publicized.[56]

But in another vote, the committee considered adding a warning to the guidelines for prescribing antidepressants based upon what they had heard at the hearing. In spite of the many conflicts of interest, the committee was deeply divided. Several committee members pressed for a warning. One of them drafted a proposed warning that read, "In a small number of patients, depressive symptoms have worsened during therapy, including the emergence of suicidal thoughts and attempts."[57] This would have alerted doctors and patients to the possibility of suicidal or violent impulses without saying the drug *caused* them. Knowing of the phenomenon, regardless of its precise cause, doctors could attempt to deal with it, for example, by modulating the dose, adding a sedative, or stopping the drug.

Here, again, Dr. Paul Leber of the FDA weighed in. "We almost have that [kind of a warning] in labeling now," said Leber. He was referring to a statement in the precautions section of the product information for antidepressants stating that "the possibility of a suicide attempt is inherent in depression." Committee members argued with Leber: This was not the same as warning doctors that suicidality could emerge or worsen after drug treatment was initiated. Leber raised concern that even a general warning for antidepressants would hurt Prozac in particular: "It is sort of a no-win situation for Prozac, because it has been in the public eye."

Despite the conflicts of interest, one-third of the panel members voted for a warning, while two-thirds voted against one.[58] This was the deeply divided vote, the strongly held, one-third minority opinion in spite of the many conflicts of interest. This vote was not highly publicized after the hearing. Those interested in the matter only learn about it by obtaining a copy of the transcript of the hearing from the FDA through the Freedom of Information Act.

Why were the stakes so high for Prozac, for the soon-to-be released Zoloft and Paxil, and for psychopharmacologists, the subspecialists of psychiatry who only prescribe pills and do not provide psychotherapy? Why was there so much concern about creating public doubt about the safety of psychiatric drugs? So much concern that even a warning was voted down?

Presumably Prozac's advocates were afraid any change in the prescribing guidelines for antidepressants, even a general warning, would have caused further public relations problems for the pharmaceutical industry. Public fear was already running high. Prozac was alleged to be associated with suicides, murders, murder-suicides, and even mass murder-suicides like Joseph Wesbecker's shooting spree at Standard Gravure. Numerous lawsuits had been filed in deaths associated with Prozac. Given how high-profile the issue had already been, any suggestion that antidepressants could cause severe agitation that needed to be controlled with sedatives would only raise more questions. Pharmaceutical companies spend hundreds of millions of dollars developing and launching a drug like Prozac. By 1991, Prozac was already the number-one best-selling antidepressant, with sales near $1 billion a year.[59] The stakes were indeed high. So the pharmaceutical industry and drug advocates decided to defend Prozac at all costs, despite the risks to individual and public safety.

In retrospect, one of the most striking features of the FDA hearing was how the concerns of patients and doctors were written off as "anecdotes" and silenced in the name of "science." "Anecdotes" was hardly an adequate description for the frightening, personal (rather than anecdotal) experiences of patients; the detailed firsthand accounts of their doctors published in medical journals; and the rechallenge studies linking Prozac even more clearly to suicide and violence (which, although they were not yet published, were mentioned by Teicher at the hearing but received little discussion). Although a few doubts were raised about the quality of Lilly's data, the committee members could have no idea how "flawed" the data would turn out to be according to experts with more time to scrutinize it.

Indeed, internal FDA memos obtained through the Freedom of Information Act reveal that long before the hearing, the FDA's own reviewers had determined that the data from Lilly's clinical studies, which the pharmaceutical company focused on at the hearing, were inadequate to the task. In a September 11, 1990, memo a full year before the hearing, Dr. David Graham, section chief of the FDA's Epidemiology Branch, wrote that Lilly had reviewed data from their clinical studies with the FDA, and had prefaced the review "with the acknowledgment that these trials [studies] were not designed for the prospective evaluation of suicidality. In these trials, patients with current suicidal ideation were excluded."[60] Those who became suicidal were only evaluated through "non-probing, open-ended questions" and a checklist rating scale "which included one question on suicide." Lilly's numerical data, in particular, were derived from this simple, checklist question. Graham said of this relatively superficial assessment, "The capacity of these trials to identify and describe the quality and intensity of suicidality was low."

Graham also performed a re-evaluation of the study, which Teicher later tried to call attention to at the FDA hearing with the slides he was unable to show. In Graham's memo, he raised concerns similar to Teicher's. While the study had been cited by Lilly as evidence that Prozac is not associated with a higher incidence of suicidality, in fact, said Graham: "the actual data . . . raise some potential questions. . . . Treatment-emergent [i.e., new] suicidality was more frequent among" patients receiving Prozac than among those receiving older, tricyclic antidepressants. "The relative risk of suicidality was 3.3. . . . Interestingly, the proportion of patients with treatment-emergent suicidality on Prozac in this study was similar to that reported by Teicher" in his original article calling attention to the problem.

Graham concluded, "The firm's [Lilly's] analysis of suicidality does not resolve the issue. The firm acknowledged that its clinical trials were not designed to study this and that the quality and specificity of data to be gleaned from these trials to address suicidality were poor. . . . Because of apparent largescale underreporting, the firm's analysis cannot be considered as proving that Prozac and violent behavior are unrelated."

If the FDA and Eli Lilly had these kinds of reservations about Lilly's data from Prozac's clinical studies, why was the pharmaceutical company allowed to focus on these data to carry the day at the FDA hearing? If the FDA had some of the same concerns Teicher tried to raise, why wasn't he allowed to show his slides?[61]

Equally disturbing are internal Eli Lilly memos written by Dr. Leigh Thompson, Lilly's chief scientific officer, in 1990 at the height of public concern about Prozac's causing suicide and violence. Teicher and Cole's original article on the subject provoked a strong reaction not only in the United States but in Europe as well, especially in England. On February 7, 1990, Thompson wrote: "Anything that happens in the UK [Britain] can threaten this drug in the US and worldwide. We are now expending enormous efforts fending off attacks because of (1) relationship to murder and (2) inducing suicidal ideation. The appropriate level of response is indicated by Dan Masica [Lilly's director of neuropsychiatry] himself and Charles Beasley [an in-house Lilly psychiatrist] immediately flying to Boston to talk to [the] authors of [a] paper on suicidal ideation [i.e., Teicher and Cole]. We have numerous 'foes.' . . . The FDA is very very skittish. . . . We must not allow one day to elapse on followup, flying to, investigating, etc. everything about Prozac. . . . Every significant event about Prozac has been a show stopper with 12th floor meetings. . . . There cannot be a fumble of even minor proportions on this one, because political pressure and perception and public news, not science [that is, Lilly's definition of "science"] could cause us to lose this one!!!!!"[62]

Later the same day, Thompson wrote: "I am concerned about reports I get re UK [British] attitude toward Prozac safety. . . . I hope Patrick [Patrick Cechane, medical director of Lilly's British affiliate] realizes that Lilly can go down the tubes if we lose Prozac and just one event in the UK can cost us that."[63] In yet another memo written on November 5, 1990, as Lilly tried to managed the crisis, Thompson said, "What are our priorities? I'd suggest that priorities are: (1) protect Prozac. . . ."[64]

But most disturbing are Thompson's descriptions of Lilly's relationship with Dr. Paul Leber, the director of the FDA's Division of Neuropharmacological Drug Products. Leber's division had originally approved Prozac and was now responsible for investigating the drug's causing suicide and violence. In a February 7, 1990, memo, Thompson described Leber as "a fan of Prozac" who "believes a lot of this is garbage."[65]

On July 18, 1990, Thompson wrote, "Paul Leber called yesterday; I contacted him at 6:15 am this morning and [had a] half-hour conversation, very very pleasant."[66] Thompson said that Leber "asked that we fax nothing to him unless he has agreed to it before hand." The concern about faxes, apparently, was that others might gain access to them. According to

Thompson, Leber said, "someone has found that mailbox and it makes a second route of information."

On September 12, 1990, Thompson wrote a memo indicating that Leber was under pressure within the FDA to add a warning to Prozac's official product information long before the FDA hearing on the matter. According to Thompson, Leber was "being pushed by Temple [Leber's boss, Dr. Robert Temple, the Director of the FDA's Office of Drug Evaluation I] . . . to change the label."[67] Leber had called Thompson to say "that he was having a meeting with Bob Temple 'in the next couple of days'" to discuss the matter of suicidality. Leber asked Thompson to prepare a report that he could take to the meeting with Temple. Thompson's memo, marked "URGENT!," said the report must get "in Leber's hands very very quickly." Wrote Thompson, "I am now very concerned that Temple et al. may force a label change even before we get there on 25 Sep [apparently an upcoming meeting between Lilly and the FDA on September 25th] or, next worse, have this a fait accompli when we arrive. That report MUST move swiftly through approval and to Dr. Leber's hands—*he is our defender* [italics added]."

The crisis was apparently averted. The FDA did not require a change in Prozac's label in the fall of 1990. The advisory committee hearing did not occur until a full year later. Of course, the FDA named the members to the advisory committee, with their many conflicts of interest, and scheduled four doctors to make formal presentations on behalf of Eli Lilly but did not schedule Dr. Teicher to present. At the hearing, Leber, Teicher, and Dr. Daniel Casey, the advisory committee's chairman, were in a three-way conversation when Casey declined to let Teicher show his slides. Leber did not intervene on Teicher's behalf. Later in the hearing, when three committee members were pressing for a warning in the official product information of antidepressants, Leber raised concerns that any warning would be "a no-win situation for Prozac."

Over the years, Leber has been criticized for his role in the FDA's handling of other controversies in his division. One controversy was adding a warning to the labels of major tranquilizers when they were found to cause permanent, disfiguring tics. A warning was added only in 1985 after the issue received intense media coverage. This was more than thirty years after the first major tranquilizer, Thorazine, was introduced.[68] Still another controversy was Leber's handling of concerns about the dangers of the sleeping pill Halcion. In his 1998 book, *Prescription for Disaster,* Thomas Moore, of the George Washington University Medical Center, reported that in a "bitter internal struggle" at the FDA, Leber backed Halcion "despite the objections of his own medical reviewer, concerns from FDA safety monitors, numerous critical magazine and television stories, and petitions from outside experts."[69] In the late 1990s, Leber left the FDA. He is the director of a consulting firm called Neuro-Pharm Group that specializes in advising pharmaceutical companies looking to develop and gain FDA approval for new psychiatric drugs.

The Wesbecker Trial

Nowhere is the cover-up of the dangers of these drugs more dramatically illustrated than in the Wesbecker trial. In the fall of 1994, representatives of Eli Lilly stood in a Louisville, Kentucky, courtroom facing twenty-seven survivors and family members of the deceased in Joseph Wesbecker's murderous rampage with an AK-47 at the Standard Gravure printing plant in Louisville five years earlier.[70] Two months before Wesbecker's assault, twenty-nine-year-old Angela Bowman had given birth to a son. Now the young mother sat in a wheelchair in the Louisville courtroom, paralyzed for life. But she was luckier than her coworker Sharon Needy, who had died, leaving three children. Three of Wesbecker's fellow pressmen—Mike Campbell, Andrew Pointer, and John Stein—walked into the courthouse supported by canes because of injuries from the shoot-out.

As it happened, in the fall of 1994 the American public's attention was riveted to another courtroom drama, the O.J. Simpson trial. Like most other news at the time, the Prozac trial received scant attention. But the trial's transcripts survive as a public record of extraordinary revelations.[71] The Wesbecker case was like many civil liability suits that have become a familiar feature of the American landscape in recent decades. Among the more prominent have been suits against asbestos companies, manufacturers of silicon breast implants, and tobacco companies. These lawsuits give attorneys unprecedented access to a bureaucratic corporation's internal workings, politics, and documents. Company executives, consultants, and researchers are forced to testify under oath. The results are often shocking disclosures. In this instance, profoundly disturbing relevations emerged regarding Prozac's dosing schedule, the use of sedatives, and how suicidality was handled during the drug's clinical testing.

Prozac's dosing schedule was an issue early in the drug's history. When Prozac was originally tested on patients in the 1970s, some patients became anxious and agitated when started on it.[72] Later, in the mid-1980s, the question arose whether or not to test 5- and 10-milligram doses in the drug's large-scale clinical testing. But according to the testimony of Eli Lilly's chief medical officer, Dr. Leigh Thompson, Lilly statisticians "massaged" data to make a lower dose "look not quite as good as 20 milligrams."[73] Lilly's CEO at the time, Richard Wood, personally intervened in the matter. Wood does not have a medical degree. Instead, he has an MBA. Yet, an internal Eli Lilly memo stated, "Upon his recommendations we will exclude the 10 milligram Prozac dosage regimen" from the testing.[74] The 5-milligram dose was also not tested.

What was the advantage of marketing only a 20-milligram dose of Prozac? Seventy percent of Prozac prescriptions are now written by primary-care doctors. In the decade before Prozac, the most commonly prescribed antidepressants were tricyclics, which require slowly raising the dose and monitoring the side effects through often weekly appointments for the first month or two that a patient is on them. Busy primary-care doctors had never been comfortable with the complexities or the time requirements for prescribing the tricyclics. By contrast, Prozac could be prescribed in the 20-milligram dose to patients with a follow-up in six months to a year. The availability of graduated doses, 5- and 10-milligram pills, would have undermined this advantage over all other antidepressants available at the time.[75] Likewise, had the FDA decided to add a warning on suicide and violence to the label of antidepressants, this would have necessitated closer monitoring of patients, markedly reducing Prozac's unique appeal for primary-care clinicians.

Another memo makes clear that dosing problems were brought to Lilly's attention again not long after the drug went on the market. In a July 1988 memo, Dr. Thompson refers disdainfully to "tremendous pressure from gurus and practicing psychiatrists to make ten milligrams or even five milligrams available" for patients who become anxious and agitated when started on the higher dose.[76]

The need for sedatives to offset Prozac's stimulating effects was also recognized in the earliest testing of the drug on laboratory animals and patients where agitation and aggression were serious problems. As early as 1979, one of the coinventors of Prozac, Dr. Ray Fuller, wrote, "Some patients have converted from severe depression to agitation within a few days. . . . In future studies, the use of benzodiazepines [Valium-type sedatives] to *control agitation* will be permitted [italics added]."[77] As a result, in Prozac's large-scale, clinical testing, Lilly's protocols allowed researchers to add a sedative for any patient who became anxious, agitated, or sleepless. Indeed, sedatives were used liberally to mask these side effects. Is it not, then, remarkable that sedatives were not suggested as an adjunct to Prozac in its prescribing guidelines? But again, I believe this was not done because it would have made the use of Prozac more complicated and less likely to be readily prescribed. It would have interfered with the simple, one-dose-fits-all-patients strategy.

Dr. Nancy Lord, an authority on testing new drugs for FDA approval, testified, "To simply sedate them, [to] make those things [anxiety, agitation, and insomnia] less of a problem and then not report them [not warn doctors and patients in the prescribing guidelines] was improper. . . . they regularly, systematically, and in a large portion of the people used tranquilizers, sedatives, to calm people down. It happened in very high percentages of the people in the study."[78]

The use of sedatives in the Prozac testing was not something relatively innocuous, like allowing aspirin if a patient had a fever. Nor was Prozac the seventh or eighth drug in a clinically established class of drugs. Rather, it was the first in a new class. Since Prozac acts on the brain, to allow liberal use of other drugs that act on the same organ "completely obscured what this product was doing to people's minds," said Dr. Lord. Among the specific examples she cited from the Prozac studies were a patient who wanted to "jump out of a window" and another who developed "paranoid delusions."

During the testing, Lilly's own researchers protested these practices. Two of Lilly's inhouse staff, Dr. Dorothy Dobbs and Dr. Lee, protested the indiscriminate use of sedatives. Dr. Dobbs had worked at the FDA for five years prior to being hired by Lilly as their liaison with the federal agency. Dr. Dobbs testified that both she and Dr. Lee called attention to the fact that there were "too many people on too much concomitant medication."[79] Dobbs tried unsuccessfully to institute "cleaner" protocols barring the liberal use of sedatives. Having worked at the FDA, Dr. Dobbs was concerned that the underfunded, short-staffed agency would miss this serious problem in their random spot checking of the data. At the Wesbecker trial, Dr. Dobbs agreed that the heavy use of sedatives is "scientifically bad," would "confound the results," and would "interfere with the analysis of both safety and efficacy."

Suicidal patients were largely excluded from the studies, as were severely depressed patients or those with other, serious diagnoses, such as manic depressive illness.[80] Still worse, patients who became suicidal were not recorded as such. According to Dr. Lord, during the studies "suicidal ideation" was routinely labeled (or coded in the databases) as "depression."[81] In other words, instead of being monitored separately, suicidality was ascribed to the patient's underlying condition—that is, depression—obscuring the phenomenon.

In Germany, Claude Bouchy, head of a Lilly-affiliated company testing Prozac in Europe, balked at Lilly's labeling practices. He raised "great concerns" when Lilly executives requested that suicidality be labeled, coded, as "depression." In a sharply worded memo to Lilly he said, "I do not think I could explain to the BGA [the German FDA], to a judge, to a reporter, or even to my family why we would do this especially on the sensitive issue of suicide and suicidal ideation, at least not with the explanations that have been given our staff so far."[82]

In the mid-1980s, the German food and drug administration notified Lilly that they were not going to approve Prozac "because of their concern with suicidality and agitation," said Dr. Lord.[83] She continued, "They [the Germans] said that people became agitated before the antidepressant effects came on, and that increased the risk of suicide. They wrote a memo concerning untoward damaging effects and Lilly then went over there and looked at the data again and pulled out cases that they didn't think were suicide. . . . How are they to know? The investigator [researcher] thought it was a suicide attempt. They said, well we don't think it is." Difficulties in other European countries were handled in a similar way.

Summarizing Lilly's approach, Dr. Lord said, "It looked like they did everything possible to kind of tone down the problems with the drug rather than give them a rigorous, systematic, and comprehensive evaluation to define what the problems were and then put it in the package insert so that doctors could be warned not to use the drug in certain types of patients, or to use it more carefully."[84] Asked how she thought Lilly's practices affected their analysis of the data, Lord said: "It renders it *worthless.*"[85] Of course, it was the data from Prozac's clinical studies that Lilly so aggressively presented at the FDA hearing as the "only scientifically valid approach" by which to evaluate Prozac's safety.

In the midst of the German uproar, American officials at the FDA asked Lilly what the Germans were concerned about. The timing was bad for Lilly, coming just a few days before the FDA was due to give preliminary approval of Prozac in the United States. The Germans were alarmed about "unacceptable damaging effects" owing to agitation and suicidality. But at the Wesbecker trial, the lead attorney for the victims said that Lilly misled the FDA, telling the agency that the Germans were concerned about "organ damage" relative to "2.1."[86] Organ damage is a medical term for injury to a specific organ—for example, the liver or pancreas. How did "unacceptable damaging effects" become "organ damage"? Lilly's moderator of Prozac's clinical testing from 1984 to 1990, Dr. Joachim Wernicke, testified that he was responsible for the FDA's "confusion" because he himself had been "confused." What organ was "2.1"? Dr. Wernicke admitted he failed to tell the FDA that "2.1" was the German code for suicide. Had he been "confused" about this, too?

Evidently not. Even though the FDA had specifically asked Lilly for information about what the Germans were concerned about, he testified, "I don't believe that I needed to point the FDA to that."

Still later in his testimony, Wernicke was asked a series of questions about the use of sedatives and Lilly's statistical practices. Wernicke was vague and evasive, particularly with regard to data on deaths that occurred during the testing. Eventually he was asked, "You had a number of deaths all along but you hadn't analyzed your database to know what number of deaths you had and how to analyze the statistics on those deaths; is that what you're telling the jury?" The Lilly scientist was unable to refute the point.

As if these problems were not enough, the Wesbecker trial hinged on even more damaging evidence. From the outset of the trial, attorneys for the survivors and victims' families sought to introduce evidence regarding two other drugs, Oraflex and fialuridine. Lilly's testing or marketing of these two drugs overlapped with the testing or marketing of Prozac in the 1980s and 1990s. Attorneys for the survivors said the stories of Oraflex and fialuridine would demonstrate that the problems with Prozac were not specific to the drug but rather part of a larger pattern in which Eli Lilly was "a company with a history of flagrant disregard for the safety of the potential patients that are getting their drugs."[87]

Lilly developed Oraflex in the 1970s. Oraflex was an anti-inflammatory agent used to treat aches and pains—for example, due to arthritis. Lilly introduced the drug in 1982 with a massive advertising and marketing campaign portraying Oraflex as a dramatic scientific breakthrough, just as they would later do with Prozac. Lilly issued 6,500 press kits nationwide and sent doctors and scientists on tour talking about Oraflex.[88] Although some expressed skepticism about Oraflex's new stature as a wonder drug, the campaign was a dramatic success: Oraflex sales skyrocketed. In response to the media blitz, prescriptions jumped from 2,000 per week to 55,000.

But in August 1982, Oraflex was withdrawn from the market just three months after it was introduced because of severe complications and many deaths. A Justice Department investigation concluded Lilly misled the FDA. The investigation linked Oraflex to the deaths of more than one hundred patients.[89] Eventually, Lilly was charged with twenty-five counts related to mislabeling side effects. Lilly's chief medical officer at the time, Dr. William Shedden, was personally cited in some of the counts and faced possible imprisonment.[90]

After Lilly pleaded guilty to the charges in 1985, the federal government fined the multibillion-dollar-a-year pharmaceutical company $25,000. Dr. Shedden pleaded "no contest" and did not go to jail. He left Lilly and went to work at another pharmaceutical company. Shedden was replaced by Dr. Leigh Thompson, who testified about "massaging" data at the Prozac trial. Dr. Sidney Wolfe, head of the Public Citizen Health Research Group, said of the Oraflex fine, "the public will remain cynical as long as corporate criminals escape harsh punishments for crimes that would result in prison sentences for individuals."[91] The eventual cost to Lilly of the Oraflex scandal was more extensive. Some 1,500 lawsuits were ultimately filed against the company because of complications from the drug, including deaths.

Then, in the early 1990s, Lilly was developing another drug, fialuridine, for the treatment of hepatitis B. A liver infection, hepatitis B affects 300 million people worldwide. Hepatitis B's chronic complications can lead to liver failure, cancer, and death. Doctors and researchers have long sought a cure for the disease. But fialuridine's testing was abruptly halted by the FDA in 1993 after five patients died and others developed severe injuries in a small, early study of just fifteen patients. A government investigation was "scathing" in its criticism of Lilly, according to reports.[92] The FDA said the head of the study, Dr. Jay Hoofnagle, had not adequately informed patients of the risks of entering the study. In many instances, researchers continued the medication even after patients complained of its ill effects. In the fialuridine scandal, Lilly was again charged with not properly reporting side effects during the drug's clinical testing. Dr. Roger William, associate director of the FDA's Center for Drug Evaluation and Research, said, "There was a pattern here, a series of lapses with regard to the reporting and the following of protocol."[93] According to the *Los Angeles Times*, "The FDA said the pattern of minimizing the drug's potential risks began long before the drug trial and actually was established during the early years of its development."[94]

During the Wesbecker trial, attorneys for the survivors repeatedly asked Judge John Potter for permission to introduce the Oraflex and fialuridine evidence.[95] Arguing in the judge's private chambers, they said Lilly "got caught not reporting deaths with Oraflex. In that case they did exactly what they're doing here [with Prozac]. They said it was part of the underlying disease process or it was something that was related to the underlying condition of the patients."[96] With Prozac, too, minimization of the drug's side effects went back to the earliest days of the drug's development. Eliminating large-scale testing of 5- and 10-milligram doses, excluding seriously ill and suicidal patients from studies, liberally using sedatives, mislabeling suicidality as "depression," and Lilly's statistical manipulations were all part of this larger pattern. Attorneys for the survivors wanted to show the jury that "the FDA has redone their regulations to require stricter reporting of adverse events [side effects], and stricter because of Lilly's conduct, specifically because of the conduct of Lilly."

Lilly's lawyers fought fiercely against allowing the Oraflex and fialuridine evidence, saying it would be too "prejudicial." On the basis of technical rules of evidence, they argued Lilly was in court to defend Prozac, not the other drugs. Initially, Judge Potter ruled in Lilly's favor. In a costly tactical error, however, the Lilly attorneys proceeded to parade a series of scientific and academic experts who, one after another, praised the company's exemplary record of drug safety and testing to the jury.[97] Indeed, Lilly's chief scientific officer, Dr. Leigh Thompson, told the jury that the FDA praised Lilly's system: "The FDA has repeatedly said that we, Lilly, have the best system for collecting and analyzing and reporting" side effects.

Eventually, the survivors' attorneys protested. Asking Judge Potter again for permission to introduce the Oraflex and fialuridine evidence, they insisted they deserved "the right to rebut" Lilly's "gratuitous evidence that this company is the best in the business: It's got the best researchers; it's got the best this, the most ethical that, the most upstanding, world-class type of people, over and over and over again. . . . We believe we have the right to rebut this evidence that they are . . . holier than thou . . . with getting things reported and complying with FDA regulations."[98]

This time, Potter was inclined to agree. Comparing Lilly's situation to someone with a long history of drunk driving and traffic violations who claims to have a flawless record when accused again, the judge said, "When a person gets on the stand and says, 'I've never run a red light; I've never had a traffic ticket; I'm the world's safest driver,' [he] probably shouldn't have said it. But once they get up there and say it, can't people say: 'Isn't it true, ma'am, that you've been arrested for drunken driving or you've got a speeding ticket,' or whatever it happens to be?"[99] Potter considered the matter overnight, and the next morning he granted the survivors' attorneys permission to present the Oraflex evidence to the jury. The judge said Lilly had "opened the door" to the Oraflex evidence, they had "injected the issue into the trial" with all the testimony about their exemplary record.[100]

Lilly's lawyers protested vehemently, even threatening the judge with a motion for a mistrial.[101] Judge Potter held his ground. Pushed by Lilly's lawyers, he said pointedly, referring to the glowing testimony of Lilly's chief scientific officer, Dr. Leigh Thompson, about the company's record, "I wonder if the jury wouldn't view his accolades for Lilly differently if they realized that, shortly after he came there, Lilly was the subject of an investigation by the Justice Department and then later pleaded guilty, and he may well have gotten his promotion because his predecessor was looking at thirteen years in jail." Lilly insisted they could go to the Court of Appeals or the Supreme Court for a second opinion. The judge said he would give them time to do so; he would delay the Oraflex evidence while they considered an appeal. But he refused to back down.

Having received permission to use the hard-won evidence, a day later attorneys for the survivors made a stunning reversal: Returning to Judge Potter's private chambers, they announced that "after a great deal of consideration," they had decided to close "without the introduction of any further evidence" in an effort to "facilitate getting this case to the jury as rapidly and expeditiously as possible."[102] Instead, they reserved the right to introduce the Oraflex evidence in a second, punitive damages phase of the lawsuit. In fact, the attorneys were posturing, covering up a secret agreement negotiated once Judge Potter approved the survivors' introducing the damaging Oraflex evidence. The secret deal only fully came to light years later, after one of the survivors was forced to reveal it in divorce court and a subsequent investigation by the Attorney General's Office confirmed the behind-the-scenes settlement.[103]

But for the remainder of the trial, the attorneys for Lilly and the survivors engaged in what Nicholas Varchaver later called a "shadow play" in a 1995 article in *American Lawyer* entitled "Lilly's Phantom Verdict."[104] Suspecting a secret arrangement, Judge Potter asked if the parties had struck a deal. Both sides denied it, says Potter.[105] So, in what later turned out to be a charade, they continued as adversaries in front of the jury. Soon afterward, in December 1994, the jury rendered a verdict in favor of Prozac and Lilly.

After the verdict, Lilly's lawyers announced triumphantly to the media that they felt this was "a complete vindication of the drug."[106] Continuing to hide the relationship that now existed between the two parties, they postured: "We had very good lawyers against us. The plaintiffs' team worked very hard and really made something out of nothing. There was never anything in any of this record to really implicate Lilly."[107] Across the country, headlines announced the verdict. One newspaper reported that "a jury's verdict clearing Prozac of inciting a Louisville man to mass murder has lifted a cloud over the antidepressant and may even boost sales of Eli Lilly and Company."[108] The *New York Times* quoted Lilly's CEO saying that it had now been "proven in a court of law . . . that Prozac is safe and effective."[109]

The survivors, who had all secretly reached a huge settlement with Lilly, were equally disingenuous. Most declined to speak with the press. But one of them, Mike Campbell, a pressman who had worked closely with Wesbecker, said, "It's not so much the money, although it would have been useful. It's the certainty we all have—all of us who knew Wesbecker well—that it was this drug that made him do it . . . that more people will have to suffer until a case is proved against Eli Lilly."[110]

Of course, the Wesbecker verdict vastly decreased the likelihood of anyone's proving a case against Lilly. More than 150 Prozac lawsuits had already been filed by December 1994. Had it not been for the Wesbecker verdict, no doubt many more would have been, just as some 1,500 lawsuits were eventually filed against Lilly in the Oraflex debacle. Lilly's public relations director, Ed West, said, "There's nothing like a victory in court to dissuade the rest."[111] After the trial, he commented on the suits already in the pipeline: "I would assume that some of these would either be dismissed or just dropped. When you peel it all back, you get into a question of money. If it becomes apparent it's very difficult to win big money in Prozac suits, this probably sends some message."[112]

But big money had been paid in the Wesbecker suit. After the trial, rumors of an enormous, behind-the-scenes settlement swirled in Louisville.[113] The settlement first came to light when one of the survivors, Andrew Pointer, was forced to divulge it as part of his divorce.[114] The exact sum is unknown because it is protected in divorce documents, which are sealed because of Lilly's insistence on secrecy. But Pointer's attorney, Cecil Blye, says, It's "a tremendous amount of money. It boggles the mind." Still, Lilly may have thought the settlement was a bargain given their enormous costs with Oraflex. In just one of the 1,500 Oraflex cases, a jury awarded $6 million to the son of an eighty-one-year-old woman who died while on the drug.[115]

According to the terms of the agreement, the Prozac money is being paid in installments over years.[116] The survivors agreed not to divulge the settlement: If any of the survivors broke the silence, payment of the remaining installments to all of them could stop.

After the trial, Judge Potter became even more suspicious that Lilly and the survivors had reached a secret agreement. Three months after the jury rendered its verdict, he called the lawyers for Lilly and the survivors back to ask again if there had been a deal. Both parties refused to answer.

In April 1995, Judge Potter filed a motion to hold a hearing into the matter.[117] He was not looking to reopen the case but merely to determine whether or not a settlement had occurred. If so, he would change the official record from a jury verdict in Lilly's favor to "dismissed as settled." To

Judge Potter's dismay, Lilly now fought *him*, trying to block or delay any hearing for as long as possible. Because of their agreement to keep the deal secret, the survivors' attorneys cooperated with Lilly in attempting to block Judge Potter's investigation.

But the judge persisted. Defending his right to hold a hearing, he wrote to the appeals court, "Lilly sought to buy not just the verdict but the court's judgment as well [by misleading him]. This is where a 'freely negotiated settlement' ends and the court's duty to protect the integrity of the judicial system begins."[118] Judge Potter lost to Lilly in the first round, in his petition to the appeals court. Undaunted, he took his case to the Kentucky Supreme Court.

In May 1996, the Kentucky Supreme Court ruled in Potter's favor, saying that "there was a serious lack of candor with the trial court and there may have been deception, bad faith conduct, abuse of the judicial process or perhaps even fraud."[119] Commented one appellate judge, Michael McDonald, "The system has been tampered with by trial counsel. Isn't that why we're here?"[120] Said Professor Richard Uviller, who teaches legal ethics at Columbia University School of Law, "I've never heard of such a thing. . . . You can't have it both ways. You can't have a settlement and still continue as adversaries."[121]

In a 1996 book summarizing the trial and some of its aftershocks *The Power to Harm: Mind, Medicine, and Murder on Trial*, John Cornwell describes the secret deal as "unprecedented in any Western court."[122] Cornwell is a British journalist who was sent to cover the trial for the London *Sunday Times*. He is also the director of the Science and Human Dimension Project at Cambridge University in England. For the book, he interviewed attorneys for both the survivors and Lilly, one of the survivors, jurors, Judge Potter, and Lilly's director of public relations.

Cornwell says both sides in the trial knew the Oraflex evidence would be "explosive," implicating Lilly in a larger pattern of abuses during clinical testing: "Lilly had clearly believed that the Oraflex evidence would put the trial at risk for them, with far-reaching consequences for Prozac and the reputation of the company and its products. Not only would sales of Prozac be badly hit in the United States and around the world, but the long-buried issue of Oraflex would once again be resurrected, fueling further bad publicity. But why not simply make a deal to settle and end the trial? The facts indicate that Lilly wanted it both ways. They wanted to quash the Oraflex evidence and, at the same time, they badly wanted the vindication of a jury verdict in their favor. A mere settlement would only indicate that there was indeed a problem with Prozac."[123]

Similarly, in his analysis of the trial in the September 1995 issue of the *American Lawyer*, Nicholas Varchaver states: "Interviews with four jurors suggest that Lilly barely escaped with a victory—and that the omission of the Oraflex evidence may have been key."[124] Varchaver notes that in Kentucky, Lilly needed only nine of the twelve jurors to vote in its favor in order to win. Even though the Oraflex evidence was withheld, Lilly narrowly escaped with just the minimum nine votes. "With the vote so close," says Varchaver, "a strong piece of anti-Lilly evidence—like the Oraflex evidence—might have changed one mind and hung the jury." Varchaver quotes one juror, Judith Felker, who voted for Lilly, as saying, "I remember somebody saying [Lilly] was a reputable company. I think if it hadn't been [reputable], we would have heard about other lawsuits beforehand."

Clarifying another of the bizarre twists in the Prozac scare of the early 1990s, John Cornwell quotes a source close to the case regarding the Church of Scientology: "You had this group, these Scientologists, who were a fringe group opposed to any kind of psychiatric treatment, opposed to any kind of psychotropic medication. They got hold of this issue [suicide and violence associated with Prozac] quickly, especially after this article by Dr. Teicher came out. What Lilly did was absolutely ingenious, and probably the brainchild of this guy Ed West [Lilly's director of public relations]. They said, 'This is not an issue over whether or not Prozac is safe, this is just this fringe group attacking a pharmaceutical manufacturer.' Then the Scientologists played into their hands."[125] In this way, Lilly was able to distract attention away from the real issues.

The Kentucky Supreme Court ruling granted Judge Potter's court "authority to conduct [an] investigation and hearing to determine whether its judgments [the jury verdict] accurately reflected the truth."[126] In September 1996 Potter asked the Attorney General's Office to allow a lawyer to be appointed as a friend of the court to investigate the behind-the-scenes dealings in the Wesbecker trial. The Attorney General conducted an investigation and issued a report in March 1997.[127] As part of the investigation, the Attorney General's Office interviewed lawyers on both sides of the Wesbecker trial. The investigation confirmed the secret agreement and exposed many more details.

In return for the victims' not introducing any more evidence, including the explosive Oraflex evidence, Lilly struck an unusual "high-low" agreement.[128] According to the terms of the deal, Lilly would pay the victims, regardless of which way the jury decided. If the jury decided for Lilly, the pharmaceutical company would still pay the "low" figure. If the jury decided for the victims, Lilly would pay the "high" number. In an unusual twist, however, payment was contingent on the jury's reaching one or the other verdict. If the jury was hung or a mistrial declared for any other reason, then no payment would be made. Furthermore, the survivors agreed not to appeal the jury's decision.

The exact sums Lilly agreed to pay have still not been divulged, but even the "low," which Lilly ultimately paid, is apparently a "mind boggling" sum.[129] One attorney familiar with the case points out that the unusual high-low agreement created a huge disincentive for the victims' side to really press their case, to go all-out for a win, because if they fell short and wound up with a hung jury, they would get nothing. Because the "low" was a huge number and tied to the jury's reaching one or the other verdict, the incentives shifted in favor of "losing" to be sure the victims and their attorneys went home well compensated. Because they agreed not to appeal the decision, this was their only chance. "Losing" was a sure bet; going for a "win" was a gamble in which all could be lost. Of course this perverts the incentives normally present in a fairly fought jury trial.

After the Attorney General's investigation, in the spring of 1997, Eli Lilly quietly agreed to the official record in the Wesbecker trial's being changed from a jury verdict in their favor to "dismissed . . . as settled."[130] Until now the public has had the impression that Eli Lilly has prevailed in lawsuits brought against them on the fiercely contested issue of Prozac's causing suicide or violence. This is largely because the original jury verdict in the Wesbecker trial was widely publicized. Now that the official record has been changed, we know Lilly has paid large sums to settle Prozac lawsuits. In fact, Lilly settled the original test case, the Wesbecker case; the settlement was just kept secret for a long time. In the Attorney General's investigation, Lilly acknowledged having settled other cases as well.

What has Ed West, who boasted "there's nothing like a victory in court to dissuade the rest," had to say of subsequent developments? How has Lilly's public relations director defended the pharmaceutical company's actions? How can he spin-control Lilly's efforts to block Judge Potter from setting the record straight? After the Kentucky Supreme Court decision allowing an investigation to go forward, West said that even if the jury verdict were changed to a settlement, as it eventually was, "it shouldn't in any way reflect negatively on the product [Prozac] . . . it's a question of legal procedural wrangling."[131]

In addition to the Wesbecker settlement, Lilly has made a number of other surprising arrangements with key figures in the Prozac murder-suicide story. Several days into the trial, Lilly approached Dr. Lee Coleman, who had been Wesbecker's psychiatrist at the time of the shootings. As

Wesbecker's treating psychiatrist, Coleman was supposed to be an entirely neutral witness, not an expert for either side. In his clinic notes and a pretrial deposition, Coleman had linked Prozac to the dramatic change in Wesbecker.

But a few days into the trial, Lilly's lawyers entered into discussion with Coleman and arranged for him to "review" material they provided relevant to the case, highlighted with yellow marker for his convenience.[132] Coleman later acknowledged that he would be charging Lilly's lawyers $200 an hour for the review and related research of his own, although no "formal arrangement" with regard to payment had been reached. At the Wesbecker trial, in front of the jury, Coleman softened his testimony linking Prozac to Wesbecker's behavior by comparison with his earlier testimony in his pretrial deposition.

In yet another surprise, Lilly's expert-witnesses disclosure statement for the trial lists Dr. Anthony Rothschild as one of the pharmaceutical company's experts.[133] Dr. Rothschild had published one of the important rechallenge studies showing that patients who became suicidal on Prozac had the same reaction if later put on the drug again. By the time of the Wesbecker trial, Rothschild had become one of Lilly's potential expert witnesses.

And in another development, Dr. David Healy of the University of Wales College of Medicine reports that six months after the FDA hearing on Prozac's safety, "when Lilly found out that two Taiwanese doctors [Drs. Ru-Band Lu and Huei-Chen Ko] planned to publish a study showing that patients who were prescribed Prozac were significantly more likely to develop suicidal ideation and make suicide attempts than patients who were prescribed Maprotiline (a drug that was already associated with a high rate of suicide attempts), they took steps to suppress the study rather than allow it to appear and undergo scientific scrutiny. After a whirlwind bout of corporate visits and meetings, the doctors agreed to not submit their study for publication."[134] An internal Eli Lilly memo written on April 8, 1992, by Dr. Allan Weinstein said of the trips, "Mission successful. Professor Lu will not present or publish his Prozac vs. maprotilin suicidality data."[135] Says Healy, "Part of their [the two doctors'] motivation may have been Lilly's promise to provide them with funding for a large and lucrative study, the results of which have never been published." Exactly how often Lilly has made these kinds of arrangements is not known.

Healy continues, "In another example of suppression of research, when a Belgian doctor, Dr. Robert Bourguignon, intrigued by reports of the relationship of Prozac to suicide, began to conduct a survey of Belgian doctors regarding their experiences with suicidal ideation and Prozac (along with some other side effects), Lilly sued him, and persuaded a Belgian court to issue a cease-and-desist order to prevent him from continuing with his research. While Dr. Bourguignon eventually prevailed in court, and published the results of his study in the peer-reviewed journal *The Lancet*, . . . Lilly's actions speak loudly."

Healy himself has continued to publish on the subject of suicidality and violence associated with Prozac. He has published numerous articles and several books, including a recent one on the Prozac-type antidepressants, *The Antidepressant Era*, published by Harvard University Press. In court declarations, Healy reports Lilly has been guilty of "bald mischaracterization" of his statements and work. Healy says Lilly's "refusal to mount or countenance further investigation" of Prozac's causing suicide and violence "must say something about their perceptions of what the likely outcome would be."

The Story of Joe Wesbecker

The dangers to society of the inappropriate use and management of serotonin boosters and the attempt to cover them up are sadly illustrated in the Wesbecker case, which echoes far too many others that have occurred since the introduction of these drugs in the late 1980s. Joseph Wesbecker was born to impoverished young parents in Louisville, Kentucky, in 1942.[136] A year after he was born, Wesbecker's father died on the job, leaving Wesbecker in the care of his sixteen-year-old mother, Martha. From there, his childhood was a story of poverty, neglect, and alleged abuse, punctuated by periods of relative calm, as he was shuttled between his mother and a series of living arrangements, including an extended stay in an orphanage.

In spite of his early disadvantages in life, as a young man Joe Wesbecker worked hard to master the trade of rotogravure printing press operator. Rotogravure presses are huge, three-story-high, 150-foot-long machines used for the high-speed printing of hundreds of thousands of copies of newspaper supplements, magazines, and advertising flyers. The 1,000-ton presses are a mass of wheeling arms, rollers, pins, and cutters. At Standard Gravure, seven of theses huge presses operated at mind-numbing speed and noise in a windowless brick warehouse. The presses use inks and solvents which, after being inhaled for eight-to-sixteen-hour shifts, leave the pressmen in a state approximating drunkenness. This can be dangerous around the high-speed machinery, and some of the pressmen had lost fingers.

Through intelligence and hard work, Wesbecker earned his way up to the highest rank in his trade, a much-sought-after journeyman's card. In the 1960s, he married, had two sons, and bought a house, in what looked like the American dream. But in the 1970s and 1980s, the printing business was subject to many pressures: mergers and acquisitions, automation, downsizing, and re-engineering. The presses Wesbecker operated were sped up threefold, from 20,000 papers per hour to 60,000, while Standard Gravure's manpower was cut from 600 to 85 employees. Those workers who remained put in grueling overtime and weekend shifts while enduring a six-year pay freeze. In the mid-1980s, Standard Gravure changed hands. The workers themselves made an unsuccessful bid to buy the company. Instead, an ambitious young entrepreneur, Mike Shea, bought it for $22 million. Shortly after the sale, the employees learned Shea had used $11 million from the workers' pension fund to defray half of the purchase price. Naturally, many of them felt embittered. As tensions mounted, arguments and fights broke out among the workers. Many began to carry guns to work, making threats to one another and the management. Wesbecker was among those known to have guns. Said one pressman after the shootings, "Standard Gravure was a time bomb waiting to go off."[137]

An angry Wesbecker felt he was being "jerked around" by the Standard Gravure management and foremen. In particular, he felt unduly singled out for long shifts in the high-pressure helmsman's seat of a press. Since the reduction in staff, only one helmsman, rather than two, operated a press, and Wesbecker had come to dread it. As one coworker described the job, "You're driving that machine like you're driving a car. You're cramped with no space to move. You're surrounded by panels of switches, rows of flashing lights. Everything is coming at you in every direction. You screw up and there's thousands of dollars' wastage right there. The sound, the vibration, is like being inside a jet engine; you're saturated, you're breathing in a spray of solvents. You come home from being [in the helmsman's seat] . . . and you go on tasting and feeling and hearing that machine inside you."[138]

As the tension spilled over to his home life, Wesbecker and his wife of almost twenty years divorced. A second marriage quickly suffered the same fate. He began seeing psychiatrists, was diagnosed with severe depression, made a suicide attempt, was hospitalized, and was put on multiple psychiatric drugs. Psychiatrists and the Louisville Human Relations Commission appealed to Standard Gravure to assure Wesbecker he would not have to work so many shifts in the helmsman's seat, but the company refused.

Wesbecker told coworkers and friends the foremen were making him run presses "just to prove they could make him do something he didn't want to do."[139] One coworker suggested the company exploited his ability. Wesbecker began telling friends he was a victim of "industrial sodomy."[140]

Because of his deteriorating condition, Wesbecker went on disability in the spring of 1989, but his struggle with Standard Gravure continued.[141] He felt cheated by the company because of cuts in his disability payments and the company's contribution to his health insurance premium. Wesbecker feared he would not have enough money to live on, would be forced back to work, and would once again be assigned to the dread job of being in charge of presses.

In the period before the shootings, Wesbecker's psychiatrist was Dr. Lee Coleman. The psychopharmacologist treated Wesbecker in twenty-minute sessions that took place less than once a month. Wesbecker was not receiving psychotherapy to give him emotional support or to provide help with understanding his problems. Indeed, Coleman later acknowledged learning nothing in detail from Wesbecker about his life history, tragic childhood, or failed marriages.[142]

In August 1989, as Wesbecker became more depressed over his struggle with Standard Gravure, Coleman switched his antidepressant to the new drug Prozac. Eli Lilly sales representatives had been touting Prozac in their frequent visits with Coleman.[143]

A month later, in mid-September, when Wesbecker returned for follow-up, Dr. Coleman noted a drastic change. Wesbecker was severely agitated, sleepless, had "tangential thoughts" (rambling, disconnected thinking, a symptom of psychosis), and "weeping in the session," which had never happened before. Coleman wrote in Wesbecker's record that he thought Prozac was the cause of the dramatic change. In later testimony during a pretrial deposition he said, "I knew that Prozac in some people could cause nervousness, could cause agitation, could cause sleep problems, plus I had started him on it three or four weeks before. When you start a new medication and something different happens, you tend to support that it's the medication that is causing it within that period of time."[144]

Coleman told Wesbecker he should stop the Prozac immediately and come into the hospital, but the patient pleaded, "Don't take me off the Prozac. I feel it's helped me."[145]

"Well, how has it helped you?"

"It's helped me remember this incident of sexual abuse at work."

"Remember? What was it you had forgotten, Mr. Wesbecker?"

"I forgot . . . I forgot they forced me at Standard Gravure to perform sex with one of the foremen. The foreman forced me to perform oral sex on him with my coworkers watching. That was the price to take me off the folder [helm of the press]."

In fact, Wesbecker was out of touch with reality. He had not been given any assurance that he would be free from operating presses. In his agitated, psychotic state, his earlier statements about "industrial sodomy" and being forced to "do something he didn't want to do" had become performing oral sex on the foreman in front of onlooking coworkers. In a cruel irony, Wesbecker refused to go off Prozac because he thought it helped him "remember" the "sexual abuse at work." He also refused to go into the hospital.

Over the next several days, Wesbecker continued to be severely agitated. Echoing Dr. Coleman's observations, his friends described him as "real agitated," not sleeping, uncharacteristically unkempt, and "pacing" endlessly. Although he had suffered some of these symptoms in the past, his ex-wife, Brenda, who saw Wesbecker on the morning of the shootings, said, "He was more nervous than I'd ever seen him." His son James said that "he wasn't really the same person."

Three days after the appointment in which Dr. Coleman urged him to stop the Prozac, Wesbecker entered Standard Gravure with an AK-47 and opened fire. As he walked through the offices and plant, survivors of the shootings say, he looked like a zombie, an automaton. "I saw a man that was totally gone. . . . He looked totally dehumanized." "When he looked out towards us, he looked like he was in another world. . . . he looked through us . . ." as he fired the rounds of ammunition. At the end of the murderous rampage, Wesbecker took his own life, putting a gun to his head and pulling the trigger.

As I researched Wesbecker's case, I was struck by the similarities between his infamous story and the reactions I and other psychiatrists have witnessed in patients. Within weeks of starting Prozac, a dramatic change had occurred in his clinical condition: He was psychotic and severely agitated, with thoughts of suicide and violence. Like other patients, even when informed that Prozac could be causing his deterioration, Wesbecker refused to give up the drug. In a psychopharmacology format, patients are told they have biochemical imbalances and genetic defects for which medication is the best hope. Especially when so many other drugs have not helped, who wants to give up hope in the wonder drug that has supposedly worked for millions of others? By the time a patient's thinking is as disorganized as Wesbecker's, realigning his expectations of medication is extremely difficult.

Wesbecker's zombie-like, automaton state at the time of the shootings is again just like what other patients describe. Earlier I discussed Anna, who took a serious overdose shortly after starting Prozac, while in the care of a previous psychiatrist. Anna vividly describes feeling as if she were outside herself, observing her actions as she methodically took dozens of pills, "horrified" but powerless to stop herself. Was this how Wesbecker was feeling during his rampage or a short while later as he put a gun to his own head?

Wesbecker's delusion was similar to that of Sunita, my patient who became psychotic and suicidal shortly after starting Prozac. In her deteriorated state, Sunita thought a professor was forcing her to perform oral sex in front of a class, just as Wesbecker thought he had been forced to perform oral sex on his foreman. These are psychotic metaphors that patients need help understanding. When I started seeing Sunita, she was a frightened, timid, isolated, overly hardworking young woman who came to see me distraught over her mother's death from breast cancer. Sunita's parents lived in India, so her grief was complicated by the long distance. Her father, who was still living, was a severe alcoholic who had been physically and psychologically abusive. As described earlier, shortly after her mother's death, Sunita switched the focus of her studies to the premed requirements.

When she became psychotic on Prozac, in addition to the oral sex, Sunita thought she was being "brutalized," that her bloody body parts were strewn in trees about the campus. Sunita slowly recovered from her psychotic break without antipsychotic medication, which she refused after her experience with Prozac. In psychotherapy, Sunita realized that she had never really wanted to be in the premed classes. All her life, her parents wanted one of their two daughters to go to college in the United States and to attend medical school. Since her older sister was not a good student, Sunita was the parents' "only hope" of having one of their children get this "ticket to success."

Sunita eventually realized she "signed on" to the premed requirements in her grief over her mother's death. She wanted to give her deceased mother and grieving father "this thing they had always wanted." But all along she felt intensely ambivalent about going to medical school. She felt "trapped" into doing it by her mother's death and her abusive father's persistent demands. She came to see her professors, premed advisers, the college, and even me as conspiring to "hold her to this task," because we had, unwittingly, been supportive and encouraging.

That fateful spring, as the anniversary of her mother's death approached and these barely conscious feelings came to a head, Prozac tipped Sunita over the edge. In her agitated, psychotic state, she felt "brutalized" by everyone. The loss of her own center and direction in life became symbolically represented in her body parts being strewn around the campus. Now the task her professor held her to was performing oral sex on him in front of the class.

An important part of Sunita's long-term therapy was my strong support of her dropping the premed track over her father's vigorous protests. She switched back to what had been her original interest, history. She ultimately did very well academically and went on to graduate school.

Joe Wesbecker did not have the benefit of psychotherapy. He never came to understand the symbolic meaning of his delusion. In the years before the shootings, he said the management at Standard Gravure were putting him in charge of presses "just to prove they could make him do something he didn't want to do." He also referred to himself as the victim of "industrial sodomy." In his agitated, psychotic state, industrial sodomy and being forced to do something against his will became symbolically represented as performing oral sex in front of his coworkers. Of course, the likelihood that the foreman had so much power he could force Wesbecker to do this and an entire crew of men to watch is extremely unlikely. Throughout the long depositions and trial, no evidence emerged of sexual abuse at Standard Gravure. This was a psychotic, sexualized metaphor for his workplace tensions.

Finally, like other patients who have become suicidal and violent, Wesbecker was started on a 20-milligram dose of Prozac a day. Here, Dr. Coleman was following the prescribing guidelines for the new drug. In these early years, few psychiatrists had any idea that some patients should be started at a lower dose. Being treated in a psychopharmacology setting, with his life in a shambles, started on a relatively high dose, and already anxious before he began the drug, Wesbecker was a setup. He was in the worst possible combination of circumstances when he started Prozac.

At the Wesbecker trial in 1994, just as they had at the FDA hearing on Prozac's safety in 1991, Eli Lilly's bevy of experts engaged in an academic, splitting-hairs debate over whether or not Prozac could be *proven* to be *the* cause of Wesbecker's mass murder–suicide. Casting the argument in black and white, they attempted to pose the either-or question: Was Wesbecker's tragic childhood the cause? Or was it the stress at Standard Gravure? Or was it Prozac? Lilly's marketing and promotional material reduce human behavior to chemical imbalances remedied by pills. In this biological model, one's fate is determined by neurochemistry, not personal history. But in *The Power to Harm,* John Cornwell points out that at the trial, Eli Lilly did a stunning about-face. Lilly insisted it was Wesbecker's history that caused him to pull the trigger; Prozac and its effect on his brain chemistry had nothing to do with it.

In fact, because of Wesbecker's prior psychiatric history, Lilly went to great lengths to have this be the test case that went to trial. Many of the other lawsuits in the pipeline involved suicide and violence in reasonable, stable people who, before they went on Prozac, had no psychiatric history. Lilly knew these would have been much more difficult cases to win. During the later investigation of the trial, Lilly was forced to admit it had settled a number of earlier suits, making way for Wesbecker's to be the test case.[146] Indeed, Lilly acknowledged settling earlier cases with Paul Smith, one of the lead attorneys for Wesbecker's victims and survivors.

Of course Lilly's use of the Wesbecker case to blame patients rather than the drug was a strategy to distract from the real issues. The truth is that life history, current stresses, and the effects of drugs can never be completely separated. Anyone who has sat with psychiatric patients knows this. Anyone who has witnessed patients have this anxious, agitated, suicidal, violent reaction recognizes that the drug is simply an addition to the mix. But for some patients, it is *the* dangerous addition to the mix, putting them over the edge.

Dr. Mark Pollack, a psychopharmacologist and professor of psychiatry at Harvard Medical School, tests new drugs and provides consulting services for seven manufacturers of new antidepressants introduced to the market since the late 1980s: Eli Lilly, Pfizer, SmithKline Beecham, Solvay, Parke-Davis, Bristol-Myers Squibb, Wyeth-Ayerst, and Glaxo-Wellcome.[147] In a presentation on the management of antidepressant-induced side effects at a 1997 Harvard Medical School conference on psychopharmacology, Pollack said the following regarding serotonin boosters's causing suicidality and violence: "My read of people who have experienced this in talking to some of the patients, some of it may have been that these patients were anxious or agitated to begin with and when they were started on medication their dose was rapidly increased rather than loaded [gradually raised from a low starting dose]." A little earlier in the talk, Pollack said of Prozac's making patients anxious or jittery, "I think part of the reason why Prozac developed a reputation of being a particularly stimulating antidepressant causing a lot of anxiety is that they [Eli Lilly] went first and they wanted, for marketing reasons really, for ease of use, to adopt a one-dose-fits-all-patients strategy. So they started everybody . . . at 20 milligrams a day. And for an anxious or agitated patient, for panic patients, this often *blew them out of the water* [italics added]."[148] One could not find a better description of what happened to Joe Wesbecker. I saw exactly the same thing happen to my patients. Dr. Teicher, who originally called attention to this problem, summed it up in exactly the same way at the FDA hearing on Prozac's safety: "We know that some of these drugs can produce a worsening or exacerbation in anxiety, at least initially, and sometimes they can induce panic attacks. You add a panic attack to a patient who is already depressed and that may be the *straw that broke the camel's back,* so that in those cases you may have patients who go out and commit suicide who would not have committed suicide otherwise [italics added]."[149]

Teicher's research group, Rothschild, Van Putten and Wirshing, Hamilton and Opler, and countless other psychiatrists, therapists, patients, and their families have witnessed this reaction. It should not be a trade secret only discussed among privileged insiders. Indeed, it turns out that many insiders have known for some time that the one-dose-fits-all-patients was, from the beginning, a marketing strategy. In *Listening to Prozac,* Peter Kramer wrote in a footnote at the back of his 1993 book, "The manufacturer of Prozac made the brilliant marketing decision at first to manufacture only one form of Prozac, the 20 milligram capsule. Then all doctors could be taught to dose their patients with one pill a day—so simple, as the pharmacists say, that even an internist [primary-care doctor] can do it. This marketing decision was one factor in the enormous popularity of Prozac."[150]

Remarkably, the prescribing guidelines for serotonin boosters have *still* not changed. Twenty milligrams of Prozac or Paxil and the equivalent, 50 milligrams, of Zoloft or Luvox, are still the recommended starting dose for depressed patients.[151] Many psychiatrists and most primary-care doctors are not aware of the dangers for depressed patients who are anxious or particularly sensitive to the drug. Ultimately, under pressure, Eli Lilly introduced a lower-dose, 10-milligram capsule of Prozac but they charge the same price. This discourages the use of lower starting doses, because patients already have a difficult enough time with the high price of the medication (roughly $3 a pill). Because suicidality and violence with serotonin boosters have not been thoroughly studied, we have even less information on the occurrence of these side effects with Zoloft, Paxil, or Luvox than we do with Prozac. There are isolated reports of other serotonin boosters being associated with suicide or violence, but adequate information is lacking.[152]

In the product information for Prozac, there is still no warning that the drug can trigger suicide or violence. There is still no recommendation for a concurrent sedative in some patients. European countries do have warnings about agitation and suicidality, together with guidelines for coping with them. For example, the German prescribing guidelines for Prozac warn of suicidality and suggest the use of sedatives. But American doctors are still left, in spite of the great dangers, to reinvent the wheel and exchange this critical information with colleagues by word-of-mouth.

How often is the reaction happening? Because the issue has been white-washed, there is no way to know. We do know prescribing serotonin boosters to teenagers is soaring. Have the drugs contributed to the escalating suicide rate among young adults? There are published reports of suicidality occurring in children to whom these drugs have been prescribed.[153] One of the more tragic is a fifteen-year-old adolescent who committed suicide by hanging, two weeks after starting 20 milligrams a day of Prozac. Prescribed the drug for obsessive-compulsive disorder, the teenager had "little or no preexisting depression," according to the report published in 1990 in the *American Journal of Psychiatry*.[154] In the last decade, around the country, communities have been shocked by brutal, senseless murders and murder-suicides. How many of these sensational tragedies might have been due to serotonin boosters? Should doctors and families, left guilt-ridden over events of suicide or violence committed by a patient or family member, be considering the possibility that a serotonin booster may be responsible? How often might Prozac, Zoloft, Paxil, or Luvox have been the missing clue, the secret that would help explain suicides or murder-suicides that have been devastating to families, caregivers, and communities?

PART II

Balancing Medications
with
Alternative Approaches

5

Behind-the-Scenes Forces
Understanding the
Prozac Phenomenon

By now you may be concerned about some of the side effects described in earlier chapters. The question arises: If serotonin boosters are problematic, what are the alternatives? Fortunately, many natural alternatives are available, from the herbal antidepressant St. John's wort to twelve-step programs to psychotherapy. Not only are the alternatives effective in clinical practice, research has clearly demonstrated them to be as effective, if not more so, than drugs.

In the 1980s and early 1990s, landmark studies—one headed by researchers at the National Institute of Mental Health and another at the University of Minnesota—compared psychotherapy with medication in the short-term treatment of depression.[1] In the studies, more than 300 patients received three to four months of treatment with psychotherapy, antidepressant medication, or a combination of the two. Roughly two-thirds of patients responded to psychotherapy or medication. Published in the *Archives of General Psychiatry* in 1992, the Minnesota study reported, "No differences in overall responses were observed" between the treatments. Patients who received medication in addition to psychotherapy did not do markedly better than those treated with psychotherapy alone.

Other studies have looked at the long-term outcome of different treatment modalities, following patients for up to four years. These long-term follow-up studies demonstrate a clear-cut advantage of psychotherapy over medications. In a study in Edinburgh, Scotland, published in the *Journal of*

Affective Disorders in 1986, depressed patients received nine months of treatment with psychotherapy or antidepressant medication.[2] After the treatment phase, patients were assessed every six months for two years. At the end of two years, only 23% of the patients who had been treated with psychotherapy had relapsed. By contrast, 78% of those treated with only medication had had a return of depression. Similar studies of the treatment of anxiety disorders have shown psychological interventions more effective in the long run than medications.[3] Because of the high relapse rates when patients are treated with just medication, psychopharmacologists frequently recommend that patients stay on them indefinitely. But as we saw in earlier chapters, staying on drugs long-term inevitably entails risks.

Not just psychotherapy but other alternatives to medications have also been carefully studied. A 1994 issue of the *Journal of Geriatric Psychiatry and Neurology* was devoted to seventeen research papers on the herbal antidepressant St. John's wort.[4] Studies have shown that St. John's wort is as effective as prescription drugs for mild to moderate depression. Similarly, clinical studies have compared the herbs kava and valerian favorably with Valium-type sedatives for the treatment of anxiety.[5]

In order to understand the overall benefits and disadvantages of Prozac-type medications versus those of the alternatives, one first needs to put these medications in perspective. Why are these drugs called "antidepressants" when they are prescribed for so many other conditions? How are new drugs developed and approved? Why are serotonin boosters often emphasized instead of the natural alternatives in many medical settings, especially managed care settings? Only with this background can one understand what the drugs do and do not offer, when one should take them and when not, and how to balance medications with the natural alternatives.

The Role of Psychopharmacology

When I was a Harvard Medical School student many years ago, psychopharmacology was in its infancy. Psychopharmacology was a new subspecialty within psychiatry, treating patients exclusively with medications. Psychopharmacology is also called biological or medical psychiatry, and psychopharmacologists are sometimes referred to as "medication doctors." To me psychopharmacology's narrow chemical prescription for healing people in troubled states seemed oddly out of sync with the essential psychological nature of many psychiatric symptoms.

One of my first encounters with this new subspecialty was when a fellow medical student and I observed a pioneer psychopharmacologist interview a patient in the emergency room. A fifty-eight-year-old man, the patient had come in distraught because earlier in the day his daughter, whose apartment he was living in, had threatened to evict him.

Some twenty-five years before, the patient had walked out on his wife and children, running away with his secretary to Seattle. He divorced his wife, paid no child support because his wife had family money, and had virtually no contact with his young children. After twenty-five years, his second wife, the secretary, threw him out, tired of supporting him and his extramarital affairs. Almost "destitute," he returned to the East Coast and took up residence with his dutiful daughter. After six months, she was tired of supporting him and told him he would have to help around the apartment or, better yet, get a job.

Throughout the interview, the patient kept offering his daughter's phone number at work, "just in case" we "wanted to let her know" that he was in the emergency room. With this, my fellow medical student and I thought the patient repeatedly tipped his hand, that he came hoping we would help manipulate his daughter by impressing upon her how distraught he was over her display of impatience. But this went over the psychopharmacologist's head. Ticking through rote checklists of questions instead of mining psychological clues, he did not ask, "How do you think your daughter would feel if she knew you were here? Would you like me to call her? What might that accomplish?" A profound lack of communication developed as the patient furtively sought to accomplish his mission while the psychopharmacologist methodically went through his checklists.

Finally, the psychopharmacologist came to the checklist for depression. "Have you had trouble falling asleep?" "Has your appetite been decreased?" At first the patient answered with a hesitant "yes," not really sure what was going on with these questions about bodily functions. But then he seemed to grasp that these were the symptoms the doctor considered evidence of grave distress. With increasing gravity, he answered a resounding "yes!" to every symptom. The psychopharmacologist lightened up a bit. He cast knowing glances to us, the two medical students observing quietly.

Exiting the room to discuss the case, he explained that the patient was severely depressed, so depressed he needed to come into the hospital right away to start medication. My classmate and I were dubious as we returned to the expectant patient, who immediately looked incredulous at the idea of hospitalization. "But I have to get home," he insisted. "My daughter will be home from work soon and I haven't done any of the chores she gave me."

She could visit in the hospital, the doctor explained. Indeed, she would need to bring him a toothbrush, pajamas, and a fresh set of clothes. Alarm flashed across the patient's face. This was more than he had bargained for. He was not depressed, he protested.

As the two struggled, the psychopharmacologist tried to save face. "You have a biological illness. You're not fit to go home," he insisted.

"You're nuts!" the patient finally declared, thundering to his feet, not looking at all depressed. "I have to get home to feed my cats!" he shouted in disgust and stormed out of the room, leaving modern psychiatry bewildered.

While this story has a certain irony and humor, it is, in fact, quite poignant. The patient did not get what he came for. He neither accomplished what he thought he wanted—assistance in manipulating his daughter—nor what might have truly helped him, which was some insight into his strained relationship with his daughter. While his story is amusing because he escaped the clutches of medical authority, most patients are medicated, often needlessly, having been convinced they have a "biological illness" that renders them unfit to go home without a drug. The story underscores the problem with the psychopharmacology model of treatment, with its overemphasis on superficial symptoms and quick-fix medications at the expense of more thoughtful psychological interventions.

Psychopharmacology's Disease Model

Psychopharmacology rests on a "disease model" of psychiatric symptoms. This is the application of an extreme medical or biological model to psychological syndromes. In all likelihood a few severe psychiatric conditions such as schizophrenia, manic depressive illness, or psychotic depression have a strong biological component. But to treat all psychiatric symptoms as though they were exclusively biological is unacceptable reductionism.

Medical and psychiatric patients come to see doctors because of symptoms. But symptoms in and of themselves are not necessarily indicative of a disease. In medicine, strict criteria exist for calling a condition a disease. In addition to a predictable cluster of symptoms, the cause of the symptoms or some understanding of their physiology must be established. This knowledge elevates a diagnosis to the status of a recognized disease. For example, "fever" is not a disease, it is merely a symptom. In the absence of a known cause or physiology, a cluster of symptoms that one sees repeatedly in many different patients is called a syndrome, not a disease.

Psychiatry is unique among medical specialties in that all of its diagnoses are merely syndromes, clusters of symptoms presumed to be related, not diseases. We do not yet have proof either of the cause or the physiology for any psychiatric diagnosis. This is why the official names for psychiatric diagnoses in the American Psychiatric Association's *Diagnostic and Statistical Manual (DSM)*—such as major depressive disorder, obsessive compulsive disorder, or manic depressive disorder—use the term "disorder." Here the word "disorder" is being used for syndrome. The diagnoses are called disorders because none of them are established diseases. We do not yet have a major depressive disease or even a manic depressive disease.

In the absence of any verifiable diseases, in recent decades, psychopharmacology has not hesitated to construct "disease models" for psychiatric diagnoses. These models are hypothetical suggestions of what *might* be the underlying physiology—for example, a serotonin imbalance. Through the 1970s and 1980s, a curious circularity invaded psychiatry, as "diseases" began to be "modeled" on the medications that "treat" them.[6] If a drug elevated serotonin in test tubes, then it was presumptuously argued that patients helped by the medication must have serotonin deficiencies even though we lack scientific proof for the idea. In the past decade, as part of promoting the new antidepressants, these "disease models" were presented to patients as if they were established facts. Writing in the November 1997 issue of the *Archives of General Psychiatry*, psychopharmacologist Lewis Judd of the department of psychiatry at the University of California at San Diego described depression as "a disease of the brain."[7] Patients are often explicitly told they have such a disease, usually to justify treating them with medication. But when one looks closely, all the disease models are built on three pseudoscientific cornerstones: superficial checklist diagnoses, putative "biochemical imbalances," and alleged genetic determinism.

Checklist Diagnoses

Psychiatric patients used to be helped through understanding and support, sometimes with medications, but mostly by getting to know them in depth. Typically, when first consulting with a doctor, patients have no idea what is really bothering them. Neither does the doctor. Indeed, even an experienced psychiatrist needs to guard against the hubris of thinking he or she understands the patient's predicament too quickly.

Psychopharmacologists do not emphasize talking to patients. Instead, they emphasize rapidly diagnosing patients and prescribing drugs. The lens through which patients are examined is the *Diagnostic and Statistical Man-*

ual (DSM), now in its fourth edition.[8] Published by the American Psychiatric Association, the current *DSM* is a compendium of checklist diagnoses: cursory, superficial menus of symptoms in which a minimum number (for example, four of eight or three of twelve) is needed to make a particular diagnosis. The symptoms used to assess depression include decreased energy, poor performance, and changes in sleep, appetite, and activity level. The emphasis is on physical, behavioral symptoms rather than emotional states. These checklists take what are essentially psychological conditions and define them as though they were *merely* physical symptoms rather than viewing the physical symptoms as merely manifestations of a psychological state. In the process, the forest is lost for the trees. Any attempt to help patients understand themselves and to effect real change is lost in the rush to diagnose and medicate them.

As another example of what a disservice this approach can be to patients, consider the case of Hamlet. Suppose Hamlet were to come to a psychopharmacologist or, as would be more likely, to be brought in by his "concerned" mother and stepfather. Recall that Hamlet is the prince of Denmark, suffering excruciating grief over his father's death. Further, he suspects (rightly so, as it turns out) that his mother and stepfather conspired to kill Hamlet's father in order to install the new husband-king. With his severe pessimism, endless philosophical ruminating ("To be or not to be, that is the question. . . ."), and visual hallucinations (his father's ghost), Hamlet would be diagnosed with major depression, paranoia, and psychosis. Instead of supporting Hamlet's exploring and, ultimately, discovering the truth, the psychopharmacologist would heavily medicate these dreadful "diseases." When Hamlet resisted, as suspicious patients often do, he would earn the added indignity of borderline personality disorder, be hospitalized, and be medicated against his will, most probably with a "drug cocktail" consisting of a serotonin booster, a sleeping pill, a Valium-type antianxiety agent, a major tranquilizer, and an anticonvulsant. Fortunately for Hamlet and posterity, he was in the hands of Shakespeare and not a psychopharmacologist. Hamlet's example may sound far-fetched, but it truly is the reality of the current climate for many psychiatric patients.

As sales of the serotonin antidepressants took off in the 1990s, even the *DSM* checklists became cumbersome. Researchers began publishing articles describing psychiatric diagnoses as "spectrum disorders." In *Listening to Prozac*, Kramer calls the spectrums "penumbras."[9] According to Kramer, vague conditions like low self-esteem or perfectionism fall within the "penumbra" of depression. The danger of this kind of thinking is that before long any symptom can qualify for the diagnosis: Having trouble sleeping? You're depressed. Try Prozac. Shy? You're depressed. Try Paxil. Of course, the ultimate emancipation was throwing off the shackle of any symptom: Feel well? You could feel better-than-well. Try Zoloft.

The Mystique of a Biochemical Imbalance

Another cornerstone, probably *the* cornerstone of disease models of psychiatric syndromes, is the concept of a biochemical imbalance. To examine this construct, let's look at two biochemical imbalances in general medicine. When I was practicing general medicine, I once had a patient who was brought to the emergency room by her distraught husband and family because she was "berserk, out of control." This normally decorous, middle-aged woman was disoriented, talking nonsense, combative, and lewd—to the mortification of her family. Admitted to the hospital, she had to be restrained in bed and observed round-the-clock because she wanted to escape out the seventh-story window. Although her symptoms were behavioral, they were characteristic of delirium, not psychosis, although the two are often confused.

A battery of laboratory tests is used to diagnose the cause of delirium. Eventually, one of the patient's blood tests came back abnormal. The concentration of sodium in her blood was dangerously abnormal, wreaking havoc on her brain function. Treatment consisted of intravenously infusing fluids to restore her sodium balance. Within hours, the patient's abnormal behavior cleared and on retest her sodium was normal. The cause of the imbalance? It turned out her pharmacy had accidentally doubled the dose of one of her blood pressure medications, leading to the problem. Although this patient's condition was behavioral, it was strictly a biochemical event, a sodium imbalance complete with characteristic symptoms, a definitive diagnostic test, rational therapeutics, full resolution of the symptoms, and a definitive retest showing everything was back to normal.

Diabetes is another biochemical imbalance in general medicine. Here the symptoms are weakness, hunger, and weight loss in spite of eating well, together with excessive urinating and constant thirst because of fluid loss. The physiology of the disease, discovered in the 1920s by a team of Canadian doctors, is that the body does not adequately metabolize ingested sugars. In particular, the regulation of sugar metabolism by the hormone insulin is defective. The definitive test and biochemical imbalance is a high blood sugar level. Treatment in severe cases is insulin injections, which restore sugar balance. The symptoms clear and retest shows the blood sugar is normal.

Nothing like a sodium imbalance or blood sugar imbalance exists for depression or any other psychiatric syndrome. But in an act of remarkable reductionism the disease model acts *as though* there were such a simple, biochemical explanation for psychiatric symptoms. Indeed, doctors frequently tell patients they need to take a serotonin booster "like a diabetic takes insulin." In fact, even in diabetes, where something is known about the physiology, only about 10% of patients have conditions severe enough to require insulin.[10] For the rest, their less severe diabetes can often be managed with milder agents, diet, and lifestyle changes. What if doctors tried to make all diabetics dependent on insulin?

In recent decades, we have had no shortage of alleged biochemical imbalances for psychiatric conditions. Diligent though these attempts have been, not one has been proven. Quite the contrary. In every instance where such an imbalance was thought to have been found, it was later proven false. Two particularly infamous ones are noteworthy. In the mid-1970s, a hormonal imbalance was said to indicate depression.[11] This was an abnormality in the daily, cyclical rhythm of cortisol release by the adrenal gland. This "biochemical imbalance" was diagnosed with a complicated assay called the dexamethasone suppression test, or DST, which required multiple blood tests during the day. For a time, in the late 1970s and early 1980s, the DST was hailed as a medical breakthrough: the first reliable, quantifiable abnormality in psychiatry.

For several years, psychiatrists used the DST to diagnose "biological" depressions. Then suddenly the DST turned out not to be specific for depression at all, since it could be abnormal in many other conditions. Indeed, the DST could be abnormal in people who were simply stressed but had no psychiatric diagnosis. Psychiatrists quickly abandoned the DST as a laboratory test for depression.[12] Unfortunately, unlike the "medical breakthrough," the debacle did not receive the same kind of coverage in the popular press, and a large section of the general public goes on thinking there are established biochemical imbalances for psychiatric ailments.

Even earlier, in the 1960s, psychiatrist Joseph Schildkraut thought he had discovered that an imbalance of the neurotransmitter adrenaline caused depression, after he found abnormalities in the metabolites of adrenaline in the urine of depressed patients.[13] At the time, an adrenaline imbalance was believed to underlie depression, because prescription antidepressants like amphetamines (speed) and tricyclics affected adrenaline in test tubes. Schildkraut's work was hailed as a medical milestone. He hoped to develop urine tests that would differentiate different kinds of adrenaline imbalances.[14] The result would be increased diagnostic precision and the development of new drugs aimed at specific types of depression.

Schildkraut's dream never materialized in spite of two more decades of research. His urine tests never made it into clinical use. Unfortunately, despite the inadequacy of this simplistic explanation for depression, Schildkraut's approach was resurrected in the 1990s, with a deficiency of adrenaline being replaced by a deficiency of a newly popular chemical, serotonin.

A serotonin deficiency for depression has not been found. A pioneer in the search for one is the Dutch psychiatrist Herman van Praag. In his 1993 book *"Make-Believes" in Psychiatry,* van Praag traces the history of the search for a serotonin imbalance.[15] Initially, in the mid-1960s, van Praag and other researchers found a deficiency of a close chemical cousin of serotonin, called 5-HIAA, in the cerebrospinal fluid of some depressed patients.[16] The work was suggestive of a serotonin deficiency but far from conclusive. Later researchers found similar suggestive but inconclusive deficiencies in patients with a wide range of diagnoses, including anxiety, personality disorders, and schizophrenia. For a time, researchers thought the deficiency might be indicative of suicidality rather than any specific psychiatric diagnosis.[17] Eventually, however, this too proved not to be the case, as it was found in patients who were not suicidal but simply irritable, hostile, and aggressive.[18] In the end, the deficiency proved neither diagnostic nor specific for any psychiatric condition. Still, patients are often given the impression that a definitive serotonin deficiency in depression is firmly established.

Still worse, it turns out that a deficiency of 5-HIAA, the actual chemical that was being measured, would not necessarily have indicated a deficiency of serotonin. Rather, a 5-HIAA deficiency could have indicated *either increased or decreased* serotonin. Says van Praag in *"Make-Believes" in Psychiatry,* "The available data do not allow a judgment as to the question of whether low CSF [cerebrospinal fluid] 5-HIAA [the chemical being measured] in aggression disorders reflects *a decrease or an increase* in 5-HT ergic [serotonergic] functioning [italics added]."[19] In his critique of the contemporary scene, van Praag calls inadequately substantiated claims like serotonin deficiencies "make-believes" in psychiatry. Too often psychiatry makes believe that hypothetical concepts are more firmly established than they really are.

Even if a biochemical imbalance were found in some depressed patients, this would not necessarily mean that it was the cause of the problem. Suppose one day you were standing on a street corner waiting for the bus home when someone came along and robbed you at gunpoint. Your assailant heaps abuse and death threats upon you as he absconds with your money, jewelry, and other valuables. You are left traumatized and panicked at the thought that he will return for you. If you ran to the nearest medical clinic, you might well be diagnosed with a biochemical imbalance. All kinds of stress hormones and chemical signals would be coursing through your brain and body. But these biochemical events would be the result of your psychological distress, not the cause. They would be the cart, not the horse. This would not be anything like a sodium imbalance causing behavioral disturbances. If a biochemical imbalance is ever found, it should come as no surprise that psychological states have physiological correlates. Instead, in the past decade, hypothetical biochemical imbalances have been presented to the public as established fact. The result is an undue inflation of the drug market, as well as an unfortunate downplaying of the need for psychological treatments for many patients.

Genetic Determinism

Yet another cornerstone of disease models closely related to biochemical imbalances is the idea of genetic inheritance. A number of times in recent decades, prominent headlines have announced how the gene for manic depression was found. One of these was a particularly prestigious study done by researchers at the Massachusetts Institute of Technology, Yale University, and the University of Miami and published in the international scientific journal *Nature*.[20] Each time, the announcements were hailed as extraordinary medical breakthroughs. But none of the studies stood the test of time. Upon close scrutiny, all of them had to be retracted.[21] Unfortunately, the retractions did not receive the same publicity, so many people are left to believe that genes have been found for a great many mental states and that more related discoveries are being proven at regular intervals.

No claim of a gene for a psychiatric condition has stood the test of time, in spite of popular misinformation.[22] The studies of psychiatric syndromes are called "linkage" studies, tracking whether or not a psychiatric diagnosis runs in families with an established gene, such as that for blood type, which is called a "marker" gene.

One problem with the studies is that they rely on what geneticists call serial, rather than parallel, data in family trees, or pedigrees. Serial data is quite fragile. If someone in a pedigree is misdiagnosed, then the entire structure of inference lower down is thrown off. This is especially problematic if the individual is high in the pedigree. This partly explains why even the most impressive-looking studies have not stood the test of time. In the case of the study published in *Nature*, the addition of two rediagnoses and a small number of persons to the pedigree caused the original findings to collapse.

Another problem is the poor quality of diagnoses for people higher up in the pedigree. Since they are deceased, these individuals cannot be interviewed to reliably diagnose them. Often they are characterized as "Aunt Jane had a nervous breakdown" or "Uncle Bob was mentally unstable." Although more recent methodologies have attempted to address this problem, as yet they have not produced significant results. So-called twin studies, of twins reared apart, are even more problematic, because not even a marker gene is involved. They are not linkage studies. Rather, twin studies are closer to simple pedigrees looking at whether or not a condition runs in families.[23]

In the absence of a definitive gene, calling diagnoses that run in families "genetic" is a huge hypothetical leap. Religious affiliation and political party are the two traits most reliably running in families. Would anyone claim these are genetic? Renowned geneticist and Harvard professor Richard Lewontin has been an outspoken critic of the poor designs, terrible statistics, and exaggerated claims made in "genetic" studies. In a superb book, *Biology as Ideology,* Lewontin says, "The fact is, not a single study of personality traits in human populations successfully disentangles similarity because of shared family experience and similarity because of genes. . . . The argument confuses the observation [that a condition is running in families] with its explanation."[24]

Lewontin quotes Nobel Prize–winning biologist David Baltimore, who was aghast when a journal as prestigious as *Nature* was forced to retract the manic depression study because it was later found faulty.[25] Asked Baltimore, "Setting myself up as an average reader of *Nature,* what am I to believe?"

"Nothing," answers Lewontin: The studies are propaganda in the "ideology of biological determinism." Detailing the extraordinary financial ties between modern science and commercial interests, from funding of research to stock options in start-up biotech and pharmaceutical companies, he says, "Once again, what appears to us in the mystical guise of pure science and objective knowledge about nature turns out, underneath, to be political, economic, and social ideology."[26] Lewontin points out that while insulin and something about the physiology of diabetes have been known since the 1920s, in spite of decades of research, the genetics of diabetes is still poorly understood.[27] Experts insist diabetes is far too complex to be explained by a simple genetic cause. If a simple genetic explanation is unlikely for diabetes, just think how unlikely it is for depression. Indeed, with a condition as vaguely defined as depression, it is highly unlikely a single causative gene exists.

Undaunted, some doctors act *as though* depression and other mental states have been proven to be genetic. As part of conveying this impression, "family history" is emphasized in evaluating patients. Even if a patient lacks a family member with depression, a relative—even a distant relative—who might be described as vaguely "moody," "eccentric," "irritable," or "alcoholic" will be noted as "depressed" and the patient described as having a family history of depression. With such a loose definition, almost anyone might be thought to have inherited depression. Says Leston Havens, professor of psychiatry at Harvard Medical School, "Why I could get a 'family history' from a stone! Even they have relatives who've rolled downhill a few times, you know."[28]

Family history is taken terribly seriously by many doctors and unsuspecting patients. Often it is the deciding factor used to convince hesitant patients to go on medication. In fact, psychological damage, not genes, may be what is "inherited." As yet, we have no definitive data to differentiate these possibilities. In the meantime, patients are often seriously misled.

Since a genetic basis for psychiatric syndromes has not been proven, other equally unsubstantiated disease models have been proposed. Rapidly gaining in the public consciousness is a hypothesis known as "kindling." The kindling model is based on experiments in which epilepsy is induced in monkeys.[29] When an electrode is inserted in a monkey's brain, the delivery of an electric current triggers seizures and scars the surrounding brain tissue. Initially, the scarring is insufficient to produce spontaneous seizures— that is, epilepsy. Eventually, however, a point of no return is reached: The scarring is so extensive the monkey becomes epileptic. Comparing seizures to fires in the brain, the epilepsy is said to have been "kindled" by the repeated trauma.

Psychopharmacologists first analogized kindled epilepsy to manic depressive illness, although this is pure speculation. Now the model has been extended to depression and other psychiatric conditions. In *Listening to Prozac*, Peter Kramer compares life stresses, each episode of minor depression, to the scientist's needle repeatedly singeing the brain: "If we accept the analogy between mood disorders and kindled epilepsy, this is how we will see manic depression, and perhaps all depression: It is a progressive, probably lifelong disorder."[30] The conclusion? Drugs should be given as early as possible to "protect" people from progression of the "disease." Proclaims Kramer, "The goal is to prevent the hard-to-reverse deterioration that occurs as the illness progresses. . . . Early and prolonged intervention is crucial."

Nowadays, a notable number of patients come to psychiatrists fearful that their bad moods are burning the hole of lifelong depression into their brains. Because of their strong belief in the biological model of psychiatry, some psychopharmacologists tell patients this is the case even though it is hypothetical. Frightened, patients request medication to protect them from the dreadful prospect.

Still another hypothesis is that viruses cause psychiatric syndromes. This model stems from research showing a seasonal pattern in the births of schizophrenics. If schizophrenia were genetic, the birth rate should be evenly distributed throughout the year. To explain the seasonal pattern, researchers speculate schizophrenia may be caused by viral infections occurring during pregnancy, arguing that different viruses occur at different times of the year. Although it is unproven, the viral model has now been extended to other psychiatric syndromes and to personal characteristics that are not psychiatric conditions. Indeed, an article entitled "A New Germ Theory" in the February 1999 issue of the *Atlantic Monthly* suggests that everything from depression to homosexuality may be caused by viruses.[31]

Genetic determinism, kindled epilepsy, and psychopathic viruses are all part of a misguided tendency to view psychiatric syndromes as exclusively biological rather than as having more complicated psychosocial origins. Almost inevitably the treatment then offered is drugs.

If the foundations of disease models are so insubstantial, where do persistent notions of biochemical imbalances come from? On what basis are claims made that depression, obsessionalism, shyness, eating disorders, addictions, and all the other "diseases" treated with the Prozac group are due to a serotonin imbalance in particular?

Test Tube Studies of Blenderized Rat Brains

One cannot measure serotonin levels in the brain of any patient. Nor can one measure serotonin at specific synapses. Synapses are the spark plugs between nerve cells, junctions where they exchange chemical messages and where drugs are said to work. Blood levels of serotonin are of little use. Not only is blood drawn from an arm far removed from the brain synapse, 95% of serotonin in the human body is in the stomach and other tissues, not the brain. Therefore, blood levels of circulating serotonin bear little relation to what is going on in the nervous system. Some studies of the effects of drugs on serotonin are performed on human blood cells, but again, these cannot provide much of a picture of what is happening in the brain.

To circumvent these major problems with human subjects, pharmaceutical companies turned to animal models. A rat can be killed and its brain thrown into a blender and mashed to bits. In test tubes, fragments of the smashed brain reconstitute into little spheres, which researchers call synaptosomes, a name evoking synapses in patients, although the ground-up bits of rat brain may have little in common with them. The effect of drugs on serotonin levels in the synaptosomes is measured in test tubes, although the results may bear little relation to the complexity of what the drugs do in the living human brain.

These test tube studies show that Prozac, Zoloft, Paxil, and Luvox raise serotonin levels. This is where the hypothesis of a serotonin imbalance comes from: extrapolating to humans from test tube studies of blenderized rat brains. Obviously, this is faulty logic, pseudoscience again. This is almost like saying that someone whose headache is relieved by aspirin has an aspirin deficiency. The truth of the matter is: No one has anything but the vaguest idea of the chemical effects of these drugs on the living human brain.

The idea of "selectivity" also comes from these test tube studies. In the official product information on a drug, pharmaceutical companies typically report the results of test tube studies on up to half a dozen neurotransmitters. The product information for Prozac reports on four neurotransmitters in addition to serotonin. The Prozac group preferentially affect serotonin by comparison with the other neurotransmitters they are compared with. Thus they are said to be "selective" for serotonin. But this small number of neurotransmitters in the test tubes are a small percentage of the more than a hundred known neurotransmitters in the brain, with new ones being continually discovered. We have no idea how the drugs affect the other hundred even in test tubes, let alone in the brain.

Even if the drugs did preferentially affect serotonin neurons (nerve cells in the brain), there are hundreds of thousands of serotonin neurons, extending to and influencing virtually every region of the brain. [32] Each serotonin neuron branches over 500,000 times as it makes contact with innumerable other neurons. Through this intricate circuitry and myriad delicate balances, neurons are constantly talking to one another, reciprocally influencing one another in endless feedback loops. One of the most important of these balances is the serotonin–dopamine connection, which has been implicated in so many of the major categories of side effects discussed in the first half of the book. To talk about "selectivity" in regard to smashed brains in test tubes where fragments of dead cells no longer influence one another is irrelevant; to talk about it in regard to living humans is simply folly.

Thoughtful scientists and clinicians have seriously questioned the concepts of serotonin imbalances, deficiencies, and selectivity. At a 1997 Harvard Medical School conference, Dr. Andrew Nierenberg, director of the depression research program at the Massachusetts General Hospital and a professor at Harvard, reviewed the disease models of depression. Nierenberg then said, "The dark side of all of this is that we have many elegant models but the real fact is that [when it comes to] the exact mechanisms by which these things work, *we don't have a clue* [italics added]."[33]

Dr. Jerrold Rosenbaum, chairman of the department of psychopharmacology at the Massachusetts General Hospital and also a professor at Harvard, agreed: "After all these years, when someone's asked how antidepressants work, the expert answers 'I don't know' and now the people who are less expert are talking about norepinephrine [the form of adrenaline found in the brain] and serotonin."[34] Given these statements from up-to-date, highly qualified researchers in the field, what the public has been told in the past decade is truly astounding. While the alleged "selectivity" of the drugs makes good marketing copy, implying that they target a depression center in the brain, no such center is known to exist.

Eventually, scientists may discover real proof that a small percentage of patients have genetically determined, biological symptoms. But we are a long way from any such knowledge. When patients are told otherwise, they are being seriously misled.

The Development and Testing of New Antidepressants

At the time when cocaine elixirs and amphetamines were popular prescription antidepressants, pharmaceutical companies and doctors could make whatever claims they wanted on behalf of their miracle cures. No requirement existed for proving a drug's efficacy. One typical advertisement for prescription amphetamines (speed) showed a sporty-looking cowboy with a whip under the banner "Sparks Energy, Relieves Chronic Fatigue and Mild Depression."[35]

This state of affairs only changed in 1962 when Congress passed the Harris-Kefauver Amendment to the Federal Food and Drug Act. This amendment was an attempt to curb the excesses seen in the promotion of drugs like amphetamines, barbiturates, and opiates to the general public. For the first time pharmaceutical companies were required to demonstrate the efficacy of a new drug before being allowed to market it. The legislation was hailed with great hopes that it would usher in a new era of "rational therapeutics" based on the scientific method.

The requirement to test new drugs is cumbersome and costly for pharmaceutical companies, but it also offers an advantage. One of the claims made for serotonin boosters is that they have been "scientifically proven" safe and efficacious.[36] In fact, scrutiny of the studies turns up many surprising findings.

Each year, pharmaceutical companies synthesize scores of new chemicals. Many are close copies of existing drugs with slight structural changes in the hopes of finding patentable new agents. When it was first synthesized, Prozac had the inauspicious name Compound LY 110140.

New drugs are first tested on animals, rather than human subjects, to establish a modicum of efficacy and safety. With a potential new antibiotic, for example, one can infect laboratory animals and see if a test drug kills the infection without being too toxic to the host. But right away, here one has a problem when it comes to antidepressants: One cannot interview a laboratory rat to see how depressed she is and whether or not a drug makes her feel better.

To circumvent this major limitation, researchers turned again to animal "models." In these models, observable, quantifiable behaviors in animals are *presumed* to bear some relationship to depression in humans. Among the animal models used for antidepressants is screening for drugs that heighten aggression. The studies involve giving drugs to selected members in colonies of laboratory animals. Observers then evaluate the medication-enhanced animals for their aggressive behavior. Examples of the kinds of aggressive behaviors looked for are climbing in the colony's dominance hierarchy and violence toward new members who are introduced into the group.[37] Other studies involve creating brain damage that produces disinhibited aggression and screening for drugs that heighten the aggression even more.[38]

Such experiments are not pretty. Most patients would probably be upset to think their drug was originally selected for its ability to heighten aggression in deliberately brain-damaged animals or to make animals more violent toward strangers. Most doctors, too, are unaware of how the drugs they prescribe were selected. These kinds of screening tests were once used to test amphetamines. In some instances, new drugs are tested with an amphetamine, to see if the test drug augments the amphetamine's effects.

The initial clinical studies of a new drug are small-scale: the drugs are administered to as few as fifteen to twenty patients. These small-scale studies give researchers some familiarity with how patients respond to the drug and establish safe doses. Only then does large-scale clinical testing begin.

Large-scale clinical tests are multicenter studies involving hundreds of patients at different sites around the country. Each study is numbered and called a "protocol," for example Protocol Number 14. Most studies are "randomized"—that is, patients are randomly assigned to receive either the test drug, a comparison drug, or a placebo. The gold standard are "double-blind, placebo-controlled" protocols. Here patients are randomly assigned to either a drug or placebo group. Moreover, neither the patients nor the technician-raters are supposed to know who is on active drug versus placebo; both groups are "blind" to this information. These studies are designed to eliminate bias created by knowing who is on the drug versus the placebo, since such knowledge can easily become a self-fulfilling prophecy, skewing the data and study results. To win approval of a new drug, its advantage over placebo must be demonstrated in at least two double-blind, controlled studies.

The clinical tests of antidepressants are remarkably short, especially considering that depression can be a chronic condition. The FDA's guidelines for large-scale clinical tests recommend they last at least six weeks, although in some instances studies as short as four weeks are accepted. Typically, the studies last six to eight weeks.

When an antibiotic undergoes testing, many objective data are available regarding the condition for which volunteers are being treated, including temperature, physical examination, blood tests, X-rays, and bacterial cultures. But with depression, here again one has a major problem: No definitive diagnostic criteria exist that can be confirmed by physical examination of the patient or by laboratory tests. No test of the blood, urine, or even cerebrospinal fluid. No X-ray, CAT scan, or even electroencephalogram (EEG).

Like all psychiatric diagnoses, depression is a syndrome, meaning merely a cluster of symptoms presumed to be related. To complicate matters, the symptoms are subjective emotional states, making the diagnosis extremely vague. Depressive symptoms overlap with many other psychiatric syndromes and with fatigue caused by a host of medical conditions. Mild depression, in which patients are sad and tearful but still relatively functional, barely resembles severe depression, in which patients are incapacitated, suicidal, and even psychotic. Depression can be masked by other symptoms like eating disorders, sexual compulsions, and even cheerful fronts.

Pharmaceutical companies "solved" the complex dilemmas of diagnosing depression by focusing primarily on moderately depressed patients in studies of the new antidepressants. In the Prozac studies, seriously depressed patients, anyone suicidal, those with other serious diagnoses (like manic depression), children, and the elderly were typically excluded—even though all these groups would be prime candidates for the drug once it was approved.

Further, the subjective diagnosis of depression was turned into a seemingly quantitative number using "instruments," which prove to be cursory, superficial checklist rating scales. The scales were designed to fit hand-in-glove with the effects of drugs, emphasizing the physical symptoms of depression that most respond to antidepressant medication.[39] Examples are the Zung Self-Rating Scale for patients and the Hamilton Depression scale for technician-raters who interview patients.[40] The scales ask patients to respond to items such as "I get tired for no reason," "I have trouble sleeping at night," "I notice that I am losing weight," "I feel down-hearted and blue." Each item is scored on a numerical scale, with the lowest score indicating "a little of the time" and the highest score indicating "most of the time." On the most commonly used scale, the Hamilton, a score greater than 28 indicates severe depression.[41] Patients with Hamilton ratings in the low twenties are considered moderately depressed.

While assigning a number to a patient's depression may look scientific, when one examines the questions asked and the scales used, they are utterly subjective measures based on what the patient reports or a rater's impressions. A patient with a checklist score of 20 may be far more depressed than another with a score of 30 because of ethnic, cultural, and gender differences in how emotions are experienced and expressed. As a result, comparisons between patients are not possible. In effect, each patient is his or her own study.

This creates the next major problem: How does one define a positive response to treatment? In the case of a lung infection, one has many objective criteria that can be monitored: fever drops, abnormal respiratory sounds disappear, the dense mass in the chest X-ray clears, and cultures no longer grow the offending bacteria. But for depression there are no objective measures of success.

To circumvent this problem, researchers use a relative measure for drug response. That is, the patient's pre-drug and post-drug depression scores are compared. What exactly is the definition of a drug "response"? On the Hamilton scale, depression-free is considered a score of 6 or less for at least three consecutive weeks.[42] This is only a statistical norm using a subjective measure. But it is a higher standard than that used in most tests of new drugs. After all, the studies only last six to eight weeks. The best that is hoped for is not a recovery but just a 50% improvement. Typically, the

Hamilton scores of patients in antidepressant studies drop from an average of 24 to 12. Obviously, this means they are still quite depressed, with scores twice those indicating freedom from depression.

Thus, at the core of antidepressant studies, the essential piece of data is a patient's short-term, subjective, relative, partial response. The effective criterion, therefore, is that patients temporarily feel "a little better" on a stimulating drug. Since statistical analyses are only as good as the data upon which they rest, any conclusions drawn from such studies are no better than this meager result.

Once all the patients have been assessed in this fashion, the results for the placebo group are compared with the results for the test drug group. A surprisingly low level of statistical analysis is used by comparison with the standards in other areas of medicine and especially by comparison with the standards in hard sciences, such as chemistry or physics.

In many antidepressant studies, the drug does not outperform the placebo: an equal percentage of patients in both groups evidence a response.[43] Studies with these sorts of results tend to be ignored. When applying to the FDA for aproval, the pharmaceutical companies only have to come up with at least two studies demonstrating a "statistically significant" difference. Even in studies that demonstrate this difference, however, the results are still remarkably close. The Agency for Health Care Policy and Research in the Department of Health and Human Services recently analyzed the data from more than 80 clinical studies of the newer antidepressants. Overall, half the patients did not respond to the drugs. Moreover, among those who did, 64% of the reported benefit was accounted for by the placebo effect.[44]

Placebos are so effective in these kinds of studies because mild to moderate depression is responsive to attention and suggestion. Patients come to the studies with curiosity and hope. The medical settings and technicians have an air of authority. Raters spend time interviewing patients and develop a relationship with them. The patients come to the center frequently to be evaluated and to have their placebo pills dispensed. In short, they receive a lot more than just sugar pills. Moreover, it turns out that in many antidepressant studies, the critical standard—the double blind—is something of an illusion: If, during a study, one asks patients and raters who is on active drug versus placebo, both groups know with 83% and 88% accuracy respectively.[45] How? Because of obvious side effects. Indeed, patients and raters may openly discuss this: "I'm feeling a little shaky today," says a wide-eyed, jittery patient. "Guess you're not in the placebo group," thinks the experienced rater.

This problem arises because the placebos typically used in antidepressant testing are inert; that is, they produce no physiological effects. There are placebos available, such as low doses of atropine, that cause "side effects," but they are not ordinarily used. These placebos with side effects have no known antidepressant properties. They do cause a variety of mild side effects, however, like dry mouth. When a placebo with side effects is used in an antidepressant study, performance of the placebo climbs and the difference between the placebo and the antidepressant is virtually washed out.[46] Why? Suggestibility: People *think* they are on an active drug and there is no objective standard for any kind of measurement. For this reason, Roger Greenberg and Seymour Fisher, in the department of psychiatry at the State University of New York, argue that placebos with side effects should be required in antidepressant testing on the grounds that psychoactive drugs, which will be prescribed to millions of people, ought to be held to the higher standard.[47]

Children are even more susceptible to suggestion and the placebo effect than adults. This is why repeated studies have shown antidepressants are no more effective in children than placebos. In a 1996 review in the *Journal of Nervous and Mental Disease* of the published double-blind, placebo-controlled studies in children, Drs. Seymour Fisher and Rhoda Fisher concluded, "The evidence is unanimous that antidepressants are no more effective than placebos in children with symptoms of depression."[48] The Fishers cited several other reviews that had reached the same conclusion.

Unfortunately, despite such important evidence, the prescribing of antidepressants to children has become a common practice. Writing in the same issue of the *Journal of Nervous and Mental Disease,* Dr. Edmund Pellegrino, a professor of medicine and medical ethics at the Georgetown University Medical Center, said physicians lack ethical grounds for "ignoring authenticated evidence from scientifically conducted clinical trials [i.e., the placebo-controlled studies]" when prescribing treatments "that fly in the face of established scientific evidence."[49]

Another area for concern in antidepressant testing is testing "mills"— the establishments where the lucrative testing is carried out. In this country a surprisingly small number of testing centers and psychiatrists conduct the majority of research on new psychiatric drugs for pharmaceutical companies.[50] The same names appear over and over again in published articles on the research and in pharmaceutical company–sponsored promotion of the drugs. Seventy-five percent of the research is conducted by for-profit testing centers; only 25% is conducted at nonprofit academic hospitals, which lend an air of greater respectability overall to the testing.[51]

Over the years, repeated exposés have highlighted stunning abuses in the testing of psychiatric drugs. For example, in 1998 Minnesota psychiatrist Frank Abuzzahab was found guilty of "recklessly" entering patients into psychiatric drug studies, falsifying their records, and fabricating positive drug responses in an investigation by the Minnesota Board of Medical Practice. Said Dr. Morris Goldman, of the University of Chicago, who headed the investigation, "He would have the patient's diagnosis called one thing in the regular chart and then the person would be put on a drug study and the person's diagnosis would be called something else to fit the criteria."[52] While the patients' hospital records clearly indicated that their conditions had deteriorated while on the study drug, Abuzzahab's reports to the pharmaceutical company presented a far rosier picture. Abuzzahab was a past president of the Minnesota Psychiatric Society and the chairman of its ethics committee. He was a lead investigator in one of the four placebo-controlled studies of Prozac that Eli Lilly submitted to the FDA to win approval for the drug.[53]

One of the most highly publicized scandals surfaced in the spring of 1997. The chairman of the department of psychiatry at the Medical College of Georgia, psychopharmacologist Richard Borison, and another professor in his department, Bruce Diamond, were indicted by the Georgia Attorney General on 172 counts of bribery, racketeering, forgeries, and endangering patients in connection with clinical testing of psychiatric medications for some twenty pharmaceutical companies over a decade. During this time, the two professors published more than twenty articles in scholarly journals and built national reputations based on their "research" on depression, anxiety, schizophrenia, and Alzheimer's disease. The April 1997 *Psychiatric Times* reported that one "bribery count in the indictment alleges that Borison and Diamond paid an undisclosed sum to an MCG [Medical College of Georgia] employee in exchange for her not filing a complaint regarding a patient suicide that occurred during a clinical study."[54] From 1989 to 1996 alone, these two psychopharmacologists made more than $10 million on drug research, a rare glimpse into the profitability of testing psychiatric drugs.

In sworn depositions, employees of Borison and Diamond described how attractive young women were specifically hired to lure male patients into drug studies. These recruiters were paid thousands of dollars in bonuses and given prizes—in one instance, a new car—for exceeding patient-recruitment goals. "When there is a possibility that you are going to get a car, you're going to do whatever you can" to convince people to enter the studies, testified one of Borison and Diamond's research coordinators, Angela Touhey.[55]

Many of the staff were untrained and had no medical background. They entered patients into studies, drew their blood, and adjusted the dose of their medication. Borison and Diamond specifically told the staff that they did not care to hear about the patients. "Bruce [Dr. Diamond] told me," testified Touhey, "We don't care about how the patients are doing. We just want to know how many people you have enrolled in the past week or couple of weeks."

The pressure to recruit patients and get results comes from pharmaceutical companies with which Borison and Diamond were consistent favorites and by which they were awarded lucrative research contracts. In a November 1998 exposé on psychiatric drug testing in the *Boston Globe,* reporters Delores Kong and Robert Whitaker stated, "The companies need to get patients into their trials quickly, and they will pay researchers handsomely for doing so. But they also expect the researchers to deliver. Researchers who do not meet their patient quotas are not likely to get a contract for the next project."[56]

Indeed, Newell Unfried, vice president of a for-profit testing center called Alliance for Multispecialty Research, says, "The pressures are enormous." Pharmaceutical companies rate "every physician in clinical research on their patient recruitment. There is pressure to get these patients." Increasingly, testing centers advertise for study subjects in newspapers and on television. In some instances, subjects are paid to participate in the studies.

Doctors Borison and Diamond pleaded guilty to the theft, bribery, and racketeering charges brought against them by the Georgia Attorney General. They were each fined $125,000 and were sentenced to prison. At the time of their highly publicized indictment, Eli Lilly pulled all studies still in progress with Borison and Diamond, reassigning them to other centers. Regarding the many studies the pair had completed over the years for Lilly, however, a spokesperson said the company was confident that none of the data provided was compromised in any way.[57] But Dr. David Hess, chief of neurology at the hospital where Borison was the chief of psychiatry, told investigators, "This whole thing was very dirty. It was basically a numbers game. These patients are purely used for the greed of the researchers.... [It] was very apparent to me what was going on."[58] While some insist that the repeated exposés are not representative of the testing of psychiatric drugs, others note that many of the most disturbing practices highlighted in the exposés—such as the exorbitant sums of money involved, employing staff with little training or clinical experience to evaluate patients, and advertising for subjects rather than using real patients coming into doctors' offices seeking treatment—are not uncommon in psychiatric drug testing.

The efficacy and safety of serotonin boosters is anything but "scientifically proven," given the many problems with their clinical testing: the short duration of clinical studies, the lack of objective criteria, the use of subjective rating scales, the acceptance of partial drug "responses," the use of inert placebos, questionable double blinds, high placebo response rates, and statistical manipulations. With the protocols used by drug manufacturers, almost any stimulating drug would pass as an "antidepressant." This would be true for cocaine elixirs, prescription amphetamines (speed), amphetamine-like drugs such as Ritalin (which is prescribed as an antidepressant), thyroid hormone (also prescribed as an antidepressant), caffeine pills, or even nicotine. Indeed, a study, published in the September 1996 issue of the *Journal of Clinical Psychiatry*, demonstrated that nicotine is an effective "antidepressant."[59]

At the height of the controversy over whether or not Prozac made some patients suicidal and violent, Eli Lilly claimed their clinical testing of the drug was the "only scientifically valid" data available. It is ironic that such strident claims of being scientific have been made on the basis of testing that is so unscientific, riddled with so many flagrant violations of the scientific method and careful scientific reasoning. David Healy of the North Wales College of Medicine observes that "these studies are not scientific studies; they are simply studies required for [FDA] registration purposes aimed at demonstrating that in some population an effect can be demonstrated."[60] There is little effort to investigate why the drugs have the effects that they do, no effort to test them thoroughly on representative samples of all the different kinds of patients who will ultimately be prescribed the drugs, and scant attention to long-term safety. In short, the testing satisfies a minimal regulatory requirement. It is not genuine science.

How "Antidepressants" Work Clinically

When starting a serotonin booster, many patients report feeling nervous or jittery and have difficulty sleeping. Most often patients describe these effects as feeling "caffeinated." Say many patients, "It's like I've had several cups of strong coffee." Indeed, people often have to cut back on their caffeine intake—coffee, tea, or soda—because the combined effects of the serotonin booster and caffeine are overstimulating. For most people, the caffeinated feeling is an early response that wears off in two to four weeks. This is because the nervous system adapts to the medication, compensating to some degree for its effects. After this early phase, the increased energy the drug provides becomes more evenly modulated. But even after the initial jitteriness wears off, some patients still notice a subtle but distinct "hit" every morning as the drug takes effect. Typically, this occurs within an hour of taking the medication. The discernible "lift" in energy level lasts for the morning or the better part of the day.

Prozac is the longest-acting serotonin booster. It lingers in the blood for weeks even after it is stopped. Beyond the early, adaptation phase, this tendency to linger cushions the effect of each individual dose, modulating the elevation of the patient's energy level over time. Zoloft and Paxil are much shorter-acting, lasting only a day or two, but still providing some cushion. Wellbutrin (also known as Zyban) is one of the shortest-acting of the new antidepressants, lasting only hours. In part because its effects wear off quickly, Wellbutrin is often taken several times a day. In this regard, Wellbutrin resembles short-acting amphetamine-type drugs, such as Dexedrine or Ritalin, which are also taken several times a day.

As with any energizing drug, people vary widely in their sensitivity to the stimulating effects of serotonin boosters. Some patients adjust very quickly. They may notice mild jitteriness for a day or two, or nothing at all. Years later, many patients forget they felt anxious or tremulous when they first started the drug until they are asked specifically or reminded by a recurrence of the same side effects when the dose is increased.

Some patients report that serotonin boosters help to focus their attention. This allows people to concentrate better on whatever task is at hand. From factory workers, to laborers, to students, to Wall Street brokers, people say the drugs aid their concentration, especially for boring, repetitive tasks. Some patients report feeling clearer-headed and sharper-thinking: "It's like a fuzziness around the edges of everything goes. Instead of getting lost in endless possibilities, I just seem to be able to function in a more straightforward way."

A corollary of the focused attention is that patients report a decrease in distracting, obsessive, usually negative thoughts. For some patients, this is the most salient effect of the drugs: "I used to spend my days obsessing about things I'd said or thought I'd done wrong. It didn't matter how trivial a trigger was, one thing would always lead to another and I'd end up beating myself up, thinking I was a terrible person whom no one liked. Zoloft just seems to cut the thoughts off. It's not that I never have them, but one thing doesn't lead to another. It's almost as though I can watch the thoughts rise up and then stop, just cut off before they get too bad." For many these downward spirals of obsessive self-criticisms held them back, socially, academically, or at work. Without them and with newfound energy, they feel more confident and assertive, even aggressive.

Finally, these drugs can have a mood-brightening effect. They make some people feel less irritable, better able to tolerate the bumps and scrapes of life, more tolerant, even "complacent." In light of the hype surrounding the drugs, many patients are surprised to find that they are not really "happy pills"—few people feel that their mood is constantly buoyed by them. When patients on these drugs do feel sad, however, they are less vulnerable to sudden or dramatically plummeting moods. It is as though the drug puts a floor under them, holding them up, limiting how far their mood can slide.

Some people describe a general "numbing" of their feelings. People who were crying a lot find they literally cannot cry. Some even seek out wrenching films and are distressed to find their emotions cannot break through: "Before I went on Paxil I was a basket case, crying all the time. Now I can't cry even if I want to, when everybody else in the movie theater is and it would be appropriate." Some find this numbing effect disturbing; they feel there is a kind of "blanket suppression" of their emotions. A few people even report feeling disconnected from themselves, as though they are observing themselves interact with other people. This reaction is usually very disturbing to patients.

Individual variation causes an incredibly wide range of responses to serotonin boosters. For almost any reaction, no matter how common, one hears of equally intense but opposite reactions.[61] While many feel jittery when first starting the drug, a few are immediately calmed. Although a decrease in obsessive, negative thoughts is common, a small number of patients develop obsessions. Some patients say their thinking becomes clearer, but others report the opposite: their thinking becomes clouded and they have difficulty with their memory. As discussed in Chapter 3, while the majority of people report markedly diminished sex drive, a few become hypersexual.

This wide range of responses is sometimes confusing. It has even been exploited by drug advocates, who use the anomalies to distract from the average, typical response. In spite of the wide variation, many patients report that the drugs give them more energy, focus their attention, decrease negative thoughts, and brighten their mood.

Patients who are former amphetamine or cocaine addicts spontaneously report that their serotonin boosters are like "mild versions" of these street drugs. Say many patients, "So long as I didn't do too much coke, if I just did a few lines, I would feel in such a good mood. It was only when I did too much or if I smoked it or shot it up instead of snorting lines that I would feel really racy and strung out. Prozac is like the milder effect, like just a line or two."

Over the years doctors have referred to antidepressants by many different labels. These have included "mood brighteners,"[62] "psychostimulants,"[63] and "psychic energizers."[64] Many psychiatrists use the term "controlled hypomania" for the set point at which they aim to adjust people's moods with the Prozac-type antidepressants.[65] That is, they raise the dose until the patient is hypomanic. Of course "manic" means "high." The prefix "hypo" means "a little." Thus, the explicit goal is to make people "a little high."

One might ask how serotonin boosters can have any similarity to cocaine and amphetamine (speed), which we think of as stimulating people to excess. The answer is the dose, or strength, at which the drugs are prescribed. Remember, cocaine and amphetamine, too, were once the most popular prescription medications—the Prozacs—of their day. Except in particularly sensitive individuals, *at prescription doses* all stimulants have similar effects: heightening energy, focusing attention, and brightening mood. As a result, prescription doses are calming even though the drugs are "stimulants." The energizing, mood-brightening, calming, and attention-focusing effects of stimulants have been demonstrated in repeated studies of normal, healthy volunteers.[66] There is nothing "paradoxical" about this response; this is simply the effect of stimulants when given at prescription doses.

Only at much higher doses or in sensitive individuals do the drugs have the overstimulating, disorganizing effects we nowadays associate with the word "stimulant." Higher doses are achieved either by taking larger amounts orally or, more often, by crushing the drugs and snorting them through the nose or shooting (injecting) them intravenously. These routes of administration deliver the drug to the brain much more quickly for a faster, greater high. Cocaine and speed are not the only drugs abused in this way. Patients involved in the underground drug culture report that the new antidepressants are also crushed into powdered form and snorted in lines, just like cocaine or speed, or they are shot intravenously for a more intense effect. According to patients, the two antidepressants most commonly abused in this way are Prozac and Wellbutrin (Zyban).

Corroborating the stories I have heard, Dr. Daryl Inaba, director of the drug detoxification and rehabilitation program at the Haight-Ashbury Free Clinic in San Francisco, said in an interview on "Prozac 'Abuse'" published in the February 23, 1994, *Anderson Valley Advertiser* (California): "From its early use in our clinical situation, patients mentioned that it had an arousal effect. . . . We've had some testimonies from clients who claim they inject Prozac and others who take it to get high. . . . A lot of people are taking Prozac now and claiming they're 'better than normal.' That's a scary phrase. What is 'better than normal'?"[67] Discussing the more stimulating of the new antidepressants, Inaba said, "They're getting pretty close to cocaine and speed." Responded the interviewer, "Cocaine for squares." That is, prescription drugs for people who would never consider taking illicit ones. Of course most patients are unsuspecting that their medication may be a stimulant. Had cocaine or amphetamines been discovered in the 1990s, the same kinds of pseudoscientific rationalizations for their effects—including disease models of depression and biochemical imbalances alleged to be due to neurotransmitter deficiencies—could have been invented for these drugs.

Lack of awareness about the effects of stimulants at prescription doses and the lack of clarity in the term "antidepressant" are two of the most fundamental misunderstandings on which the artifice of psychopharmacology has been built. The term "antidepressant" is misleading because it implies a definitive treatment for a definitive condition, neither of which is the case. Patients are better served by the truth: These drugs are stimulants for people who would otherwise be fatigued, distracted by negative thoughts, or have difficulty concentrating. With their energizing, attention-focusing, mood-elevating, and calming effects, serotonin boosters would make almost anyone feel better so long as they did not experience distressing side effects. This is why the drugs are such all-purpose psychoanalgesics, effective for everything from depression to anxiety to chronic pain syndromes to PMS. This, also, is why they make people feel "better than normal."

Of course, the effects of cocaine, amphetamines, tricyclics, the Prozac group, Wellbutrin, and other antidepressant drugs are not identical. They differ according to many variables, including their specific effects on the brain (which are still poorly understood), how long-acting they are, the dosage prescribed, and the sensitivity of individual patients. But all of these drugs have a core of stimulating properties—increasing energy, focusing attention, and brightening mood—which is essential to their clinical effects. All of them can "paradoxically" make people fatigued or lethargic, especially after weeks or months of use.

At the height of the popularity of prescription amphetamines, in 1975, Harvard psychiatrist Lester Grinspoon wrote an influential book called *The Speed Culture*. With remarkable foresight, Grinspoon predicted, "Drug companies probably will continue to produce increasingly sophisticated and disguised amphetamines, and these 'new' drugs undoubtedly will be greeted with initial enthusiasm by the medical establishment until it is recognized that any drug with amphetamine-like central nervous system stimulating properties almost invariably is just as toxic, potentially addic tive, and therapeutically limited as Benzedrine or Dexedrine [amphetamines]. . . . Only the medical jargon describing the alleged 'diseases' has become more sophisticated."[68]

In the 1980s, between the fall of amphetamine antidepressants and the introduction of Prozac, psychiatrists prescribed a class of agents called tricyclic antidepressants. In retrospect, tricyclics were a footnote in the history of antidepressants, never attaining the popularity of their predecessors or successors. When Prozac was introduced, it was much more stimulating than the tricyclics. Whereas doctors had become used to prescribing tricyclics at bedtime, Prozac needed to be taken in the morning because otherwise its stimulating effects would make it too difficult for people to fall asleep. This notable change was explained to doctors by introducing a euphemism: Prozac needed to be prescribed in the morning because it was "activating." In a series of papers in academic journals, psychiatrist Charles Beasley described Prozac's "activating" effects.[69] Beasley is an in-house researcher at Eli Lilly.

Initially, doctors, including myself, used this explanation and the word "activating" with patients. After hearing many people describe the effects of serotonin boosters, however, psychiatrists soon realized "activating" was a euphemism for "stimulating." The Prozac group are now often referred to by psychiatrists as "stimulating antidepressants." The very short-acting Wellbutrin (Zyban) is openly referred to by some psychiatrists as "stimulant-like," a term connoting "amphetamine-like."[70]

It turns out that in the 1980s when the FDA was reviewing Eli Lilly's application for approval to market Prozac, the agency noted that the drug behaved like a stimulant. As part of the review, Prozac's safety was evaluated by an FDA psychiatrist named Richard Kapit, who, in a 1986 memo, stated, "Unlike standard tricyclic antidepressants, Prozac's profile of adverse effects [i.e., side effects] more closely resembles that of a stimulant drug. . . . Among treatment emergent signs and symptoms, the most common effects produced by Prozac included nausea, insomnia, and nervousness. Indeed nervousness was the most common adverse symptom cited by long-term Prozac patients who eventually discontinued therapy due to an adverse reaction. In addition, Prozac is known to suppress appetite and produce weight loss" like other stimulants.[71]

Thus, the term "antidepressant" is virtually meaningless and seriously misleading. It is, as Grinspoon predicted, the latest disguise, the latest jargon for prescription stimulants. A further loophole in our system of drug regulation allows a drug, once it is approved, to be legally prescribed for any condition; therefore a drug approved as an "antidepressant" can be prescribed for everything from shyness to PMS to feeling "better than normal," or for whatever else a physician wishes to try it. At this point, any pretense to "rational therapeutics" is lost.

The Role of Managed Care in the Prozac Phenomenon

By now, a great many people look on managed care with deep skepticism, because they have some experience, direct or indirect, with one of its basic goals, which is to deliver medical care as cheaply as possible. Doctor-patient appointments become "products," counted like widgets coming off an assembly line. The goal is to keep "productivity" up and costs down. Patients are "customers" to be wooed with sophisticated marketing and then given as little as they will tolerate. Doctors find themselves cogs in the wheel, at odds with insurers who know little or nothing about clinical care. Managed care contracts include what are unofficially referred to as "gag rules," policies that prohibit doctors from telling patients the truth about the limited treatment options being offered to them. In recent years, President Clinton has championed legislation to weaken gag rules, but insurers circumvent the effects of such legislation by simply terminating clinicians who do not "cooperate."[72] Unfortunately, in order to survive, nonprofit hospitals and physician groups are forced to play by the same rules. Nowhere have the effects of managed care been more pervasive than in the delivery of mental health care. While managed care policies have cut the value of general medical insurance benefits by 7.4%, mental health benefits have been cut much more drastically in half.[73]

Dora was in her late sixties when she first consulted me for a second opinion about her treatment. Two years earlier, she had retired from being a schoolteacher. At first she enjoyed her newfound freedom, especially the extra time she had to spend with her grandchildren. But as the fall and winter wore on, she began to miss her work and to feel that she had too much time on her hands. Eventually she became mildly depressed.

At her HMO, Dora's doctor told her mild depression was a disease, a biochemical imbalance for which one takes Prozac. In less than twenty minutes, he gave her a prescription for a year's supply of the medication with no follow-up appointment. Initially, the drug made Dora feel more energetic, even "jittery." But after several months, although she did not exactly feel depressed, she developed a "bone-weary fatigue" on the medication. At the one-year mark, instead of just renewing her prescription, she called her doctor's office. The secretary instructed her to leave a message on his voice mail that she was running out of medication. To Dora's dismay, without even talking to her to see how she was doing, the doctor called in another year's worth of the drug to her pharmacy. Shortly thereafter, Dora decided to get a second opinion and consulted with me.

Born in Hungary, Dora was a delightful, gracious woman who still had a strong accent. When she was nine years old, her Jewish family fled Budapest as Hitler's army invaded the city. Unfortunately, the family was quickly captured. In a horrific scene, in the struggle with the soldiers, both Dora's parents were shot to death in front of her. She and her sixty-six-year-old grandmother were transported to Auschwitz. A month after entering the concentration camp, her grandmother went to her death.

After the war, Dora emigrated to the United States, married, raised a family, and taught for thirty years. All her life she worked hard to survive and to put the horrible Holocaust memories out of her mind. As we talked over the following months, it became clear that after she retired, with more time on her hands than she was used to, these memories returned and made her depressed. Painful feelings often surface when people have less structure in their lives, fewer activities to distract them.

At times during our work Dora was extremely sad, but after just six months of psychotherapy, working through the painful recollections and gradually easing off the medication, she was no longer depressed. She felt relieved both to be talking about the secrets from her past and to no longer be dependent on medication. How could her HMO have failed to inquire even minimally into her psychological state and life history? Are Holocaust memories really a "disease," a "biochemical imbalance" that should be "corrected" with a pill?

In countless cases like Dora's in recent years, the managed care industry has pressured primary-care providers not trained in psychiatry to treat psychiatric syndromes, especially depression, to reduce costs. To do the job, primary-care clinicians are trained to follow simple algorithms—treatment "protocols"—which are cookbook formulas for how to prescribe medication according to checklists. Especially where the compensation of primary-care providers is tied to keeping costs down, this results in a drastic reduction in services. This is true whether the insurer's doctors work in a staff-model HMO or in more loosely organized, office-based "networks."

The most pernicious financial arrangement is called capitation. In capitated systems, the doctor is paid a fixed amount per year per patient. If the doctor spends less than the allotted amount, she keeps the difference. If she spends more, the money comes out of her earnings. This makes the doctor the real insurer and the "insurer" a mere middleman skimming the profits. In a capitated system, a doctor has to keep referrals to specialists, and costs in general, down. She is literally paying for the referrals, and if she makes too many, she will lose money. This creates an inherent conflict of interest that most doctors do not like. But insurers insist on it. In another type of financial arrangement, a significant percentage of a doctor's income is withheld and only paid as an end-of-the-year "bonus" if the doctor has met the insurance company's requirements for cost cutting and efficiency, a key measure of which is keeping referrals to specialists at a minimum.

This policy of having primary-care doctors treat a significant percentage of mental health patients was facilitated by the introduction of serotonin boosters with their one-dose-fits-all-patients, ease of use, and their broad applicability for dozens of conditions, not just depression. With these easy-to-prescribe pills, managed care insurers pressed primary-care doctors to limit the treatment of depression and other psychiatric conditions to drugs with no regard whatever for the long-term consequences for patients. Now primary-care clinicians prescribe 70% of all antidepressants, much of it under duress from managed care.[74] A recent Rand study found that the majority of primary-care physicians spend less than three minutes counseling depressed patients.[75] As we have seen in many cases, prescriptions are frequently written for a year's supply with renewals by telephone voice mail. These drugs are far too potent for such a cursory approach.

Primary-care clinicians are not happy with this state of affairs but feel they have little choice. In a recent survey sponsored by the Robert Wood Johnson Foundation, 72% of primary-care doctors expressed frustration because of their inability to obtain quality mental health services for their patients.[76] The inability to access services is due to severe cutbacks in mental health staffing and the unwillingness of insurers to facilitate referrals. Some 5,000 doctors nationwide were questioned about a variety of medical specialties. Only 18% expressed frustration over accessing other specialists. The psychiatry number "jumped off the page," said Dr. Robert St. Peter, one of the researchers who conducted the survey: "Primary care physicians are identifying this set of services as significantly more difficult to get than other kinds of specialty services" because of restrictions imposed by managed care administrators.

Most primary-care clinicians do not feel they have the training to adequately serve psychiatric patients. They resent the heavy use of medications to mollify patients. Many say managed care has particularly discriminated against psychiatric patients and services because they are vulnerable. The privacy concerns of psychiatric patients make it difficult for them to protest managed care's practices in an individual, let alone an organized way. One primary-care doctor told me she was extremely distressed over a patient who committed suicide after being started on medication but before psychiatric services could be arranged. "I was devastated," she said, "after a patient I started on medication hanged himself before psychiatry was able to see him." Indeed, Dr. Leon Eisenberg of the department of social medicine at Harvard Medical School says, "Managed care and psychotropic drugs are a Satanic mix."[77]

For those patients who are referred to a mental health specialist, the controlling arm of managed care is still keenly felt. In order to limit expenditure on mental health, HMOs and managed care networks employ very few psychiatrists, and they are usually only expected to prescribe medication. Increasingly, psychiatric nurses are hired to do the prescribing, with supervision from psychopharmacologists. Clinical psychologists and social workers are often replaced with "therapists" with virtually no training who can "talk" to patients at a minimum of expense. Once again, everyone is following protocols. If the "therapist" cannot take care of someone in a few visits, they are instructed to send the patient back for another medication evaluation. Since the psychiatrists' and psychiatric nurses' positions depend on prescribing, there is great pressure to do so. Increasingly, psychiatrists' income is also subject to incentives for providing a minimum of care, which means medicating people.

At every juncture, the emphasis is on using medication to merely return patients to their baseline level of functioning and nothing more. To accomplish this, often ingenious biases are built into the system. Unlimited appointments for medication evaluations and checkups are typically allowed, whether with a primary-care clinician, a psychiatrist, or a psychiatric nurse. Even the medications themselves are fully covered, subject to a small co-payment. By contrast, psychological evaluations and psychotherapy are severely limited. This limitation is accomplished by requiring prior approval, reapproval after every five psychotherapy sessions, onerous monitoring, and severe paperwork, which grossly violates patient privacy.

Many managed care insurance plans advertise half a year's worth of psychotherapy—approximately twenty weekly visits—in their mental health "benefit." But realistically, few patients get more than five visits per year. In the fine print of HMO pamphlets are buried euphemisms like "medically necessary psychotherapy" (criteria excluding all but psychosis and imminent suicidality) and "quality assurance" (the onerous monitoring). Why even allow five? Because this is the minimum required by law in some states.

Privately, some managed care administrators acknowledge their false advertising and deceptive practices, justifying them as necessary to "compete in the marketplace." At the same time, they disparage people who want more than five sessions, saying they have to "educate" patients out of this "health care entitlement." Never mind that the patients are innocently trying to use the twenty visits advertised as part of their insurance plan. These practices have been perfected by national managed care companies, which provide low-budget mental health coverage to over 120 million Americans.

The September 1999 issue of the *NASW [National Association of Social Workers] News* reported that a federal class-action lawsuit has been filed in New York by a group of social workers, psychologists, and psychiatrists against nine of the largest managed care companies specializing in mental health care: Green Spring Health Services, Human Affairs International, Merit Behavioral Care, CMG Health, Options Healthcare, Value Behavioral Health, United Behavioral Health, Foundation Health Systems, and MCC Behavioral Care.[78] The suit specifically charges the companies with the inappropriate, excessive use of medication for psychiatric patients as well as "coercion," "intimidation," and terminating of therapists who protest their policies.

Further lawsuits and legislative efforts will probably be necessary to force insurers to provide more adequate treatment for patients. In private discussions, insurers make it clear they will not change of their own accord. Following the negative publicity about drive-by deliveries (women having to leave the hospital less than twenty-four hours after delivering babies), a number of states enacted legislation that forced managed care companies to allow women a minimum two-day stay in the hospital. Insurers say they have little problem with this because all of them are forced to provide the same coverage. The playing field remains level: everyone's costs, and therefore prices, are driven up by the same amount. No one is at a "competitive disadvantage." The point is that change can only be brought about by forces outside the insurance industry. Otherwise, only the most ruthless market forces control health care decisions.

At times, the financial incentives in managed care can be perverse in their effects on patient care. I recently had a patient who wanted to try St. John's wort for mild depression rather than go on a prescription drug. But he was unsure he could afford the herbal antidepressant. He was an artist—a painter—barely able to make ends meet on his salary as a pastry chef. The least expensive brand of St. John's wort he could find was $40 a month, more than he could afford. If he went on Prozac, his insurer would pay for it.

I agreed to call the patient's managed care insurer to see if they would reimburse him for the St. John's wort instead. Prozac would cost the insurer about $1,000 to $4,000 a year, depending on what dose he needed. Even though St. John's wort would cost significantly less, they were unwilling to pay for this natural alternative. Why would cost-conscious managed care insurers handle mental health treatment in this way? Principally, I believe, because of bureaucratic biases toward medicating psychiatric patients with powerful prescription drugs.

In an ironic twist in the last year, the skyrocketing prescription drug costs of HMOs have made national headlines.[79] For most HMOs, drugs now exceed their total costs for all types of medical and surgical hospitalizations. The drugs costing them the most money are the serotonin boosters, because these drugs have been so thoughtlessly pushed on patients. Now that this policy has backfired financially, HMOs and managed care insurers are trying to get doctors to prescribe the older, tricyclic antidepressants, which are as effective as the Prozac group. These older drugs are generic and vastly cheaper. But with the heavy promotion of the new antidepressants, few patients are willing to accept one of the older ones. As a cost-cutting alternative, many HMOs and managed care insurers contract for a discount with the manufacturer of one of the serotonin boosters. In return for a cut-rate price, an HMO pressures its doctors to prescribe the drug as the HMO's "preferred" serotonin booster. The pharmaceutical company strikes a tough bargain and actually monitors the HMO's prescriptions to be sure it gets an increasing "market share" of patients prescribed antidepressants. Otherwise, the pharmaceutical company will not renew the cut-rate price the following year. Sometimes insurers switch their "preferred" serotonin booster from one year to the next, depending on which pharmaceutical company will give them the cheapest price. They then ask doctors to switch the drug they preferentially prescribe to patients. While this is obviously ill advised with existing patients, it is often set as a goal with new ones.

Even if they are unwilling to pay for psychotherapy or natural alternatives like St. John's wort, insurers should not interfere with doctors' expressing their professional opinions to patients to explain, for instance, that many treatments are more effective and safer in the long term than drugs. Then patients can make their own choices about whether or not to pursue such treatments, even if not covered by their insurance. But managed care insurers discourage doctors from speaking frankly to their patients: the truth raises too many questions about why they refuse to pay, especially for helpful psychological interventions. So instead patients are misled into thinking they have genetically determined biochemical imbalances, "diseases," for which medications are the sole answer. What well-informed consumers of mental health care have come to realize is that nowadays it is a conflict of interest for insurers to advise them about mental health treatments, because they do not want to pay for alternatives to medication. Sadly, this can apply as well to their doctors, restrained by their insurers, following the insurers' protocols. The result is that patients need independent consultation, a second opinion, from clinicians who have no affiliation with their insurers.

Pharmacy Nation

In addition to psychopharmacology and managed care, the third major player in the Prozac phenomenon has been the pharmaceutical companies themselves. Over the years, the prices of the drugs keep going up. One year numerous patients brought to my attention the fact that the price of Prozac, Zoloft, and Paxil went up by 50%, increasing from about $2 to $3 a pill. In fact, the increase had not happened abruptly. Pharmacists report that while drugs like the Prozac group are under patent, their price goes up at regular intervals by about 3 to 5%. The patients just happened to notice it all at once when the price approached $3 a pill. The cost of drugs in the United States is much higher than in most of the rest of the world, where governments—often through the buying power of their national health services—negotiate prices with pharmaceutical companies. Sales of Prozac, Zoloft, and Paxil now exceed $4 billion a year. Awash with money, the pharmaceutical industry's influence on doctors, patients, and the culture at large has become pervasive.

With their funding of drug research, pharmaceutical companies buy the credibility of academic institutions. In recent decades, controversial contractual arrangements have formed partnerships between drug manufacturers and medical schools. Increasingly, the companies retain certain rights over the results of basic science research, such as any patentable products. Medical scientists are then unable to speak freely or collaborate on research in progress, because it has become subject to the secrecy of commercial product development. Publication of important research results is delayed by the long patent-application process or efforts to protect financial interests.[80] Some sponsoring companies even attempt to block publication of unfavorable results. A highly publicized example was a study of thyroid medications by researchers at the University of California at San Francisco, which was sponsored by Knoll Pharmaceutical Company. When the study did not find Knoll's Synthroid superior to three other drugs, the company delayed its publication for six years through a series of legal threats and intimidation. Indeed, Knoll only capitulated to publication of the study in the *Journal of the American Medical Association* after the case received intense media attention.[81]

In an example involving a psychiatric drug, in the 1980s Upjohn pharmaceutical company sponsored a study in which its Valium-type antianxiety agent, Xanax, was compared to behavior therapy for the treatment of panic attacks. The study was conducted by a group of researchers headed by Dr. Isaac Marks in London—one of the world's leading authorities on behavioral treatment—and Dr. Richard Swinson in Toronto. Published in the *British Journal of Psychiatry* in 1993, the study found behavior therapy superior to the drug, especially in the long term.[82] But, in an accompanying commentary published in the same issue of the psychiatric journal, the researchers reported that while Upjohn initially supported the study generously, the funding "stopped abruptly when the results became known. Thereafter, Upjohn's response was to invite professionals to critique the study they had nurtured so carefully before. The study is a classic demonstration of the hazards of research funded by industry."[83]

As a result of their enormous financial clout, pharmaceutical companies exert a pervasive influence on the agenda of biomedical research. When news broke that Eli Lilly was considering petitioning the FDA for approval to market a peppermint Prozac for depressed children, drug proponents acknowledged that we do not have adequate research documenting either the efficacy or safety of these drugs for depression in children.[84] Indeed, as described earlier, repeated studies have shown antidepressants are no more effective than placebos in depressed children. Studies of the long-term effects of the drugs on the developing nervous systems of children are lacking.

Undaunted, drug proponents insist that "while waiting for more research to be done," we need to "hold our breath" hoping for the best, and prescribe the drugs to children. But there is a precedent here. We have been prescribing amphetamine-like drugs, such as Ritalin, to children for six decades, since the 1930s. Says Ciba-Geigy in Ritalin's 1999 product information: Even though "suppression of growth (i.e., weight and/or height) has been reported with the long-term use of stimulants in children . . . sufficient data on the safety and efficacy of long-term use of Ritalin in children *are not yet available* [italics added]."[85] In a 1995 article in the *Journal of the American Medical Association*, Alan Zametkin, a psychiatrist at the National Institute of Mental Health, wrote, "Does early treatment with stimulants alter the integrity of dopamine systems at later stages of life? Until very long-term longitudinal studies are conducted, the effect . . . of stimulant treatment on the dopamine system ontogeny [development] in later life will remain unknown."[86]

In the sixty years we have had to do studies on children using stimulants, no significant long-term studies have been completed. Given the influence of pharmaceutical companies on the agenda of medical research, why should we "hold our breath" hoping that studies of the long-term effects of Prozac will be forthcoming? Given the repeated studies showing the drugs are no more effective than placebos in depressed children, why not treat children with psychotherapy, talk to them, instead of prescribing these powerful drugs?

Another area in which pharmaceutical companies wield enormous influence is medical "education." Most doctors in this country are visited on a regular basis by "representatives," salesmen from large pharmaceutical companies. In surveys, doctors list pharmaceutical salesmen as one of their most important sources of information about new drugs.[87] Salesmen and drug company "literature" are where doctors first learn about things like "serotonin imbalances" and serotonin "selectivity." Lavish advertisements in medical journals carry similar messages.

In addition, in recent decades pharmaceutical companies increasingly provide generous support for "symposia" at national and local psychiatric meetings. The symposia have names like "Recent Advances in the Treatment of Depression" or "Antidepressants: Current Clinical Issues." These conferences can include expensive dinners and gift certificates. Some symposia become traveling road shows, visiting major cities across the country. Others award continuing education credits, which doctors need to renew their licenses.

Pharmaceutical companies pay academic "experts" to give the talks for lucrative "honoraria," as "consultants" or members of their "speakers bureau." Many of the experts are the same people lavishly paid to do the clinical research on the drugs. Psychiatrist E. Fuller Torrey, director of research for the National Alliance for the Mentally Ill, told the group's annual meeting in the summer of 1998, "What gets put out is not necessarily the truth. You'd be surprised at how much money many of my colleagues are regularly taking from the pharmaceutical industry. Ten thousand dollars is not an uncommon amount to be given for giving a talk."[88] In some instances, the conferences are hosted by prestigious medical schools. Doctors attending the conferences for continuing medical education credits can be unaware that the speakers may be getting paid this kind of money to give the talks.

In a rare glimpse into the sums of money involved in consulting to pharmaceutical companies, the October 8, 1999, *Boston Globe* reported on the financial ties of Dr. Martin Keller to the pharmaceutical industry. Keller is a professor and the chairman of the department of psychiatry at Brown University. In recent years Keller has published research articles advocating long-term use of the new antidepressants—Zoloft in particular—to treat depression. Many of the articles have been coauthored with other psychopharmacologists who take a similar position. Appearing in prestigious medical and psychiatric journals, Keller's articles have the appearance of impartial academic publications. In the few journals that require an author to disclose financial ties to pharmaceutical companies, Keller lists being a "consultant," being on the "advisory board," or receiving "honoraria" from most of the manufacturers of the new antidepressants: Pfizer (Zoloft), Bristol-Myers Squibb (Serzone), Wyeth-Ayerst (Effexor), Eli Lilly (Prozac), Forest Laboratories (Celexa), and Organon (Remeron). Doctors are not required to disclose the exact dollar amounts involved. Few people would guess the payments could add up to hundreds of thousands of dollars a year. But in an unusual look at these kinds of financial arrangements, the *Boston Globe* reported that "Keller earned a total of $842,000 last year [1998], according to financial records, and more than half of his income came . . . from pharmaceutical companies whose drugs he touted in medical journals and at conferences."[89] The *Boston Globe* reported that Keller received more than half a million dollars in personal income from pharmaceutical companies. While publishing articles endorsing Zoloft, in particular, Keller received $218,000 in 1988 alone from Zoloft's manufacturer, Pfizer. "At the same time," continued the *Boston Globe,* "Keller was receiving millions of dollars in funding from the National Institute of Mental Health for research on depression and ways to treat it." The *Boston Globe* said Keller cited his prestigious NIMH-funded research in a journal article in which he made claims on behalf of drugs like Zoloft. The *Boston Globe* quoted Tufts University professor Sheldon Krimsky, who is a nationally known critic of the financial ties between academia and industry: If this case "does not represent a conflict of interest that should be avoided, then I don't know what such a conflict would be." Unfortunately, among prominent academic psychopharmacologists such a long list of financial ties to pharmaceutical companies is not uncommon.

Still another area of increasing influence is public "education." This is accomplished through myriad means, subtle and not so subtle, which now permeate the fabric of our society. The most commonly used methods are public relations, "public service," and advertising.

Large pharmaceutical companies maintain enormous public relations departments, which closely follow every development related to their drugs and proactively spin-control potentially damaging issues in the media. To cite just one example, in the fall of 1996 the *New England Journal of Medicine* published a study raising concerns about the taking of Prozac by pregnant women.[90] The study, which followed almost 500 pregnancies, found no increase in the rate of major structural abnormalities in newborns whose mothers had taken Prozac during the pregnancy. But an unusually high incidence of three or more minor malformations were observed in newborns exposed to Prozac during the first trimester. Headed by Christina Chambers and Kenneth Jones in the department of pediatrics at the University of California at San Diego, the study raised concern that the high rate of minor malformations in newborns "indicates that Prozac therapy during the first trimester of pregnancy has an effect on embryonic development. This finding raises the possibility of an associated defect in the development of the central nervous system [i.e., the brain] that may [only] become evident when the infant is older." When mothers took Prozac during the third trimester, infants had lower birth weights and shorter birth lengths, which the researchers suggested were due to the drug's appetite-suppressant effects. Of even greater concern was a higher incidence of premature delivery and neonatal complications requiring that infants be admitted to special-care nurseries.

Publicly, Eli Lilly took the position that Prozac should not be prescribed to pregnant women because this population of patients has not been adequately studied for the risks involved.[91] Knowing the research would make national headlines because of the large number of women on Prozac, however, the day before the study was published media outlets were flooded with a press release entitled "Health Wire" originating from Indianapolis, Indiana, Lilly's hometown.[92] The release criticized the article, saying that "independent" mental health experts questioned its validity. The press release provided the names of nine medical experts around the country who could answer reporters' questions and potentially be quoted in media reports of the *New England Journal of Medicine* article. Prominently quoted in the release and topping the list of experts was Dr. Lee Cohen of the Massachusetts General Hospital, a vocal defender of the use of serotonin boosters during pregnancy. By chance, the same month as the "Health Wire" press release, I attended a Harvard Medical School conference at which Cohen spoke. Tucked inside the conference syllabus was a "faculty disclosure statement" in which Cohen reported receiving funding—"grants" and "speaker's bureau" fees—from Eli Lilly (Prozac), Pfizer (Zoloft), and SmithKline Beecham (Paxil).[93] His financial ties to all three manufacturers of the biggest-selling serotonin boosters were not disclosed in the press release, which heavily quoted Cohen and suggested reporters call him. The press release specifically referred to "independent" mental health experts, which connotes doctors who are not employed by pharmaceutical companies. Obviously, to call experts "independent" and not disclose these kinds of behind-the-scenes financial arrangements is seriously misleading.

With their bevy of medical experts, the manufacturers of serotonin boosters spin-control countless, daily issues in the general media. These have included suicide and violence, personality change, sexual side effects, and withdrawal syndromes, as well as medication use during pregnancy.

Increasingly, pharmaceutical companies also liberally support public "education" about "advances" in psychiatry and medication treatments. National Depression Awareness Day began in 1991 and has grown into a huge media event. Media outlets receive glossy press kits well in advance of the day, generating countless newspaper and magazine articles, radio announcements, and television coverage. The media outlets provide the coverage as a free public service. On the day, in early October, thousands of sites in hospitals, corporations, and universities around the country provide free depression screening to anyone interested. The screening, which takes less than 5 minutes, consists of a modified version of the Zung self-rating scale for depression. People are then encouraged to watch a videotape that describes how treatable depression is.

In recent years, at many sites, National Depression Screening has grown to three months, October through December, during which people can telephone 800 numbers available twenty-four hours a day and take the Zung by touch-tone phone. Indeed, year-round screening is available in some locations. The automated, interactive program, which takes less than four minutes, inquires into ten different symptoms by asking the caller to rate statements such as "I have trouble sleeping through the night" or "I get tired for no reason." After each question, the caller is instructed, "Press 1 for none or a little of the time. Press 2 for some of the time. Press 3 for a good part of the time. Press 4 for most of the time." At the end of the questions, the caller's score is analyzed by computer and he is told how severe his symptoms are. Early on, a recorded operator-like voice informs the caller that you may think your symptoms are "a personal inability to cope with the pressures of life, but most often these symptoms are the result of clinical depression, an illness which responds extremely well to treatment." The 800 numbers are even individualized for special populations and will immediately link the caller to facilities like employee assistance programs, university health services, hospitals, or insurers.

This screening is operated by a nonprofit organization called the National Mental Illness Screening Project. But who pays for the expensive event, including elaborate press kits, screening kits for the test sites, and the months of 800 numbers with sound-bite psychiatry? An "educational grant from Eli Lilly and Company."[94] A consultant who helps pharmaceutical companies design such projects and find cooperative doctors to launch them told me they are called "public service with a profit motive." Indeed, every fall the depression screening infuriates many thoughtful psychiatrists, psychologists, and social workers, who call it "Dial-a-Prozac." One of the cruel ironies of the 1990s was that just as insurers cut already minimal mental health benefits for patients, pharmaceutical companies came bearing gifts.

In his superb 1997 book, *The Antidepressant Era,* psychiatrist David Healy describes the educational initiatives of pharmaceutical companies as shaping the medical marketplace. Observes Healy, "It may often be far more effective to sell the indication [i.e., what the drug is indicated for, such as depression] than to focus on selling the treatment."[95] Pharmaceutical companies have learned to market psychiatric illnesses "in the expectations that sales will follow."[96]

Healy points out that for the marketing of psychiatric diagnoses, they are often redefined to include much milder forms and, therefore, include many more people. This has been particularly true for depression, obsessive compulsive disorder, and social phobia. The term depression was formerly reserved for severe cases. The official term is currently "major" depression. But, we now have a "mild" version of "major" depression even though this would seem to be a contradiction.

The definition of obsessive-compulsive disorder (OCD) has also been dramatically expanded in recent years to include milder and milder cases. This has coincided with the marketing of new drugs, like the Prozac group, for the condition. At a Harvard Medical School conference on psychopharmacology in the fall of 1998, Dr. Ross Baldessarini said: "OCD when I went to school was a rare disease, especially severe OCD. Now they tell me it's two percent of the general population. Maybe. . . . But without drugs like Prozac to offer I don't think anybody would be terribly interested in OCD, quite frankly."[97]

Most recently, the definition of social phobia has gradually shifted towards something much more common. Social phobia was an obscure, rare diagnosis for people with severe symptoms. An example of someone with social phobia was a patient who could not go to movie theaters for fear that she could not get to an exit quickly enough. But in the late 1990s, psychiatrists began receiving mailings in which prominent academic psychopharmacologists suggested a new name for the condition: social anxiety.

Obviously, this term is less stigmatizing and could include a much larger number of people who describe themselves as self-conscious socially. The mailings were sponsored by SmithKline Beecham, the manufacturers of Paxil which soon became the first drug approved by the FDA for this condition. In the general media, the development was described as Paxil for shyness. So social phobia became social anxiety which, in turn, became shyness as another rare diagnosis was suddenly "discovered" to be commonplace coincident with the marketing of a drug for it. By comparison with other branches of medicine, diagnoses in psychiatry are uniquely vulnerable to this kind of manipulation.

The enormous profits of pharmaceutical companies are often justified on the basis of the costs of developing new drugs. But in a 1997 article in *Washingtonian* magazine, Thomas Moore of the George Washington University Medical Center stated, "Like tobacco and beer companies, the pharmaceutical industry spends more for advertising and promotion than for manufacturing or research. This means billions are available to polish the image of products—and to combat critics."[98]

And for the first time in decades, pharmaceutical companies are advertising heavily direct to the public. The 1962 Harris-Kefauver Amendment to the Federal Food and Drug Act imposed strict regulations on pharmaceutical company advertising. The requirements brought to a halt the aggressive marketing of notorious drugs like amphetamine antidepressants and barbiturates. But in the mid-1990s, the FDA liberalized the requirements pharmaceutical companies have to meet. The result has been a surge of advertising drugs direct to consumers.

Many doctors are uncomfortable with this development. In the May 15, 1999 issue of the *British Medical Journal,* professors Michael Wilkes and Jerome Hoffman of the UCLA Emergency Medicine Center in Los Angeles urged British physicians to resist the trend in the United States.[99] In an editorial entitled "Direct to Consumer Advertising of Prescription Drugs, An Idea Whose Time Should Not Come," Wilkes and Hoffman said: "Such advertising is a powerful tool, designed to create a demand, in order to maximize profits. . . . [It] has little to do with educating patients or relieving suffering. It will, however, inevitably drain healthcare dollars, dramatically increase unnecessary prescribing, and strain patient-doctor relationships. . . . Ultimately, of course, consumers pay for these promotions, whether it be the fortune spent on promotions to doctors (estimated to be about as much in the United States as is spent for all medical school and residency training combined) or the potentially even greater spending on direct to consumer advertising."

Wilkes and a group of colleagues had earlier conducted a study of prescription drug advertisements which showed "many claims prove to be inaccurate or misleading." The study was published in the June 1, 1992 issue of the *Annals of Internal Medicine*.[100] For the study, Wilkes' group asked medical experts to review 109 advertisements from the country's ten leading medical journals. Using the FDA's guidelines for pharmaceutical company advertising, the reviewers "indicated that 92% of advertisements were not in compliance in at least one area" of the FDA's guidelines. Wilkes' group speculated "that the FDA is unable or unwilling to enforce adequately its rules relating to drug advertising. It has been suggested that enforcement is hampered by a combination of budgetary restraints, limited manpower, and lack of regulatory authority to penalize pharmaceutical manufacturers for violating rules." In an accompanying editorial, Dr. David Kessler, then commissioner of the Food and Drug Administration, said: "As the study by Wilkes and coworkers indicates, the problem of misleading drug advertisements is real. . . . Prescription drug advertisements sometimes distort information in ways that may be difficult to detect by even the trained observer."[101]

For their advertising campaigns in the general media and professional journals, the manufacturers of the new antidepressants have developed themes, catchy slogans like those used in cigarette or beer ads. Effexor advertisements have the theme of reclaiming one's life. One ad shows a playful, laughing mother and young daughter running up the stairs. Beneath the rheumy photograph is a note written in crayon, "I got my mommy back." Another ad shows a rugged father and son with the note "I got my dad back." Still another shows a happy husband and wife leaning into each other in an affectionate hug. Below, two wedding bands are pictured intertwined beneath a note that reads, "I got my marriage back."[102]

Zoloft advertisements have a "Zoloft moment" theme. In one advertisement, a young couple happily swing their son in a zesty playground. The verse: "A great day for Dad. A great day for Mom. A terrific day for the family. Make it happen. The Zoloft Saturday." Another ad shows a woman who has just woken up but is impeccably groomed, dressed in a white terry robe. Her charming cat is perched on a shelf above her bathroom sink. The woman is so happy she is tickling the cat's chin with her toothbrush. The verse: "A new day. A brighter outlook. Make it happen. The Zoloft Morning."[103]

Eli Lilly's advertisements depict Prozac as a sunshine pill. Across two elaborate full-color pages, a dark rain cloud of depression contrasts with a sunburst of Prozac. In another variation, a shattered eggshell contrasts with a sunny Prozac flower.[104] Beneath the Hallmark card–like drawings, half a dozen paragraphs wax poetic about Prozac's ability to remedy serotonin deficiencies. The large-print, simplistic text gives the impression the drugs are eminently safe, not "habit-forming," and cause only "mild side effects." Only on the third, back page, in barely readable fine print, does one find "suicidal ideation [thoughts]" for the controversy over Prozac's inducing suicide and violence; "anorgasmia" for the drug's severe sexual side effects; "extrapyramidal syndrome" for the group of four closely related neurological side effects; and "buccal-lingual-masticatory [cheek-tongue-chewing] syndrome with involuntary tongue protrusion" for disfiguring tics.

This escalating war of trivializing jingles now permeates the fabric of our pharmacy nation. In the psychiatrist's office, the influence of these simplistic messages is difficult to overcome. In recent years, endless "public service" programs and advertisements designed by marketing executives are trying to usurp the role of doctors providing patients with more balanced information. As we will see in the next chapter, for moderately to severely depressed patients, antidepressants have real benefits, jump-starting them on the road to recovery. But powerful psychoactive drugs ought not to be promoted like consumer products with the aim of selling as many as possible. Writing in the *International Journal of Risk and Safety in Medicine* in 1998, Drs. Giovanni Fava and Elena Tomba lamented the "unprecedented power which the pharmacological industry has come to exert over clinical research and the dissemination of information. . . . Psychiatric researchers readily find themselves skating on thin ice: either they become salespeople (and—regrettably—the main trend of many [professional] meetings is apparently to sell the participants to the sponsors [pharmaceutical companies]) or they must set out boldly to protect the community from unnecessary risks."[105]

Patients need to be informed of the behind-the-scenes forces influencing their treatment. When told they have serotonin deficiencies that will be corrected by Prozac, Zoloft, or Paxil, few patients are aware this is speculation, a way of marketing the drugs, not an established scientific fact. When offered an "antidepressant," most patients are unaware the drug is an all-purpose psychoanalgesic, a stimulating medication prescribed for dozens of other conditions too. Many patients are unaware the reason they are offered medication and not psychotherapy is that their managed care insurer does not want to pay for safer, more effective treatment. Looking at an enticing, glossy advertisement for Prozac, patients often do not realize how misleading its message is. Instead of these misleading messages, patients need to understand the appropriate role of medication in balanced, comprehensive treatment.

6

Unraveling Depression
Stifled Anger and Sadness

Over the centuries, dozens of approaches to depression have evolved, many of them full of wisdom, compassion, and humanity. Each has its own strengths and weaknesses. The best way to overcome depression is to use a combination of these approaches to simultaneously address multiple facets of the condition in an effort to speed recovery. When trying to decide what is the appropriate balance of prescription medication and natural alternatives, the most important question is whether depression is mild, moderate, or severe. Potent prescription drugs should be reserved for moderate to severe cases; for mild to moderate depression, psychotherapy and other alternative approaches have proven as effective in the short term as medications and more effective in the long term.

Jenny: A Case of Mild Depression

Jenny was a twenty-four-year-old sales clerk in Harvard Square who came to see me because she was distraught after her boyfriend Paul broke up with her. Jenny had been dating Paul for two years when he abruptly ended their relationship, leaving her shocked and confused. A wan-looking young woman with tears streaming down her cheeks, she said, "I don't understand what's happened. We'd been living together for a year. I thought everything was going fine. Two weeks ago I came home from work and all his stuff was gone. His friends helped him to move out."

Jenny felt "haunted" by the half-empty apartment. "His TV is gone.

His leather chair is gone. The coat closet is empty. Everywhere I turn I'm reminded of him," she said inconsolably.

Jenny said her family and friends were "fed up" with how "obsessed" she was with Paul: "He's all I think about. I want to know what he's doing every minute of the day. I talk to him three or four times a day."

Even though Paul had moved out in such a callous manner, Jenny was angry with herself, not him: "'What did I do wrong?' I keep wondering. Maybe I didn't give him enough space. He always wanted to spend time with his friends and I liked to tag along. Maybe I hung around him too much."

"You *were* his girlfriend," I countered, gently.

"Maybe it's my weight. I was so happy with him the last two years I put on ten pounds. I knew I should have lost it."

"If he broke up with you over ten pounds, I don't think he was worth having in your life."

"But I miss him so much." Jenny heaved a sigh between sobs.

Jenny's self-reproach was characteristic of women who are obsessed with a boyfriend who has broken up with them. She was sleeping fitfully, waking several times a night preoccupied with Paul. Whenever she talked about him she could not help crying. In spite of how distressed she felt, her work was going well. Indeed, her work was an "escape" from how awful she felt, a welcome "distraction."

While Jenny was mildly depressed, her ability to function was fully intact. In many ways it is a shame to use the word "depressed" in relation to her case. She was simply distraught over a breakup. Of course, there was the concern that her condition might worsen. Nowadays, however, because of the overdiagnosing of depression to support the liberal use of antidepressants, Jenny would be a prime candidate for the diagnosis and for medication. Yet her case was easily solved with short-term psychotherapy.

Psychotherapy

The cornerstones of psychotherapy are insight and emotional growth. Psychotherapy aims to shed light on the relationship between the conscious and unconscious psychological realms. One's mood and behavior are seen as influenced not only by one's present circumstances but also by past experiences and unconscious emotional forces. Becoming aware of previously unconscious emotions and finding patterns in one's behavior effect recovery from acute depression and make one less vulnerable to depression in future.

As Jenny and I talked, it became clear that Paul had not treated her well even prior to the insensitive way in which he broke up with her. He first began seeing Jenny in secret, while still in a relationship with his previous girl-friend. During their relationship, on at least two occasions he was unfaithful to Jenny. Paul worked part-time or not at all. Most months Jenny paid their rent, phone, food, and other bills. In spite of this, Jenny seemed only to admire Paul. She described him as exciting, outgoing, and fun-loving. She rationalized his poor treatment of her as "immaturity" and "maybe a little selfishness."

A month into our work, Jenny came to her session more upset than ever. During the week, her "worst fear" was confirmed: Paul had begun dating another girl months before he broke off their relationship. Once again, instead of being angry with him, Jenny only felt worse about herself: "Now all I can think about is what she must be like."

"What do you imagine?"

"I imagine she's prettier than me. Paul must find her more attractive and interesting. She's probably smarter. Everything I imagine about her is bet-ter than me," said Jenny in tears. "When I believed him that he just wanted a break from the relationship, I could imagine we might get back together. Knowing he has another girlfriend, that he chose someone else over me, makes me feel so much worse."

Not only had Paul been unfaithful to Jenny before breaking up with her, he had been lying about it ever since. Jenny learned of the other woman from a mutual friend. Paul's duplicity provided the first opportunity to re-ally question Jenny's one-sided view of their relationship. Gradually Jenny began to express some anger over Paul's treatment of her. Should she con-front him about his new relationship, she wondered.

"Why not?" I encouraged her.

Slowly, Jenny "worked up the courage." When Paul again denied hav-ing a new girlfriend, for the first time Jenny was upset with him. She angrily told Paul that, in fact, she knew about the relationship. Only at that point did he admit to it. Jenny was further outraged when he acknowledged hav-ing unprotected sex for a period of time with both Jenny and the new woman.

"That's awful," I said vigorously.

"You don't do that nowadays," Jenny protested. "He put me at risk and didn't even tell me."

"The way he was treating you sexually is a metaphor for how he was treating you in general," I said.

I encouraged Jenny to see her family doctor in case there was cause to be concerned about her health. Hearing the story, he performed a full battery of tests for sexually transmitted diseases, including AIDS. Having to have an AIDS test upset Jenny and drove home the risks Paul had exposed her to. Fortunately, all the tests came back negative. Still, anxiously waiting for the results only heightened Jenny's anger at Paul over his treatment of her.

In addition to her anger, Jenny began to express considerable sadness. Genuine sadness is quite different from depression. Sadness is a clarifying, relieving emotion that helps one move on after losses. By contrast, depression is a paralyzing short circuit of self-doubt and self-recrimination. Jenny was sad to lose the good parts of her relationship with Paul. She felt bad, too, that she had misjudged him. She hoped this would not happen in future relationships.

As Jenny became increasingly angry and sad, her depression cleared. One sees this repeatedly with people who are distraught and obsessed over a breakup. They are depressed precisely because they are not appropriately angry and sad over the situation. While this is true in general for depressed people, it is particularly striking in breakups because the problem is so specific to a particular relationship and its reversal can be seen so vividly.

As Jenny became more angry with Paul and less angry with herself, she nevertheless needed to take responsibility for her own actions in the relationship. Patients do not benefit from being encouraged to get in touch with anger at other people to the exclusion of taking responsibility themselves. Jenny should not have gotten involved with Paul when he was deceiving his former girlfriend. This set the precedent for what eventually happened to her. Paul's repeatedly being unfaithful to Jenny and not contributing his fair share to supporting their apartment should also have been warning signs. In future, she needed to have higher expectations of boyfriends from the outset of the relationship.

Clinical Research on the
Effectiveness of Psychotherapy

In the 1980s, the National Institute of Mental Health (NIMH) funded a large-scale study comparing psychotherapy with antidepressant drugs in the treatment of depression. The study involved over two hundred patients at multiple sites across the country. Twelve prominent psychiatrists and psychologists led by Drs. Irene Elkin and Tracie Shea at the NIMH published the results in the November 1989 issue of the *Archives of General*

Psychiatry.[1] Overall, by the end of sixteen weeks of treatment, psychotherapy and prescription antidepressants had produced comparable results. Roughly two-thirds of patients responded to either treatment modality. Because of the large number of patients involved and the prestige of the authors, the NIMH study was considered a landmark demonstrating comparable results for psychotherapy and drugs in the short-term treatment of depression.

Since the NIMH study, numerous others have produced similar results.[2] Another well-known, large-scale study involving over 100 patients was conducted by researchers at the University of Minnesota.[3] In the Minnesota study, one group of patients received three months of treatment with cognitive therapy while another group received antidepressant medication. A third group received a combination of both. Dr. Steven Hollon headed a team of seven psychologists and psychiatrists. In the October 1992 issue of the *Archives of General Psychiatry,* they reported, "No differences in overall responses were observed" in patients treated with therapy versus drugs. Moreover, "combining cognitive therapy with pharmacotherapy did not markedly improve response over that observed for either modality alone."

To diagnose patients and monitor their progress, the studies use the same kinds of rating scales and symptom checklists used by pharmaceutical companies in the clinical testing of new antidepressants. They are therefore subject to the limitations of short-term, symptom-focused research described in the previous chapter. But when psychotherapy is tested in the same way drugs are, it performs comparably. When pharmaceutical companies and drug advocates promote antidepressants as "scientifically proven" in the treatment of depression, they typically fail to point out that psychotherapy has proven as effective by the same methods.[4]

In some studies, antidepressants do work a little faster than psychotherapy.[5] In my experience with patients, drugs begin to work within one to six weeks, while psychotherapy takes six to eight weeks. But in pharmacotherapy patients are left feeling impotent in the face of problems and reliant on drugs. Indeed, patients are often left with the idea they are genetically defective and therefore in need of medication indefinitely. Psychotherapy addresses the underlying psychological causes of depression, whereas drugs merely ameliorate symptoms and can even paper over the real problems. Moreover, psychotherapy is free of the side effects and serious risks of prescription medications. Patients come away from psychotherapy with the sense of having overcome difficulties themselves. This makes the extra few weeks that psychotherapy takes to work well worth the wait.

Acute Symptoms Versus the Underlying
Vulnerability to Depression

Short-term studies of psychotherapy or antidepressants only assess the initial phase of treatment in which the goal is relief from depressive symptoms. This typically takes two to three months to accomplish, as seen in clinical practice and repeatedly documented in the clinical studies. But good psychiatric treatment does not end once acute symptoms have abated. The longer-term goal is addressing the patient's underlying vulnerability to depression. Why had Jenny reacted as she had to Paul's breaking up with her? What was the taboo she felt against feeling anger and sadness? Why were these angry and sad feelings turned against herself instead of Paul?

For most of her childhood, Jenny's father had been an alcoholic. He gambled his paycheck away, was unfaithful to her mother, and was often verbally abusive at home. With four children and an alcoholic husband, Jenny's mother was overwhelmed. Jenny told me many stories of her mother herding the children into the car when her father was in a rage. She would bring them to the library for hours to take refuge while their father slept off a drinking binge.

As the oldest of four children, Jenny ended up in a parental role, helping her mother care for her younger brothers and sisters. Much of the time, she even took care of her mother—emotionally, at any rate—acting as her mother's confidante. Under these circumstances, Jenny's own emotions, her anger toward and fear of her father, were given short shrift. Buried even deeper were her anger and disappointment with her mother for not being able to remedy the situation. This was where she learned not to feel anger and sadness welling up in her but to stifle them in order to cope. Jenny spent several additional months in therapy working on these deeper issues so that in future she would not have the same problems again.

Family, Friends, and Church

Family, friends, and church are valuable community resources, which patients should be strongly encouraged to make use of while recovering from depression. These are people who have been in a patient's life far longer than a therapist and will continue to be there long after therapy is complete.

Jenny's family was quite supportive of her efforts to reassess not only her relationship with Paul but also her early family history. Jenny's father had been sober in Alcoholics Anonymous for six years. In addition, couples therapy had helped her parents salvage their marriage. Now doing much better, her parents had long worried that Jenny had never dealt with the earlier family history and were supportive of her doing so now.

Jenny's family were Unitarians and members of a close-knit congregation. As she and I discussed her earlier reluctance to feel anger and sadness over Paul, Jenny wondered what her minister would say about the benefits or disadvantages of succumbing to these "negative" emotions. I encouraged Jenny to meet with the minister and find out. Fortunately, the message she received from her minister was much the same as what she had already gotten both from her friends and in therapy with me.

Sometimes patients get messages from therapists that are entirely contradictory to those they get from friends and family. Some patients describe their families' and churches' explicitly telling them that anger and sadness are bad emotions, because they make one less "perfect" and therefore less close to God. When one runs into this kind of conflict, a good therapist does not simply advance another dogma to which the patient must adhere. Rather, the therapist does his best to offer an alternative view, perhaps suggesting that the former approach may be part of the patient's problem. But the patient must be free to choose whether or not, and how far, to explore her feelings.

Jenny was also fortunate to have a group of close friends who were attentive to her as she struggled with her feelings. Two of Jenny's friends, also cashiers who worked with her, originally had convinced her to seek professional help. Although they knew Paul and liked him in many ways, they did not understand why Jenny was not upset with him over the way in which he broke up with her. As she slowly got in touch with her anger and sadness, they were encouraging and supportive, taking her to lunch or dinner, drawing her out, and helping her sort through her feelings.

Late in our work, Jenny saw Paul and his new girlfriend in a mall. Her reaction, she said, was a measure of how much progress she had made: "A few months ago seeing Paul like that would have set me way back. I would have felt incredibly jealous and inadequate. Instead, I just felt sad about the way the whole thing had gone and, frankly, a little sorry for his new girlfriend. Her relationship with Paul could well end the same way mine did."

Lydia: A Case of Moderate Depression

Lydia was a thirty-three-year-old black woman whose mood plummeted after she was offered her "dream job" and the opportunity to move back to

Washington, D.C., which she had longed to do for years. Lydia and her husband, Eric, had moved from Washington to New England five years earlier. Much had changed in their lives during this time: Both Lydia and Eric had established themselves in careers and now had two young sons. As their lives evolved, Lydia found herself emphasizing work and career more than Eric did. Lydia was a medical laboratory technician who had taken on increasing administrative responsibilities in the clinical laboratory of the Massachusetts General Hospital. Eric was a fourth-grade teacher who had become the primary parent for their two sons.

Particularly after the boys were born, both Lydia and Eric wanted to return to Washington. They missed the warmer, more relaxed climate. Both their families were in Washington and they wanted the boys to grow up surrounded by grandparents and cousins. In the year before I met Lydia, she made several trips to Washington to job-hunt intensively. When the "perfect position" became open at a Washington hospital, she fought hard to win it. Not only did Lydia land the job, the hospital agreed to hold the position for her for six months so Eric could finish out the year teaching and their two sons would not have to move in the middle of the school year.

Shortly after Lydia pulled off this coup, she developed "cold feet" over whether or not she could handle the added responsibilities of the new position, where she would be supervising more people and helping the director of the lab with his research. As the weeks wore on, Lydia's mood and energy level sank. She found herself turning to food for comfort, which she described as an "old habit," and was battling the temptation for fear of gaining weight. At night, Lydia sometimes went to bed right after dinner because she felt so "exhausted." Even after ten hours of sleep, some mornings she had difficulty getting out of bed to "face the day."

"This just isn't like me," stammered Lydia, a petite black woman with close-cropped hair and fiery, determined eyes. "I usually love a challenge. How can I be upset when I got what I wanted? When everything is going so well?"

Lydia's low mood and energy level had begun to affect her ability to function. Although she was eventually getting important tasks done, she was uncharacteristically inefficient. She was letting less important things slide and worried that if her condition worsened she would become "totally dysfunctional." This fear was the reason she sought treatment.

Lydia was moderately depressed, having crashed after securing her dream job. She was more depressed than Jenny had been; her symptoms were more serious and her ability to function was impaired. Was Lydia's depression a severe form of the letdown people sometimes experience after a marathon effort to achieve a desired goal? Was it a lack of confidence that surfaced only once she secured a job that was going to be a big leap? Was she conflicted over taking on a bigger position? Did she unconsciously have mixed feelings about returning to Washington, in spite of her protests that this was "exactly what she wanted"?

Cognitive Therapy

Because she was a scientist and practical sort of person, a different emphasis in psychotherapy appealed to Lydia. Prior to consulting with me, Lydia had purchased one of the popular cognitive therapy workbooks for depression currently available. Cognitive therapy focuses on the negative-thinking characteristic of depression. The patient's persistently negative views of herself, the world, and the future are called the "cognitive triad" of depression. These negative views are maintained by specific cognitive distortions such as all-or-none, black-or-white thinking; selectively attending to negative events while ignoring positive ones; or catastrophizing, always anticipating the worst. Cognitive therapists have identified more than a dozen cognitive distortions that are considered responsible for a patient's depressed mood and compromised functioning. The goal of the therapy is to change the distortions by restructuring or reframing a patient's negative belief systems in order to effect more adaptive behavior, with an emphasis on creating practical solutions to current problems.

One day Lydia came to therapy distraught after speaking on the phone with a real estate broker from Washington. During the conversation, she had discovered how much higher housing prices are in Washington, especially in Georgetown, than in Boston. In therapy, she blurted out in shock, "I'll have to commute two hours in and out of the city to find a house we can afford." Since the phone call, Lydia had convinced herself that she would not be able to buy a house in a town with good schools, that Eric would not find a job he liked, that the move to Washington would be a disaster, and that she should never have uprooted her life this way.

Lydia and I spent the session dissecting this downward spiral of negative thinking. Following the format of her cognitive therapy workbook, she first described the situation, her feelings, and her thoughts (called her inner "dialogue"). Then she analyzed her inner dialogue looking for cognitive distortions. Next, she came up with a restructured dialogue, a more positive way of viewing the situation. Finally, she noted how this restructured dialogue made her feel. By the end of the session, Lydia felt calmer and better able to deal with the housing problem. After the session, she filled out a worksheet in her cognitive therapy book summarizing our discussion. The worksheet read:

SITUATION: Spoke with Washington, D.C. broker. Housing prices are astronomical in the few good neighborhoods.

FEELING: Helpless. Confused. Frustrated.

DIALOGUE: We can't afford a house inside the District. I'll be exhausted commuting back and forth to work. Any town where we can afford to buy will not have good schools. The boys are the ones who are really going to suffer. Eric won't be able to get a good job. It's all my fault because I wanted to move.

COGNITIVE DISTORTION: All-or-none thinking. Catastrophizing.

RESTRUCTURED DIALOGUE: We'll be okay. We'll find a smaller house with less land closer to the city. If we have to, we'll buy a condominium. Everyone is looking forward to moving. The idea wasn't just mine.

FEELING: I blew that one out of proportion! Feeling better.

Cognitive therapy helps people see the cup as half full instead of half empty. With repeated examples, Lydia began to internalize the process of deconstructing her negative thinking. She began to go through the steps on her own, nipping negative thoughts in the bud.

Changing Work and Sleep Habits

On the behavioral side, Lydia and I went over her daily schedule in detail. One of her biggest problems was oversleeping, not getting out of bed in time and then running late throughout the day. "I hide under the covers," said Lydia, "because I don't want to face the day. When the alarm goes off, I push the snooze button for an extra ten minutes of sleep. I don't just do it once. I do it four or five times every morning." As she lay in bed hiding, Lydia could hear the sounds of Eric and the boys getting ready for the day. The extra time in bed did not help in any real way. Rather, she only felt disappointed and "guilty" over missing the time with her family.

At work, Lydia often put her head down on her desk and dozed off for half-hour naps. In the evenings and on weekends she would "escape" to her bed to "steal" a nap whenever possible. Said Lydia, "The boys have never seen me this way before, sluggish and avoidant. I'm ashamed of setting such an example for them."

Irregular sleeping hours and daytime naps complicate the problems of depression. Some patients doing creative work argue that irregular hours and procrastination are important to ultimately get their adrenaline up in the home stretch for their most "inspired" work. This rationalization breaks down if depression and lack of progress set in. Under these circumstances, I urge people to give up any romantic notions of fits and starts of inspiration in favor of steady, reliable work.

Lydia and I worked out a strict routine for the first hour of her day. She moved her alarm to the other side of the room. Immediately upon getting up, she took a cold shower. She dressed in the bathroom, having put her clothes out the night before, so she would not have to return to the bedroom with its temptation of going back to bed. Once downstairs, she brought in the newspaper and read it for twenty minutes over breakfast. Adhering to this schedule religiously, within forty-five minutes of getting out of bed Lydia found herself alert and ready to approach the day.

During the day, Lydia began resisting the temptation to nap. She devised numerous "tricks" to avoid naps and push herself to make it through the day. By getting up at a regular hour and avoiding daytime naps, she found herself tired at night and sleeping more soundly.

As we talked, Lydia came up with a plan to be in the office by seven o'clock in the morning, when she could work with fewer distractions. As she set out to implement the new schedule, Lydia's boss gave her approval to come in early and leave early at the other end of the day. The laboratory secretary also "got in on the act" and began protecting Lydia from phone calls and other disruptions until at least ten in the morning. In this way, Lydia had several hours uninterrupted in which to make significant progress on the lab's annual report, budget, proposals, and other projects she needed to complete before moving. Although initially the new schedule was a struggle to put into effect, once Lydia was adhering to it she found herself "getting more done by ten o'clock in the morning than I had been in whole days!"

Lydia also needed to prioritize tasks. When her new boss from Washington sent her some research protocols to review, she initially avoided this intimidating task with the "excuse" that she needed to work on the annual report and budget for her current lab. In fact, the research protocols from Washington were more important and deserved higher priority. I worked with Lydia on setting priorities and utilizing her protected, early-morning time to address the top priority each day. She had to tolerate temporarily letting other things slide, otherwise important tasks would never get done.

People often feel depressed and overwhelmed as they finish a job or creative endeavor and need this kind of hands-on, pragmatic help to focus during the home stretch. Many times, therapists help patients through their struggles trying to finish books, theses, academic degrees, research projects, films, or other work. A willingness to get into the nitty-gritty details with patients is an important part of a collaborative therapy. When Lydia gave me a copy of her workbook at the end of therapy, I was amazed by the long, daily lists she had made of tasks to complete and their relative priority.

Combinations of cognitive therapy and behavioral changes are often called cognitive-behavioral treatment for depression. In clinical research, cognitive-behavioral treatment has become the dominant type of therapy studied, because it is particularly easy to standardize. Therapists can be trained to use manuals and workbooks with cognitive-behavioral exercises. The therapy can be replicated by researchers at different sites around the country.

Cognitive-behavioral treatment has also become popular with managed care administrators. Often, it is the only form of psychotherapy they allow, typically in conjunction with antidepressant medication, even though many studies have shown psychotherapy on its own is as effective. Rather than being seen individually, patients are often put into groups lasting eight to ten weeks for short-term cognitive-behavioral treatment.

St. John's Wort

In addition to psychotherapy, Lydia went on the increasingly popular herbal antidepressant St. John's wort. An estimated 7.5 million Americans are currently taking St. John's wort, which has been dubbed "natural Prozac."[6] Where does the herb's name come from? "Wort" is the Old English word for plant. Its yellow flowers begin to bloom around June 24, the feast of Saint John the Baptist.

St. John's wort is also known by its Latin name, *Hypericum perforatum*, and has been used as a medicinal agent for centuries. Ancient Greek physicians prescribed hypericum for depression, anxiety, and insomnia.[7] Hypericum oil was applied topically for wounds, burns, aches, and pains because of its antibacterial and anti-inflammatory effects. In this country, as recently as the mid-nineteenth century in Shaker colonies, hypericum was used to treat depression and insomnia.[8] In recent decades, St. John's wort has become a popular antidepressant in Europe. Indeed, it is the most commonly used antidepressant in Germany.

In health food stores, St. John's wort is available in a number of preparations, including liquid extracts, tinctures, capsules, tablets, and teas. Most people are familiar with tea as an herbal preparation of dried leaves, buds, and flowers, which is steeped in hot water and then strained to produce a flavorful drink. Liquid extracts and tinctures are made in a similar way. The dried plant material is steeped in an alcohol-based fluid and then strained. Extracts contain higher concentrations of the botanical agent than tinctures. To make capsules and tablets, a powdered form of the dried plant is reconstituted in a solid medium.

Patients who are health food aficionados say liquid extracts and tinctures are the most natural and therefore the healthiest forms of St. John's wort to use. However, most people take the capsules or tablets for convenience. The tea form probably does not contain high enough concentrations to achieve the doses necessary to counteract depression. In recent years, as St. John's wort has risen in popularity, most preparations are available in 300-milligram doses, which are taken three times a day, for a total daily dose of 900 milligrams. St. John's wort may take one to two months to achieve a full effect. Many people who report, "I tried it and it didn't work" only took 300 to 600 milligrams a day for two to three weeks before giving up.

Like most patients, Lydia experienced no side effects on St. John's wort—a remarkable contrast to the frequent, even dangerous, side effects of prescription antidepressants. "I don't feel drugged on St. John's wort like my friends do on antidepressants," said Lydia. "They all complain of sexual problems, nausea, apathy, or changes in their weight. Taking St. John's wort feels more like taking a vitamin." Occasionally, patients report having an upset stomach after a dose. This is easily remedied by taking it with food rather than on an empty stomach. Patients should not mix St. John's wort with prescription antidepressants because of potential adverse interactions.

The effectiveness of St. John's wort has been demonstrated in numerous clinical studies. As with synthetic drugs, these are short, typically four-to-eight-week, studies in which one group of patients receives St. John's wort while another group receives placebo pills.[9] In 1994, the *Journal of Geriatric Psychiatry and Neurology* published seventeen research papers on St. John's wort in an issue entitled "Hypericum: A Novel Antidepressant."[10] In repeated studies, roughly two-thirds of patients responded to the herbal antidepressant, which Drs. G. Harrer and V. Schulz noted are "rates that are equivalent to those achieved with standard synthetic substances."[11] In studies comparing St. John's wort directly to prescription antidepressants, the herb yielded "comparable results" with far "fewer and milder side effects" than the synthetic drugs.[12] Indeed, one study reported, "Notable side effects were not found."[13] Said another, "In no case were any undesirable side effects observed."[14] In an accompanying editorial, Michael Jenike, a psychiatrist at Harvard Medical School, wrote, "This benign side effect profile may make St. John's wort a particularly attractive choice for treating mild-to-moderate depressions."[15]

In August 1996, the *British Medical Journal* published a review of twenty-three studies of St. John's wort involving a total of 1,757 patients.[16] Headed by Dr. Klaus Linde of the Ludwig Maximilian University in Munich, the review was written by half a dozen researchers in Germany and the United States. Twenty of the twenty-three studies reviewed used a double-blind design, considered the gold standard scientifically. The results of the studies were pooled in an overall meta-analysis. The results showed St. John's wort outperformed the placebo just as synthetic agents do. In studies where St. John's wort was compared directly with synthetic drugs, it proved comparable. Overall, 64% of patients responded to St. John's wort while 59% responded to a synthetic, prescription antidepressant. Summarizing Linde's report, the *British Medical Journal* said that "head to head comparisons suggested hypericum was as effective as standard antidepressants. These findings show that hypericum is a promising treatment for depressive disorders."

While the published studies in both the *Journal of Geriatric Psychiatry and Neurology* and the *British Medical Journal* are widely quoted, it is worth noting that when St. John's wort was compared with prescription antidepressants, relatively modest doses of the drugs were used. Thus, the antidepressant effects of St. John's wort are best described as comparable with a low dose of a prescription drug. When taken at the recommended dose, St. John's wort may be roughly equal to 5 to 10 milligrams a day of Prozac in terms of its antidepressant effect. For many patients with mild to moderate depression, this is more than sufficient, and the herb's far better side-effect profile makes it preferable.

Reviewing studies comparing St. John's wort to placebo, Dr. Steven Bratman, in his 1999 book *St. John's Wort and Depression,* points out that in at least one way they are superior to studies comparing prescription antidepressants to placebo. An authority on herbal remedies, Bratman says, "Drugs cause side effects [that] . . . may allow patients to distinguish between drug and placebo. . . . Thus the influence of the power of suggestion cannot be excluded from drug versus placebo tests. This makes the legitimacy of all double-blind studies for traditional antidepressant medication somewhat suspect. However, no similar problem occurs with the essentially side-effect free St. John's wort."[17]

In spite of St. John's wort's demonstrated efficacy, psychopharmacologists have resisted it as a competitor to standard antidepressant drugs. In a piece accompanying the review of St. John's wort studies in the *British Medical Journal,* Dutch psychopharmacologists Peter De Smet and Willem Nolen criticized the St. John's wort studies.[18] The pair of psychopharmacologists attacked their short duration of only four to eight weeks, the lack of specific studies of severely depressed patients, and the lack of longer-term follow-up to detect "the possibility of late side effects." As described in the previous chapter, however, all these criticisms hold equally true of most studies used to win approval to market synthetic antidepressants. De Smet and Nolen's conclusion is inadvertently ironic: "To be accepted as an antidepressant in the strict sense . . . hypericum extracts should meet the same rigorous demands that have been laid down for synthetic antidepressants." To criticize the St. John's wort studies for the same shortcomings that are found in synthetic antidepressant studies and to give the impression that the herb has not met the "rigorous" standards of prescription antidepressants is spurious. Unfortunately, when the *British Medical Journal's* coverage of St. John's wort received widespread publicity in the fall of 1996, De Smet and Nolen's criticisms were also reported by journalists who were unaware that the same limitations also apply to studies of synthetic drugs.

Questions have been raised about the consistency of the milligram dosages found in herbal products, since there are no standards for their manufacture comparable to those for prescription drugs. In spite of this, many patients report the herb is an effective antidepressant, which has also been borne out in the many clinical studies that have been published. Although herbs like St. John's wort have been used for centuries and appear to be safe, they are perhaps best used short-term, for up to a year, in combination with other natural alternatives. With the tendency to become dependent on pills in our culture, we need to be careful not to do the same thing with herbs that we have done with prescription medication, relying on them indefinitely. Nor should one rely on herbs exclusively, since, like synthetic drugs, they are not cures but merely suppress symptoms.

No one knows the exact mechanism by which St. John's wort improves mood and energy level. The active ingredient is said to be hyperforin. In fact, St. John's wort contains more than a dozen physiologically active agents. Herbalists point out that the idea of a single active ingredient that can be extracted from a plant is a tenet of Western, allopathic medicine and is anathema to holistic clinical practice. In holistic medicine, the synergistic, balanced effects of multiple components of a natural plant product are considered crucial to its beneficial effects.

Couples Therapy

By mid-March, three months into treatment, Lydia was feeling considerably better than when she first came to see me. Her mood and energy level had improved. Her sleep and appetite had regularized. Back on track, she was getting her work done more effectively. Of course one could not separate out the benefits of psychotherapy, the efforts she had made to change her work and sleep habits, and the effects of St. John's wort. All these modalities were working in concert, naturally.

While my work with Lydia had a cognitive-behavioral emphasis, I also inquired about her family and past. The timing of Lydia's depression, which struck immediately after the prospect of moving to Washington became a reality, had always impressed me. Was Eric pushing the move more than Lydia? I wondered. Did she not want to leave her friends and contacts in Boston? Or was there something about Washington and being near her family again that caused her to feel conflicted? So far, our work had turned up nothing in this regard.

Then one day Lydia called to ask if Eric could accompany her to a session. "Sure," I said, wondering what the reason might be.

When they arrived, the couple looked quite distressed. All weekend long they had been arguing over an upcoming trip to Washington. For weeks they had been trying to decide how to divide their time between Lydia's and Eric's families. In particular, Lydia's mother had been pressing them to stay with her and Lydia's father. The last time Lydia and Eric went to Washington, they stayed with Eric's parents and only saw Lydia's family once for dinner.

"Last Friday," said Eric, agitated, "my mother told me Lydia's mother was pressing her about whose family we would be staying with. When I repeated that to Lydia she got angry with me."

"Why?" I looked to Lydia.

"Because I was so mad."

"At Eric?"

"And his mother. Why did she have to tell him my mother was lobbying her? She should have said nothing. And why did he have to repeat it to me?"

"You would have preferred him to keep it secret?"

"Yes," Lydia said, pouting but seeming to recognize this as a little unreasonable.

"But your mother's the one who started the calls. Are you mad at her too?"

"No," Lydia stammered. "But that's the question Eric's been asking all weekend."

"It's unfair," Eric interjected, angrily.

"No it's not. My mother has a right to want to see more of us."

"This is where we've been stuck all weekend," said Eric, frustrated. "Neither one of us seems to be able to understand the other's position."

For a while, things remained confused in the couples session as the two sniped back and forth at one another. Then Lydia made a comment about how much "easier" it was to stay with Eric's parents that caught my attention.

"What do you mean 'easier'?" I inquired.

"Eric's parents have a much bigger house," Lydia answered. "It's more comfortable staying with them, especially with the children."

"Are Eric's parents more comfortably off than yours?"

"Oh"—Lydia rolled her eyes—"that's an understatement. Eric grew up in an elegant, nineteenth-century townhouse in Georgetown. I grew up on the other side of the tracks, in inner-city Washington."

"Do your parents still live there?"

"Yes. They're still in the house I was born in. My life has become so different from theirs. They don't really understand. I love them dearly but . . . I feel a little estranged from them," said Lydia, welling up with tears. "I feel so guilty saying it's easier staying with Eric's parents but it's true. The issue is going to come to a head when we move back to Washington."

"You feel tension around this as you think about moving back?" I asked, thinking this might be the conflict Lydia felt over moving.

"I hadn't realized it before," she said, "but I think so."

The couples session was a watershed in my work with Lydia. In the following weeks, she had a flood of thoughts and feelings. In the process she educated me about aspects of middle-class black culture that I had not been familiar with. Lydia explained that her parents worked blue-collar jobs and lived in a poor neighborhood, whereas Eric's parents were both attorneys. Eric's family were well connected socially and members of several exclusive black clubs. They summered in Oak Bluffs on Martha's Vineyard. In one of the more surprising twists, Lydia explained that within the well-to-do black community, light skin color is highly valued.

"Have you heard of the brown-paper-bag test?" she asked.

"No," I answered.

"If your skin is lighter than a brown paper bag, that's considered more desirable than if you're darker-skinned."

"But that's just a form of prejudice within the black community," I said.

"I know," said Lydia. "I don't really subscribe to it. I'm just saying it's one more highly visible difference between Eric's family and mine."

Lydia said that since becoming better educated, more financially secure, and especially since marrying Eric, she felt her life had diverged from that of her parents. She was still extremely close to them and loved them. But she felt sad about the divide that had arisen between them. Mostly, this had played itself out superficially in disagreements over how much time they spent with Eric's parents and how much with hers whenever they visited Washington. Now she realized this was a much deeper issue she had not dealt with in the five years she had been living in Boston.

"Remember I was so upset over the call with the real estate broker?" Lydia asked.

"Yes."

"Even something as mundane or practical as that, I now think is related to this."

"How do you mean?"

"I have fairly high standards now, like Eric's. But I think, 'I didn't grow up in much of a neighborhood and I've done fine. My parents are still there. Why do we have to have so much better?'"

Lydia was not in any way angry with her parents, it was really sadness that predominated in her case. One never knows what mix of sadness and anger is at the bottom of a particular patient's depression. Hers was a good example of the strain of upward social mobility, the universal conflicts and guilt people often feel regardless of their race.

If Lydia's treatment had ended as soon as she was doing better symptomatically, the couples session might never have happened. If she had been on a serotonin booster, it might well have numbed her feelings, desensitizing her to the issues around her family, leading her to ignore them yet again. Instead, Lydia was able to deal with the issues in advance of moving. She had by no means sorted out the issues completely before she moved. However, she felt much better prepared to meet the challenge of balancing the world of Eric's family, the family she and Eric had established, and her family of origin. She was unwavering in her desire to move back to Washington. But she had not been aware of this unconscious conflict before. It was a psychological blind spot, which therapy helped her to uncover.

Lydia was in therapy for seven months, and stopped therapy when she moved. At the end of our work, Lydia gave me a copy of her cognitive therapy workbook and of the diary she kept during the time she saw me. Interestingly, once she had identified the real, underlying issue that was bothering her, the cognitive therapy exercises and long lists she made in her workbook, prioritizing what she needed to do, stopped abruptly. In her diary, she described enormous "relief" at discovering the core of the problem.

Three years later, when I contacted Lydia to get permission to include her in this book, she said that she had not needed therapy again in Washington. After the work we had done, she found she was able to deal with her family issues and had not been depressed since.

Anthony: A Case of Severe Depression

In contrast to Jenny and Lydia, Anthony was struggling to keep his head above water when he first came to see me. Just a few months earlier, Anthony had moved to Boston to enroll in Boston College Law School. Now in the middle of his first semester, he was woefully behind in his reading and not going to classes. Indeed, he came to see me because he feared doing poorly in midterm exams. Living off campus in a suburb, Anthony was isolated from the majority of his new classmates who lived near the school's urban campus. Most of the time he spent "holed up" in his apartment, avoiding school and people. When he did go out, he took long walks, feeling dejected. Apart from the walks, Anthony was getting little exercise. Normally a mountain climber and outdoorsman, since arriving in Boston he had "not set foot in a gym" and felt "in terrible physical as well as mental shape."

Prior to coming to law school, Anthony had been a top student at Fordham University. His last year of college he worked "double overtime" writing a lengthy thesis. After graduation he worked for a year in a senator's office in Washington, D.C. There he put in grueling hours helping to draft important new environmental legislation. Originally scheduled to take the month of August off, instead he worked straight through, right up until the day he came to law school, because he was so committed to the environmental project.

"In September, when I first started having trouble," said Anthony, "I thought it was because I was so exhausted. I thought I should have taken a vacation. Now, it's November and I realize the problem is much more serious."

Anthony had lost close to ten pounds in just a few months because he had no appetite. Most nights, he tossed and turned in bed for hours before falling asleep. During this time he would "beat himself up" for not doing his work and, especially, for disappointing his family. Often he resorted to drinking alcohol to sleep. He was not using small amounts of alcohol for this purpose. Rather, he was drinking heavily. The price he paid was terrible hangovers in the morning. Embarrassed, Anthony said in some anguish, "How can I be doing so poorly? I should be feeling on top of the world here at law school. I have a wonderful girlfriend. How can I have suddenly fallen so low?"

One of Anthony's most disconcerting symptoms was being "afraid of people." When I asked him what he meant, he said, "I'm afraid of everyone. My professors. My new classmates. Neighbors in the hallway. Strangers on the street. Even clerks in shops, cashiers . . . I find it painful to interact with them."

"What is it you're afraid of?"

"I feel like I have to apologize for myself, as though anybody can tell how weak and unable to function I am right now. I'm afraid to interact with anyone but my girlfriend or my few close friends. Even with them, I feel a little bit like I have to pretend. I can't let on how bad I'm feeling."

This pronounced fear of people was a striking and peculiar symptom in a young man like Anthony. Nearly six feet tall and stocky, Anthony hardly looked like someone who felt afraid of everyone, even shop clerks.

Perhaps most worrisome of all, Anthony was vaguely suicidal. "It's not that I'm about to kill myself," he said, "but I keep thinking I'd rather be dead."

"Do you feel like falling asleep and not waking up again?"

"It's more specific. I wish I could quit all of this . . . just leave everything behind. I'm a mountain climber—when I'm not depressed, that is. I keep imagining climbing Mount Everest and not caring whether I survive or not. I'm sure it's because of those people who died on Everest recently but I can't keep my mind off it."

Anthony was severely depressed. He felt hopeless, helpless, and worthless. In addition to these psychological symptoms, he had multiple physical symptoms of depression—insomnia, difficulty concentrating, loss of appetite, feeling weak and fatigued. He felt afraid of people and was avoiding social situations or anywhere he might run into people he knew, including his law school classes. He was drinking heavily. What set Anthony's depression apart from Jenny's and Lydia's was the severity of his symptoms and the fact that his functioning was severely impaired. Indeed, Anthony was considering withdrawing from law school because he was so far behind in his academic work.

Balancing Medication with Natural Approaches

For someone as severely depressed as Anthony, short-term use of antidepressant medication is a reasonable option. The key questions the patient and doctor consider in making this decision are How severely compromised is the patient's ability to function? and What are the patient's immediate responsibilities in life—that is, in the coming two to three months?

Anthony was certainly debilitated by his depression. What is more, he was under tremendous pressure to perform. In the next two months, he would have to complete several papers, another midterm, and final exams. He was quite far behind in his work and had considerable catching-up to do. Anthony wanted to finish the semester and was afraid of failing out of school. Because drugs can take several weeks to work, he had little time to ponder the decision. If he was going to go on medication, now was the time to do it. If his energy level and ability to concentrate were restored, Anthony felt, he could catch up on his work and do reasonably well for the semester.

Even with someone as depressed as Anthony, I am frank about the potential long-term consequences of taking antidepressant drugs. Most patients greatly appreciate the candor. In rare instances, patients have switched their care to doctors who are not so open.

I tell patients "antidepressant" drugs are merely stimulants to jump-start them at a difficult time in their life. A stimulant would make anyone feel better in the short run unless it causes severe side effects. Therefore, if the medication worked, I told Anthony, this would not imply he was "defective" in any way, genetically or otherwise. Medication is like a cast or crutch to aid one in healing. In and of itself, it is not a cure. Anyone depressed enough to need drugs should simultaneously be in some form of therapy to effect personal change so he or she will not become dependent on drugs for life. As part of comprehensive treatment, short-term use of drugs is reasonable if one's circumstances warrant it.

Fortunately, Anthony came into treatment wanting to be in psychotherapy. He was interested in medication because he was feeling so bad and because of the pressure he was under in law school. As is often the case nowadays, he was under pressure from his family to go on medication in order to "salvage" law school. He did not involve his girlfriend in the decision, because he knew she would have more mixed feelings about drugs.

Before starting anyone on an antidepressant, doctors usually perform a number of blood tests to rule out medical conditions like anemia or endocrine abnormalities as the cause of their low energy. On a number of occasions I have diagnosed thyroid disease or adrenal gland tumors in patients. Obviously, one wants to catch these early on and treat them medically rather than just putting someone on an antidepressant, or indeed embarking on any other course of psychiatric treatment if it is not necessary. When Anthony's laboratory tests all came back normal, I started him on 20 milligrams a day of Prozac.

Caffeine, Alcohol, and Diet

An important part of Anthony's history was that he had been drinking heavily, drowning his sorrows in attempts to go to sleep. To counteract his hangovers, he often drank several cups of coffee during the course of the day.

I urged Anthony to stop drinking alcohol. Alcohol is a powerful central nervous system depressant. In the immediate few hours after drinking, it numbs feelings and acts as a sedative. With chronic use, alcohol has a strong depressant effect. As a result, alcohol and depression are a dangerous mix. Anyone struggling with depression should avoid alcohol completely. The serotonin boosters also interact adversely with alcohol, magnifying its effects and making it more dangerous.

I also encouraged Anthony to reduce his caffeine intake. I was concerned the caffeine was contributing to his insomnia. Laboratory studies have shown just one cup of coffee in the morning affects the pattern of one's brain waves during sleep at night. Most people are unaware caffeine is such a strong drug. Anyone having difficulty with insomnia should avoid caffeinated drinks.

Since Prozac is stimulating, it too can cause insomnia, particularly in the early days and weeks on the drug, before one's nervous system has adapted to it. Many people report that the stimulating effects of Prozac and caffeine are synergistic, another reason to cut back on coffee when starting an antidepressant.

It is important to inquire about people's dietary habits, especially their alcohol and caffeine intake, when starting them on a medication. By the time he came to see me, Anthony was already on a roller coaster of taking a sedative (alcohol) at night and chasing it with a stimulant (caffeine) in the morning. If one failed to ask about these lifestyle habits and to urge patients to change them, prescribing Prozac would simply be throwing another stimulant into the mix.

Anthony readily agreed to stop drinking and to cut back on coffee. Cutting back on alcohol and caffeine are particularly important in depression but eating a healthful balanced diet in general is critical to one's mood and energy level. Many people with depression benefit from consulting a nutritionist. Health food stores often have a good selection of books on the effects of diet on mood and energy level.

In the early weeks of treatment, Anthony made a valiant effort to go to his classes and do some of the reading for his courses. While his intentions were good, the results were mixed: He would improve his showing for a few days but then not be able to sustain the effort. Unlike people who are mildly to moderately depressed, those who are severely depressed often have trouble trying to simply force themselves to perform better.

When Anthony had not responded to Prozac, I put his dose up to 40 milligrams a day. On the higher dose, he felt the Prozac "kick in." One never knows exactly what dose will work for a patient. The process is one of trial and error. Many doctors and patients tell of having to try three or four drugs at maximum dose before one finally works. This is far less likely to happen when patients are getting more than just medication, and psychotherapy simultaneously begins to work.

By mid-December, Anthony's energy level and ability to concentrate had markedly increased. "On Prozac, I feel like I've had four cups of coffee," said Anthony. "I can sit and focus my attention in a way that I haven't been able to for months." Initially, he felt caffeinated, a little tremulous on the drug, but this wore off. "I'm aware of being drugged because my sex drive is so low. I had to tell my girlfriend about the Prozac because she didn't understand why I couldn't get it up. She's not happy about it. I'm relieved to be able to work again but I wouldn't want to stay on it too long." Just before Christmas break, Anthony had another midterm, which he did poorly on because he was so ill prepared. For several weeks he made a concerted effort to catch up on his work. As the end of the semester and his final exams approached, however, he expressed concern this was "too little, too late." In most courses, he had only been to about a quarter of his classes. He knew little of what his professors had emphasized and were likely to test. Even after working hard for a couple of weeks, he still had only done half the reading.

With his exams less than a week away, Anthony had to face the stark reality that he was not prepared to take them. Postponing the exams was not an option, because the second semester's work required having mastered the first semester's material. The question came down to: Should Anthony take the exams and potentially fail them or was it a lesser of evils to swallow his pride and withdraw?

Such a decision is not easy for anyone to make, especially when he is trying to recover from depression. "I can't believe I've made it this far and can't pull it off," said Anthony, dejected. My role was to help him not view withdrawing as a complete failure. He could take a leave of absence. When he was ready, he could return.

Right up until the last minute, Anthony's parents pressed him to keep preparing for his exams in the hopes that he might be able to take them. This was understandable, since they had spent so much money on the semester, which would now be a loss. Part of the dilemma was: If Anthony withdrew, what would he do? Where would he live? Would he be able to work to support himself in his current condition?

Three days before his first exam, Anthony made the agonizing decision to withdraw. "I'm pretty sure I'd fail my exams and that would be worse," he said, looking quite pained. Eager to have him return to law school in the fall, his father suggested he stay in Boston. The plan was for him to recover and then look for a job in the spring.

Why had Anthony so completely collapsed? Was he just exhausted after working so hard during his senior year of college and the year in Washington? Was he ambivalent about a legal career? Why did he not seek treatment earlier, when he would have had more of a chance of catching up? Although on a conscious level he felt terrible about disappointing his family, on an unconscious level was this what he wanted to do? If so, why? What other reasons, as yet completely unconscious, might there be for Anthony's dramatic fall?

The first few months of Anthony's treatment were "crisis mode." Once he withdrew from law school, this changed. Now we were able to turn our attention to whatever was at the root of his problem. The Prozac had kicked in, and this, together with the relief of finally having made a decision, gradually improved Anthony's mood. The line between crisis mode and being able to work on deeper issues is not hard-and-fast. In the early months of therapy, I had begun to learn about Anthony's history but now we could turn our full attention to it.

Anthony was born in Providence, Rhode Island, and grew up quite poor. He lived in a small apartment in a dilapidated group of high-rise buildings he described as "practically a project." Anthony's father was an attorney who represented clients in the Mafia; he was a compulsive womanizer, and his frequent absences from the home were a constant source of tension with Anthony's mother. Finally, when Anthony was six years old, his parents separated. His father moved to his own apartment. He had a "never-ending stream of younger girlfriends" but did not remarry. Neither did Anthony's mother. They remained on relatively good terms, celebrated holidays together, and only formally divorced a decade after they had separated.

Anthony was in kindergarten the year his father moved out. For the first time, his mother had to work to support the family. After school, Anthony became the responsibility of his older brother Ray. Anthony looked up to Ray, who was five years his senior. Although they had many good times together, after their father left Ray became moody and unpredictable. He frequently "went off" on Anthony, beating him up "for no good reason." When this first started, Anthony tried to tell his mother about the beatings when she came home from work, but she "seemed not to get it." Not wanting to burden her any more than she was already, Anthony "adapted" to the beatings. He tried not to upset his brother and to make the best of the situation. In spite of the difficulties of those years, Anthony's view of his mother was quite positive. He felt she did everything she could in impossible circumstances. In her spare time, she would go to the park with Anthony to throw a few baseballs.

In the years after his father left, Anthony saw him only two or three times a year, at holidays, even though he lived just ten minutes away. One of the few times Anthony could count on seeing his father was Thanksgiving. "I used to love Thanksgiving, because we spent the whole day together like a normal family," said Anthony, becoming emotional. "My father would watch the football game with Ray and me. Afterwards, he'd box with us and teach us a few moves. My mother seemed happy to see us enjoying ourselves. We ate a big, leisurely meal. The first few years when I was seven, eight, and nine years old . . . at the end of the day I'd ask why my father couldn't stay. Why couldn't we be together like that all the time? Those first few years I used to cry when he was leaving. I remember my father would signal me to stop crying. He would stand a little taller and say, 'This is how it has to be. You have to be tough. We all have to accept it.' Ray was always so loyal to my father, he didn't like anyone questioning him. He'd shoot a scornful look of impatience at me. I'd want to please my father too, so I'd stop crying. After those early years, I didn't bring the subject up or cry anymore."

One of the ways Anthony coped with his situation was by becoming a top student. In addition to his native intelligence, he described himself as a "people pleaser" with a keen ability to grasp what other people wanted from him. Typically, he was able to quickly intuit a teacher's style and "mold" his thinking to it. His ability to accommodate also brought him success socially.

As he grew older, Anthony developed a "thick as thieves" group of close friends, other boys his age. "We weren't exactly a gang," said Anthony, "but we were always together, roving the neighborhood. There wasn't anything we didn't know about one another. We shared everything."

Over the years I have come to appreciate the significance of such groups in the lives of men who grew up in extremely poor neighborhoods. These small bands of close friends often take the place of supportive, intact families. Emotional displays—particularly expressions of vulnerability or anything perceived as "weak"—are avoided in this macho subculture, but otherwise these groups are characterized by powerfully loyal attachments.

His freshman year in college, Anthony went to Fordham University with one of his childhood friends. "I got into Ivy League colleges but I wouldn't go on my own," he said. Even having one of his friends for a roommate, Anthony missed the others acutely and found the transition difficult. Once again, he buried himself in his work.

As always, he adapted and even thrived. At Fordham he took up mountain climbing and developed his love of the outdoors. Through his Fordham connections he landed the job in the senator's office in Washington, D.C. "Especially in Washington, I became acutely aware of straddling two worlds," said Anthony. "The world of Capitol Hill and elegant state dinners on the one hand and the neighborhood I grew up in on the other. I even have two ways of speaking. I talk one way with my Capitol Hill friends. But when I'm in my old neighborhood, I slip into a form of street talk, which is more natural for me." In fact, I had noticed this happening even when Anthony spoke of his childhood.

Anthony said he first began to have trouble performing during his senior year at Fordham. Although his grades were still good, they fell. The year he worked in Washington, he suffered bouts of malaise during which he felt he was "going through the motions." Anthony had wanted to take another year off before law school but his father talked him out of it. "He's a lawyer," said Anthony. "He's got an answer for everything." Late in life, his father had become comfortably well off, representing prominent Mafia and underworld figures. With his new resources, he was supporting Anthony through law school. "I guess I hadn't realized how much he's pushed me. I wanted to go to Suffolk, at night, but my father said, 'How could you give up all the connections that come with the better name school?' He wants me to have the best school possible, the biggest law firm, and the establishment connections he's never had."

Increasingly, Anthony began to see himself as a "puppet" of his father: "The more I think about it, the more I don't like that Thanksgiving scene where I'm crying as my father starts to leave. He's saying, 'Hang tough,' but it really means 'Shut up. Nobody can or wants to deal with your feelings!' He was doing the same thing when he wouldn't hear me out about taking another year off or going to night school." Anthony began to see his ability to "mold" his thinking to professors' and give them what they wanted as an extension of his conforming to his father's wishes. He was upset about the abuse from his older brother, although he did not hold him ultimately responsible: "Ray was as upset as I was that my father was gone. Beating me up was just his way of dealing with it."

Exercise

As Anthony pieced together this history and his feelings about it, his mood and energy level continued to improve. In early spring he resumed exercising, one of the best natural antidotes to depression. When Anthony was severely depressed, he could not motivate himself to exercise. But as soon as he was feeling better, I encouraged him to return to it.

Health experts used to advocate an hour or more of strenuous, heavy exercise four to five times a week to maintain cardiovascular and psychological fitness. For many people, this is daunting and off-putting. In recent years, however, the recommendations have changed considerably. Repeated large-scale studies have shown moderate-intensity, aerobic exercise for just twenty to thirty minutes, four or five times a week is all that is required. Activities like jogging, bicycling, swimming, or brisk walking are ideal. Lower-intensity activities like gardening or leisurely walks are not sufficient. One of the simplest criteria for judging if an activity is strenuous enough is whether or not one breaks a sweat. One does not need to become drenched but one should break a sweat in the small of one's back.

Anthony began jogging five days a week. In part he was motivated to get back in shape because he wanted to go mountain climbing for his summer vacation. After jogging for two months, he felt the exercise produced a discernible improvement: "I feel much more limber and energetic. I've reached that point where I feel 'hooked' on exercise again. If I miss a few days I can feel my body hankering for the exercise. I get this restless feeling like I have to get out and jog."

As in Anthony's case, exercise typically takes one to two months to have a sustained, antidepressant effect. Many people feel like quitting after just a few weeks because it does not work faster. I always encourage people to persist. In addition to improving mood, exercise has a distinct beneficial effect on sleep and anxiety level. One's cardiovascular and general physical health also benefit.

In recent decades, numerous epidemiological studies have documented a positive correlation between aerobic exercise and fewer symptoms of depression.[19] These have been large-scale studies of the general population involving thousands of people followed for five to twenty years. In some instances these have been community-based studies of physical and mental health. In others, the focus has been the effects of diet and exercise on heart disease but the studies have simultaneously assessed symptoms of depression, anxiety, and insomnia. The positive effects of exercise on mood and energy level are now generally well known, although exercise is too often overlooked in the treatment of depression.[20]

Most authorities speculate that aerobic exercise works by affecting the same neurotransmitter systems affected by psychiatric drugs: adrenaline, serotonin, dopamine, and endorphins. Together, these give rise to what is called "the runner's high." But, unlike medications, the effect of exercise is entirely natural.

From the point of view of evolution, humans were not designed to live a sedentary lifestyle. Back in the primordial forest and plain, we were hunter-gatherers, actively engaged in the physical challenges of our world. Each time I see the dramatic effects exercise can have on mood and energy, I wonder: How many people use serotonin boosters to give their nervous systems a kick when their physiology has become sluggish because of too sedentary a lifestyle?

Since some of the worst long-term side effects of medications are related to total cumulative exposure, keeping the dose to the necessary minimum is important. As early as March, I reduced Anthony's Prozac from 40 milligrams to 20 milligrams a day. When he continued to do well, in May, he began taking 20 milligrams every other day. Because Prozac lasts so long in the body, this is the equivalent of 10 milligrams a day. Why not just take a 10-milligram capsule daily? This costs almost twice as much money, since Eli Lilly charges virtually the same price for the 10-milligram as the 20-milligram pill.

In the spring, Anthony got a job working on a construction crew. He enjoyed working outdoors. He was relieved to no longer be experiencing the social avoidance he had struggled with when depressed.

Anthony decided he wanted to return to law school in the fall. He applied to return to Boston College and was readmitted. In July, he and his girlfriend went on vacation mountain climbing. They drove to Idaho and went climbing in the Grand Tetons. Anthony returned to Boston saying he loved being outdoors and felt committed to protecting the environment. Indeed, he had decided he wanted to work for an environmental group like the Sierra Club after law school instead of working in a large law firm as his father hoped.

When Anthony returned to school in the fall he had more difficulty than he expected. Some of his fear of people returned, although not as severely as the year before. This actually gave him another chance to examine that fear. He now felt it was a reflection of how he felt about his father and brother at a young age. "I've been having this fear of strangers suddenly pulling a dagger on me," he said. "I've thought, 'Where does that come from?' Then I realized, in those early years after my father left and my mother went out to work, my brother's turning on me was like someone suddenly pulling a knife on me, he was so unpredictable."

Anthony was increasingly angry over his father's treatment of the family: "He had a serious problem with women, but that's not how it was presented. We had to accept that this was just him, that it was okay. We had to pretend everything was fine, that we were practically a normal family, even though he couldn't live with us because he was screwing so many women."

Anthony said he had met some of his father's underworld clients, whom he described as "bullies." Increasingly, he saw his father and brother Ray as bullies too. "Ray was an unwitting accomplice of my father all those years, beating me up and keeping me quiet." More than anything, Anthony was upset over having been "silenced," having his voice taken away: "I was upset for years after he left but I wasn't allowed to express it. In fact, he talked me out of it. With his power, his physical presence, and especially his slick talk, he convinced me I wasn't feeling so bad. And I bought into it. I had to. Now I'm incredibly angry. I guess the better way to think of it is I always have been but just wasn't aware of it."

Since Anthony's case, I have seen a number of people like him: high performers who suddenly collapse. For years he had been a shell of a person, trying to please his father, teachers, friends, and others. Once he got to law school, he could no longer "play the game." He analogized having to withdraw from law school to "having to close up shop" because he was so depleted. Now he was puzzling out how this had happened.

As the fall semester progressed, Anthony tried to broach the issues that were coming up in therapy with his family. First he spoke with his mother, who was "sympathetic to a point." She wanted to listen because she had been concerned by how depressed Anthony was the year before. She quickly came to his father's defense, however. "She can't really hear it," he said. "She's never been able to. She and my father are still intertwined. They talk on the phone almost daily. They still celebrate all the holidays together. He supports her financially. She's not able to be objective about him and what happened. I don't blame her in any way. She's always wanted the best for me. But she's never been able to stand up to him."

Anthony was even more frustrated trying to broach the subject with Ray: "He just couldn't hear it. He's so afraid of losing what little approval he gets from my father that he won't hear of anyone questioning him. He's more messed up than I am." Anthony explained that Ray had been financially backed by his father in starting a construction business and was heavily indebted to him. "It's Ray's business but my father calls most of the shots." Just a year ago, Ray walked out on his wife and children. "He's crazy. His wife was devoted to him. He has three wonderful children. He's doing the same thing to them my father did to us but he can't see it. Even my mother sees what's happening and is worried about him."

Anthony even approached his father, telling him a little about how he was feeling and why he thought he had become depressed. His father admitted he "basically abandoned the family" but said it was important for Anthony "to move on."

"That's good he acknowledged it," I said, seeing the conversation as positive. "He's not saying it never happened. It sounds like he can talk about it more than Ray."

Anthony surprised me with his vehement response. "Bullshit," he said angrily. "It was business as usual. Saying I had to 'move on' was once again putting the responsibility on me. He's too clever to deny it. He's smarter than Ray. But he's still trying to push it away, to sweep it under the carpet."

Recovering, I asked, "Did you tell him how his response made you feel?"

"No. At the time I didn't realize what was happening. He disarmed me by admitting it. He's clever in that way. But after the conversation, I was agitated for hours. I went over and over the phone call with my girlfriend before I figured out what had happened."

At other times, Anthony felt more favorably toward his father. As he was writing briefs and papers in law school, he called him to discuss legal issues. "He was first in his class at law school, where he was on a full scholarship," said Anthony. "He has an incredible memory for cases and a knack for crafting legal arguments. After law school he went to work in a big law firm but hated it. Things weren't easy for him either." Here Anthony was identifying with his father, following in his footsteps as a lawyer who was uncomfortable in large, corporate law firms.

That Thanksgiving Anthony went home to Rhode Island. He felt more tension than usual being around his family. In fact, in the middle of the day he and Ray had an ugly confrontation: "He was playing the older brother, telling me what to do all morning. I was irritable with him but he wasn't getting the message. When it came time to eat, I was carving the turkey at the kitchen counter to get a particular cut for myself. Ray came over belligerently saying, 'Don't carve that side of the turkey. The other side's not done yet.' He reached out to take the knife away from me. Without thinking, I karate chopped his arm. It was quite a scene with Ray howling and the knife flying out of my hand across the kitchen. 'Don't mess with me,' I growled. Ray was stunned. I was really ready to fight him. My father didn't know what to do. My mother scurried around saying they should treat me with kid gloves because I've been having difficulties. But I know that wasn't why Ray backed off. He didn't want to mess with me. I'm in a lot better shape than he is these days. He couldn't have been nicer the rest of the day. It was the first time I've ever stood up to him."

Listening to the story, I thought Anthony was displacing a lot of his anger at his father onto Ray. Presumably he was still too afraid of his father to have such a confrontation with him. For the time being, Ray was getting the brunt of his anger.

Anthony went off Prozac in the early fall, not quite a year after he had started it. Although he was still struggling some in law school, he was not depressed. He felt strongly about getting off the medication and dealing with the issues that were coming up. Throughout the spring, summer, and fall, we had gradually reduced his dose, keeping him on the drug through his transition back to law school. In addition to minimizing drug exposure, keeping the dose as low as possible keeps the psychological issues the person needs to deal with alive. This is called titrating, or balancing, the dose. Overmedicating people only serves to paper over issues once again.

The Christmas holidays passed uneventfully for Anthony, whose focus was on preparing for his exams. His midterm exams had gone well and at the end of the semester, he took all his final exams, successfully completing the first semester of law school. He felt enormously relieved. Flush with this success, in the break between semesters, he visited his parents again. This time he had a run-in with his father. "I told him I want to work for an environmental protection organization, not a law firm," said Anthony. "He told me I should at least try out a law firm this summer. He was pissed when I held my ground. A couple of hours later he started giving me a hard time about money. He started complaining about how much law school is costing him. He was so obvious. For the first time in my life I could clearly see him trying to manipulate me. When he told me he wasn't sure he could give me the money for second semester, I lost it."

"What happened?"

"I told him, 'Fine. If you don't pay for law school I'll go climb Mount Everest. And I won't care whether or not I survive.'"

"Mount Everest as in when you were suicidal last year?" I asked, surprised.

"Exactly."

"How did he respond?"

"He was furious. He told me I was 'shaking him down for the money for law school.' That's his Mafia street talk."

"What did you say?"

"Nothing. It was bullshit and I wasn't going to get into it with him. He was the one shaking me down. Those are his tactics. I was just fighting fire with fire for once."

The next week, Anthony's father called, still upset over the Mount Everest threat: "He went on in a long monologue. I just held the phone away from my ear and kept going about my work outlining cases."

"How did his monologue make you feel?"

"I don't care how upset he is. He's never cared how I felt. I don't deserve to be jerked around about law school just because I'm not doing his bidding. I'm not putting up with him anymore."

Within a few days, Anthony's father sent him the money, apparently finished with the dispute. But Anthony was not satisfied. Over the next few weeks he decided the Everest threat was "too indirect" an expression of his anger. "The next time I see him I'm going to tell him how I really feel. I don't want to have the conversation over the phone. I'll tell him when I see him next, over spring break."

In addition to his anger, Anthony felt considerable sadness over what had happened to him. "My world as I knew it fell apart when I was a kid," said Anthony. "All of a sudden my father was gone. Then my mother went to work. I was left at home with my brother beating me up. And the worst part was having to pretend it was all fine, which was suffocating. I look back on it and think none of it had to be like that. What a shame. It's all such a waste. My father's father treated him badly. He won't talk about it, so I don't know the details, but my mother says he was mean and nasty. I guess we all paid the price for it."

In March, unexpected news shocked Anthony's whole family. Anthony's father had a severe angina attack and was told he needed open-heart surgery, an emergency bypass operation. Before the attack, Anthony's father had not been aware of angina or any other symptoms of heart disease. Immediately on hearing the news, Anthony went to Providence to be with his family. He and his father said nothing of their recent difficulties. "I could tell he was grateful that I had come to see him before he went into surgery," said Anthony, full of emotion. Anthony waited with his mother and brother during the long operation. It was successful, and in the spring his father's convalescence and recovery were slow but steady.

Anthony completed his spring semester successfully and took a summer job doing research for a professor who specialized in environmental law. This would be a good springboard for future employment with a group like the Sierra Club. Somewhat to my surprise, Anthony remained determined to confront his father in spite of his surgery, as soon as his convalescence was over. "He could die," said Anthony. "I've got to have this conversation with him."

"Shouldn't you wait a while longer?" I asked, concerned. "What if he has a heart attack in the middle of the conversation? That would be awful and you'd feel guilty for life."

"No. I'll feel worse if I don't talk to him," Anthony insisted.

By the summer, Anthony's father had recovered enough to be working part-time. "If he's fit to work, he's fit to have this conversation with me," said Anthony. Contemplating such an emotional conversation, I wondered about the wisdom of Anthony's determination, but therapists cannot really control what their patients do. Perhaps Anthony was right. These are not decisions for therapists to make for their patients. Still, I was apprehensive the weekend he went to Providence.

When Anthony returned, he reported that the conversation with his father had gone surprisingly well. "I was really blunt," said Anthony. "I didn't spare him anything. I told him he was a failure. That he had abandoned us. That Ray and my mother and me were fucked up by it. I said he had made me stuff my emotions and had been running my life too much ever since. I told him I didn't want any more grief over going into environmental law. I said that I don't know what his problem is with women but that it's serious. He's never dealt with it or with its consequences for the rest of us. I just laid it all out."

"What did he say?"

"He said I was right, everything I said was true. This time he really tried to listen. And he apologized. I think that's what mattered most to me."

Family Therapy

Over the next several weeks, Anthony and his father spoke a number of times by phone. In fact, his father said he wanted to come to Boston to continue their conversation in person. Would it be possible, he wondered, to come with Anthony to meet with me?

When Anthony proposed this, I welcomed the idea. Shortly thereafter, his father came to Boston for a week. During the visit, I met with Anthony and his father three times. Although still recovering from major surgery, Anthony's father was still a formidable figure. In his sixties and graying, he was a tough-looking, square-jawed man who looked as if he had stepped straight out of *The Godfather.*

I felt privileged to be present for these emotional meetings. Anthony's father seemed to be making a concerted effort to face the past and settle issues with his son. One of the most poignant things I remember him saying was his description of going into the operating room for open-heart surgery.

"Lying there on the table knowing I could die," he said, "my whole life flashed in front of me. What I thought about was all the people I'd hurt, especially my family."

Anthony's father made no pretense about being able to change his problem with women "at this late date." He admitted having hurt many of the women he dated, too. "I can't make a commitment," he said to Anthony. "Your mother, Ray, and you are the only constants in my life. Really, I'm a lonely old man who hasn't spent enough time with the people who loved me."

As though not able to help himself, Anthony's father tried to interject some commentary on Anthony's working in a law firm rather than for an environmental group. Anthony was quick to cut him off. Later, Anthony said to me, "He's not going to change dramatically but he did make an impressive effort."

Like Jenny, Lydia, and Anthony, those prone to depression are often conflict-avoidant people who are on the passive, dependent end of the personality spectrum. Typically, they learned early in life to put other people's emotional needs ahead of their own. In our culture, women are particularly vulnerable to having been socialized to forfeit their emotions in the service of others—although this can happen to men as well, as Anthony's case demonstrates. These underlying personality styles are at the root of depression. Changing these patterns is the only way to reliably reduce or eliminate one's vulnerability to depression in the future.

Having "confronted his demons," Anthony "felt like a new person." He said, "Dropping out of law school and dealing with the psychological pain I was experiencing was the best thing I've ever done. My father and brother had taken away my person at the core. It's like I had masking tape over my mouth all those years. I couldn't express how I was feeling. I couldn't express who I really was."

"In my experience," I said, "when you can't express feelings, you eventually lose touch with them. You don't even know you have them. But human emotions don't just go away. Forced underground, they follow twisted, circuitous paths and pop back up again as psychological symptoms."

"When I appeared to be okay, I was actually at my worst," Anthony reflected. "When I started to feel the pain at the end of college, and especially when I got to law school, it was a wake-up call telling me something had to change. When you're in pain, it means there's a conflict. It's actually a sign of life. There's the potential to change. I was worse off all those years when I was performing and not feeling anything. The pain is the impetus to change. It's important to pay attention to it. You have to find out what it's trying to tell you."

Anthony compared the experience of having confronted his father to that of a sexual abuse victim telling her abuser, "You'll never touch me like that again." Said Anthony, "What held me back was like a dam holding back water. Once it's broken, the water can never go back again."

At the end of therapy, Anthony was truly a different person. He was not so radically changed as to be unrecognizable. His past, what had happened to him, had not changed at all. But what had changed dramatically was his awareness of how he felt about it. Anthony had unearthed deeply buried emotions that had become toxic to his body and psyche. Having accomplished this, he now experienced his emotional life in a different way. Never again would he allow his feelings to be stifled as they once were.

This transformation—the lifting of depression with the excavation of stifled emotions—is so often seen in clinical practice that many have concluded that at bottom depression *is* stifled anger and sadness pressing to be heard. Reminding me that mental hospitals used to be called "madhouses," a patient of mine who is a psychiatrist recently said, "People who are depressed are mad, as in angry, but don't realize it."

The changes Anthony made affected all aspects of his life. He learned to be more expressive and assertive in all his relationships: with his girlfriend, his professors, and his bosses. He did not become a selfish or aggressive person. He just effected a better balance of expression and understanding in his relationships.

Anthony's case happens to address an important aspect of the "functionality" mentality. Especially in managed care settings today, much emphasis is placed on a doctor's ability to simply keep people functioning, even at a bare minimum, to prop them up at almost any cost. In fact, certain losses are simply part of life, like, for instance, the necessity of Anthony's temporary withdrawal from law school. Sometimes one needs to be set back in order to ultimately move forward. Therapists must not be so committed to keeping people functioning, often at the behest of insurers, that they inadvertently perpetuate underlying problems that badly need attention.

Anthony was in psychotherapy for two and a half years. While nowadays insurers actively thwart such long-term psychotherapy, two years or more is often what it takes to restructure basic problematic elements of people's habits and personalities.

Research on the Long-Term Effectiveness of Psychotherapy

Earlier, I described studies like the landmark National Institute of Mental Health study and the Minnesota study demonstrating that early in treatment psychotherapy and medications are comparable in achieving symptomatic relief of depression. At the end of three to four months, roughly two-thirds of patients respond to either treatment alone or to a combination of the two.

But while psychotherapy and medication are comparable in the short term, research on the long-term effectiveness of the two reveals a marked difference. When patients in the NIMH study were evaluated two years later, 50% of those treated with medication had become depressed again, while only 35% of those treated with therapy had relapsed.[21] In the Minnesota study, an even greater difference emerged: 50% of the patients treated with medications had relapsed within two years, while only 18% of those treated with therapy had relapsed.[22]

Another long-term follow-up study was conducted by a group led by Dr. I. M. Blackburn at the Royal Edinburgh Hospital in Scotland. In the Edinburgh study, patients received cognitive therapy, drugs, or a combination of the two.[23] In addition to several months of initial treatment until their depressions cleared, patients were given an additional six months of continuation, or maintenance, treatment, bringing the total length of treatment closer to a year. During this time, therapy consisted of just "booster" sessions every six weeks. At the end of treatment, patients were assessed at six-month intervals for two years. The Edinburgh study was published in the January 1986 issue of the *Journal of Affective Disorders*. By the end of two years, 78% of those who had only received drugs had relapsed. By contrast, just 23% of those who had therapy had relapsed. The group that received a combination of therapy and drugs had the same low rate of relapse (21%) as the group that received psychotherapy alone, indicating that medication made no difference in the long run.

Other follow-up studies have documented the superiority of psychotherapy over drugs long-term.[24] Indeed, one study followed patients for four years. The study was headed by psychiatrist Giovanni Fava at the University of Bologna and the department of psychiatry at the State University of New York at Buffalo. Fava is one of the world's leading authorities on research comparing the effects of drugs and psychotherapy. In the study patients were first treated for three to five months with antidepressant medication until their depressions lifted. As the drugs were then tapered off and stopped, half the patients received five months of cognitive-behavioral therapy while the other half did not. Once active treatment had stopped, the patients were evaluated every three to six months for four years. Writing in the July 1996 issue of the *American Journal of Psychiatry,* Fava's group reported that by the end of four years, 70% of those who had only been treated with drugs had relapsed.[25] By contrast, only 35% of those who received cognitive-behavioral treatment had relapsed.

While the results of research on the long-term effectiveness of psychotherapy are impressive, in clinical practice therapy can be even more effective. Psychotherapy research is modeled after drug research. As such, it is forced to reduce complex therapeutic encounters and clinical progress to overly simplistic rating scales and numerical indices. Good psychotherapy is an existential encounter that can never be reduced to checklists and numbers. In its statistical analyses, even the best psychotherapy research cannot capture the real-life drama of good psychotherapy.

Dr. Fava has been a particularly outspoken critic of psychiatric drug research that equates "health" with the suppression of symptoms instead of a higher expectation of well-being for patients. In his most recent research on treatment after initial improvement of depressive symptoms, Fava emphasizes lifestyle modifications and what he calls "well-being" therapy.[26] Patients are informed that "depression is merely the consequence of a maladaptive lifestyle, which does not take life stress, interpersonal friction, excessive work, and inadequate rest into proper account." Fava focuses on lifestyle changes and resolving maladaptive behavior to effect a recovery from depression, not just symptom suppression.

Unfortunately, the high relapse rates seen in repeated psychiatric studies when patients go off antidepressant medications have prompted some psychopharmacologists to recommend that patients stay on drugs for years, often indefinitely.[27] Of course, this leaves people vulnerable to becoming dependent on the drugs, to the possibility of the sensitization of brain cells worsening their conditions long-term, and to the other severe side effects described in the first half of this book. Given the effectiveness of the alternatives, it is regrettable that so many patients are simply being maintained for years—even decades—on drugs.

In 1994, *Consumer Reports* conducted a study of which treatments best help people with depression and anxiety. The findings of the *Consumer Reports* study are in agreement with official psychiatric research showing that psychotherapy is more effective in the long term than medications in overcoming depression. Some 4,000 readers of *Consumer Reports* responded to a detailed survey asking about their experiences with mental health treatment. "Our survey adds an important dimension to existing research in mental health," said the November 1995 issue, reporting the results.[28] "Most studies have started with people who have very specific, well-defined problems [i.e., diagnosed with symptom checklists], who have been randomly assigned to a treatment or control group, and who have received carefully scripted therapy. Such studies . . . aren't a realistic reflection of most patients' experiences. Our survey, in contrast, is a unique look at what happens in real life, where problems are diverse and less well-defined, and where some therapists try one technique after another until something works." *Consumer Reports* quoted Dr. Martin Seligman, former president of the American Psychological Association, saying that "the success of therapy under these real-life conditions has never before been well studied."

People overwhelmingly reported that psychotherapy, not medication, is the crucial element in recovering from depression and anxiety. Confirming the results of psychiatric research, people reported, "Psychotherapy alone worked as well as psychotherapy combined with medication, like Prozac or Xanax [a Valium-type antianxiety agent]." Regarding the optimal length of treatment, *Consumer Reports* said, "Longer psychotherapy was associated with better outcomes. Among people who entered therapy with similar levels of emotional distress, those who stayed in treatment for more than six months reported greater gains than those who left earlier. . . . For many people, even a year's worth of therapy with a mental health specialist may be very worthwhile." Unfortunately, patients whose HMO or managed care insurer "limited the length and frequency of therapy, and the type of therapist, reported poorer outcomes."

✳   ✳   ✳

Patients often ask, What is the relationship between medications and other forms of treatment for depression? If psychotherapy works, why take medications? Conversely, if medications work, why bother with other treatments, like exercise or psychotherapy? With Jenny's, Lydia's and Anthony's cases as representative examples of mild, moderate, and severe depression and having reviewed the psychiatric research, we can now answer these questions in a thoughtful manner.

At its core, depression is stifled anger and sadness. Bottled up, without expression, these emotions have toxic effects on the psyche and the body. The result is the psychological and physical symptoms of depression. The psychological symptoms—like feeling helpless, hopeless, and worthless—represent the stifled anger and sadness turned against oneself. The physical symptoms—such as fatigue and difficulty concentrating—result from psychological distress. The physical symptoms become more prominent as depression becomes more severe.

It is the physical symptoms of depression that stimulating medication can be helpful in reversing—not as a cure for the fundamental, underlying problem but as a form of symptomatic relief to help restore a patient's ability to function. Medication should be reserved for those patients whose depression is severe and whose ability to function has been compromised. Once functioning is re-established, the goal shifts to understanding the reasons for one's depression. Therapy—whether individual, couples, family, or group—can be a painful process, but it is the only really effective way to overcome depression. In the course of therapy, stifled anger and sadness are excavated—that is, given expression. In the process, deeply ingrained habits of stifling these emotions and maladaptive patterns of behavior are broken, leaving the patient truly less vulnerable to depression in future.

7

Surmounting Anxiety
Training for Elevators,
a Patient's Story

Anxiety and depression are overlapping clinical syndromes. Many patients
have symptoms of both simultaneously. The American Psychiatric Association's *Diagnostic and Statistical Manual (DSM)* has been criticized in recent years for its massive proliferation of psychiatric diagnoses, for
pathologizing everyday life. Yet the *DSM* does not have an official diagnostic category for a combination of anxiety and depression.

Since in many cases anxiety and depression are not entirely separable,
this chapter builds on the previous one. The same general treatment principles apply to both anxiety and depression. Although today a common
response to patients with anxiety is to prescribe a serotonin booster,
often indefinitely, it is important to realize that a wide variety of alternatives are available. Short-term approaches to symptom relief should always be balanced with attention to underlying, root causes. Depending
on the particular type of anxiety, behavioral techniques are remarkably
effective.

Anxiety comes in many forms: panic attacks, agoraphobia, obsessions,
compulsions, specific phobias, or post-traumatic stress disorder. Within
each of these categories, patients can have mild, moderate, or severe symptoms. The cases in this chapter cannot cover all of these many possibilities.
Instead, they have been chosen to illustrate the range of treatment options
available for anxiety.

Roberto: A Case of Elevator Phobia

Roberto came to see me early in his senior year at Harvard College because he was phobic about riding elevators. Phobias are severe avoidance responses that occur in reaction to particular objects or settings. On numerous occasions Roberto had tried to take elevators but been unable to because he panicked. His heart raced, he became short of breath and sweaty, and he felt as if he was going to faint. Occasionally, he had anxiety about flying in airplanes or riding on subways and was worried about his phobia's spreading. Indeed, not long before coming to see me, Roberto visited a friend whose mother was a psychiatrist. She "scared" him by telling Roberto his phobia probably would spread even though it had been stable for years. Giving him a prescription for Valium, she urged him to get a complete psychiatric evaluation and go on Prozac, because his condition was "genetic." Both Roberto's father and brother suffered from the same problem. His father was afraid of riding in elevators or flying on airplanes and was on Zoloft through his primary-care doctor. His brother was afraid of elevators, subways, and airplanes. He was on high doses of Paxil and Valium through a psychopharmacologist.

Roberto said he had been phobic about riding elevators for as long as he could remember. He had decided to discuss the problem with his friend's mother, and shortly thereafter came to consult with me, because in just a few months' time he needed to go for interviews at consulting firms in New York and other cities around the country. "The first round of interviews will be on campus," said Roberto. "But then I'll get call-backs, second- and third-round interviews where they'll fly me down to their headquarters on the fiftieth floor of a Manhattan skyscraper. The interviews will last all day. I'll have to be able to ride elevators *with* people to go to lunch and dinner. I can't bolt at the elevator door like a wild pony. Not only will I have to ride elevators, I'll have to be able to do it with ease, so I can continue to carry on a conversation with enthusiasm."

Of medium height with a compact build, Roberto had a boyish look and a gregarious personality. He had grown up in a Brazilian-American neighborhood and was an avid soccer player. Roberto played center forward, a position of intense visibility and pressure to score. "I'm the one everybody always turns to when we have a penalty kick. That's pressure," he said.

"It is," I said knowingly. For several years I had been coaching my sons' soccer teams.

"I go out there on the field all alone, just me and the goalie, in front of all the fans and score. Then I say to myself, 'How can I not be able to ride a stupid elevator? It's ridiculous.'"

Roberto had many humorous stories of the "jams" his phobia had landed him in. "Just last week," he said, "I went on a first date with a woman I met at a club. When I got to her building, her apartment was on the sixth floor. 'Oh, man,' I thought, 'how am I going to get in and out of here?' She buzzed me into the lobby, where I made a dash for the stairwell. You learn to find stairwells quickly when you're afraid of elevators. I raced up the six flights of stairs because I didn't want her to notice me taking any extra time. I expected to get to the sixth floor and take a minute or two to catch my breath before knocking on her door. But when I arrived, there she was waiting for me in the hall. She looked startled when I dashed out of the stairwell huffing and puffing. 'Why didn't you take the elevator?' she asked. 'Oh,' I said breathlessly, trying to be casual, 'I needed the exercise.' She looked at me like I had two heads.

"We talked in her apartment for about half an hour and that went fine. We were going to dinner and a movie. All the while I kept thinking, 'What excuse could I make to leave ahead and meet her downstairs?' I wished I had my car or my bicycle so I could say I needed to check the lock, but I didn't. I became determined to take the elevator with her. I thought, 'This is as good a time as any to overcome this. I really like this girl. It's just six flights. I've got to do it.'

"When we were leaving, it felt like it took forever for her to lock her door, I was so nervous. My heart was pounding. Then she called the elevator and my heart sank. She lived in an old brick building in Boston. I swear the elevator was an antique. The doors creaked as they opened. The elevator had one of those black grates you slide open to get into it. When it finally came to a stop, the elevator floor was about five inches below the hall floor; they didn't line up. I imagined stepping down and the elevator plummeting in a free fall. I'm sure I went white in the face. 'Are you all right?' she asked. 'No. Ah . . . well, I really do need the exercise. I think I'll take the stairs. I'll meet you in the lobby, okay?'"

"How did she respond?"

"She was cool about it. What was she going to say? 'Are you some kind of a nut case?' Which I guess I am. We went out and had a good time. I haven't called her yet for a second date. That'll be the test. We'll see."

Even more amusing were Roberto's descriptions of working in a Manhattan bank building the previous summer.

"I worked on the forty-third floor of a skyscraper," he said.

"You did? You rode the elevator?"

"No. I walked."

"You walked?"

"Four times a day. Up in the morning, down at lunch. Back up again in the afternoon and down at night."

To do this, Roberto had to befriend the building manager and his staff, who controlled access to the stairwell: "You can't just get into the stairs in a high-rise. They have alarms for security. In the building where I worked, even the maintenance people couldn't get in on the first floor. They had to ride the elevator to the third floor, get out, unlock the door to the stairwell, and walk back down to the first floor where I was waiting. I felt so bad asking them to do this, not once but several times a day."

"Once you got inside, you walked up forty flights of stairs?"

"It was murder. This was July and August. There's no air conditioning in stairwells. I was wearing three-piece suits and lugging a heavy briefcase. I'd be sweating bullets by the time I got to the top. Forty flights of stairs, twenty a flight, that's eight hundred stairs a trip. Three thousand, two hundred stairs a day! It was like Olympic training."

"God . . ."

"When I finally got upstairs, I had to hide for fifteen or twenty minutes because I was drenched with sweat and didn't want anybody to see me. I'd go to the bathroom and use masses of paper towels to wipe off my face, hair, and neck.

"I was wearing flat-footed business shoes. They didn't have any padding. The impact of all those stairs really hurt! I started having knee problems. In July, I injured my hamstring on my right side. After work, I'd go to play basketball with my friends and be exhausted, favoring my right leg. They'd look at me like, 'Man, what's wrong with you?' When I told them I'd injured my hamstring, they asked, 'How? All you've been doing is working at a desk.' My parents were freaking out, picturing me running up and down thousands of stairs a day, ruining my body.

"The hardest thing was arranging to have lunch with people. I'd always agree to meet them at the restaurant. Then I'd sneak out a half hour or forty-five minutes ahead of them."

"Forty-five minutes?"

"It takes a long time to walk forty flights of stairs."

"Wow."

"The worst circumstance was when a group of people would spontaneously decide to go out to lunch and want me to join them."

"What would you do?"

"I really had to scramble. Usually, I'd go out to the elevator with everyone and wait until it arrived. Just as we were about to board, I'd make some excuse, that I'd forgotten my wallet or something. Sometimes people offered to wait for me but I always insisted they go ahead to get a table. It was really tough. I was always afraid my cover would be blown, that someone would see me coming out of the stairwell or one of the maintenance people would complain."

"Did anyone ever find out?"

"I told one person whom I became quite friendly with. No one else knew."

As amusing as Roberto's stories were, his phobia was a serious disability. If he could not ride elevators, he was going to be severely compromised looking for jobs. Roberto thought he would like an international career that would take him to Latin American countries. How could he manage working in the high-powered business world as long as he was petrified of riding in elevators? Returning to the interviews looming just a few months away, he said anxiously, "I don't know how I'm going to do it. Can you help me?"

"I think so." I tried to remain calm in response to Roberto's urgency. "It's a tall order in just a few months when you've had this all your life, but I think it's doable."

"Do I have to go on medication?"

"You're reluctant to?"

"My brother's like a zombie sometimes on all his medication. My father doesn't take as much, but he has a lot of reservations about it. I do too. I think that's why I've avoided seeking help."

Wanting to set things off on the right footing, I said, "I don't think there's any reason to believe your phobia is going to spread to airplanes or subways. I don't agree with your friend's mother."

"What a relief. I have to fly to all these interviews too." Given their authority, doctors have enormous power of suggestion. Why suggest Roberto's condition would spread instead of suggesting the opposite?

"Secondly, there's no proof your condition is genetic. Both you and your brother could have learned this from your father. His fear could have been a model for yours. Growing up, did you know he had this problem?"

"Yes. But it was subtle."

"Meaning?"

"If we went on vacation, even to Florida, we always drove because my father couldn't fly. We lived in New Jersey, so that meant a two- or three-day trip. With a car full of kids, that wasn't easy. But I wasn't really aware of why we didn't fly until much later in life."

"Did you know he couldn't ride elevators?"

"That I did know. I have memories of getting to elevators and my Dad freezing up. He wouldn't be able to take them and we'd all walk up the stairs."

"What about subways?"

"He never took subways either. That I was aware of too. My Dad tried to hide his problem from us. We didn't often end up in front of a bank of elevators, because he usually succeeded in avoiding it. But I do remember a few times vividly."

"You were young and impressionable at the time."

"Yes."

"I'm sure you looked up to your father. If he was afraid of elevators, why shouldn't you be? One can pick these things up almost subliminally. Don't worry about it being genetic."

"That means I can fix it myself, right, without going on medication?"

"We may need to use a little bit of medication like Valium. But it would be very little and only for a brief period of time. We'll see. Nothing long-term. No Prozac-type drug, which is what your father and brother are on."

Relaxation Techniques

As part of my work with Roberto, I referred him to a brief, four-session course of relaxation training. Relaxation, or stress-management, courses teach effective techniques for coping with anxiety using a variety of techniques: relaxation tapes, breathing exercises, meditation, biofeedback, progressive muscle relaxation, and cognitive therapy exercises for reframing anxious thoughts. While the courses vary in the particular combination of skills taught, some form of breathing exercises is essential. Much of the panic people in a hyperaroused state feel is due to rapid, shallow breathing with the upper chest. Instead, they need the calming effect of diaphragmatic breathing. Learning diaphragmatic breathing is essential to being able to talk oneself down from escalating anxiety.

The particular type of relaxation training Roberto received is called biofeedback. Biofeedback utilizes medical technology to monitor physiological measures of arousal like heart rate, breathing, or muscle tension. A small device is placed on the skin and wired to a monitor. The monitor provides a graphic display of one's breathing or other vital signs, giving instantaneous feedback regarding one's anxiety level. While a patient is being taught diaphragmatic breathing, progressive muscle relaxation, and other exercises, he can watch his heart rate or respirations displayed on the screen. This instantaneous feedback on biological functions (hence, "biofeedback") accelerates learning relaxation techniques.

Roberto learned the techniques quickly. Of course, the anxiety he felt riding elevators could not be replicated in the office as a real test. To accomplish this, his treatment needed to move into real-life situations.

Exposure

Since phobias are anxieties tied to specific objects and situations, they can often be unlearned by a treatment called "exposure."[1] In a series of increasingly stressful steps, the patient is gradually exposed to the anxiety-provoking event. The steps are worked out in advance by the patient and therapist. In each step, a portion of the patient's anxiety wears off as he acclimatizes to the situation. Eventually, the small steps add up until the patient is comfortable with the formerly phobic object or circumstances.

The first stage of exposure treatment is to visualize increasingly stressful steps. In Roberto's case, the steps were (1) going to the elevator in the lobby of a building, (2) pushing the button to call it, (3) watching the numbers light up above the door as the elevator descends, (4) watching the doors open, (5) stepping inside the elevator, (6) letting the doors close, (7) riding up just one flight, (8) watching the doors open, (9) getting out. Still more difficult was (10) imagining riding in a crowded elevator or (11) taking it up ten, twenty, or thirty flights, or more.

For a number of sessions, Roberto would lie back in the chair, imagine each of these increasingly anxiety-provoking steps, and use the relaxation techniques to calm himself. Gradually, Roberto became more comfortable as the process demythologized riding in elevators. Unfortunately, he did not have much time to spend on this stage of the treatment. Visualizing the situations was just a warm-up. The next stage—putting himself in real-life situations riding elevators—would be much more stressful as well as more productive. Given the time constraints, he had to move on to the next stage fairly quickly.

For the real-life exposure, Roberto and I made a list of increasingly difficult challenges. The behavior therapist who taught him the relaxation techniques agreed to go with him several times to ride elevators. With my encouragement, he lined up close friends who were willing to go at other times. Roberto said riding in a glass elevator would be the easiest first step.

"Why a glass elevator?" I asked.

"Because then I could see where I was going. I wouldn't have quite the same trapped feeling."

"Okay. Well, there's the Cambridgeside Galleria Mall and also the Hyatt Hotel. Both of them have glass elevators. They're not too tall. They might be ideal starting points."

Once he could ride glass elevators to the top, Roberto would move on to enclosed ones. We worked out a schedule of increasingly difficult exercises in which he needed to be able to ride one story, five stories, ten stories, twenty stories, thirty stories, or more.

"At the end of each stage," I asked, "what would be the sign that you'd mastered that level before moving on?"

Roberto thought a minute, then said, "When I visualized riding in an elevator and did the relaxation exercises . . ."

"Yes?"

"I imagined watching the panel of lights that tell you which floor the elevator is passing. It would be a real test for me to turn my back to that panel, not be able to see it."

"Because?"

"Then you have no idea where the elevator is on the journey, and that's more stressful."

"Good. At each stage, that's what you'll do to feel confident to move on to the next one."

Finally, Roberto said the most difficult challenge would be riding an express elevator that quickly ascends twenty to thirty stories before it begins stopping at the higher floors. For this, he would need to go to the financial district in downtown Boston. This final step would replicate the situation he would face interviewing in New York and elsewhere.

I did not accompany Roberto on any of these trips. The behavior therapist accompanied him on the first few, which were quite stressful. He described one incident in which the behaviorist literally pushed him into an elevator because he was a little hesitant. This made me somewhat apprehensive, but it apparently worked.

Meanwhile, Roberto began going out almost every day with one of his friends riding elevators. He had a group of loyal friends, other Harvard undergraduates, all of whom knew about his problem and were willing to help. On some days he went on his own. At each meeting, Roberto and I went over the drill for what he had to accomplish that week. Ever the jock, he referred to himself as "being in training" for elevators.

Psychotherapy

In addition to monitoring his progress, Roberto and I talked about his history. Aside from his father being a role model for the anxiety, were there any other underlying causes?

Roberto's parents had both immigrated from Brazil, coming to this country with their parents when they were young children. His grandfather started a family business, a restaurant, which his father now ran.

"It's a typical self-made, immigrant story," said Roberto. "My parents aren't rich, but they're comfortably well off. The family is incredibly close-knit. Uncles, aunts, cousins, and grandparents, we all get along pretty well."

"Do you feel under any pressure to continue the immigrant success story by becoming a Wall Street consultant?"

"I don't think I'm under pressure. My parents just want me to be happy."

"I ask because people under pressure can become resentful and symptomatic."

"That might have been true for my father. He might have been resentful when he was young."

"What happened to him?"

"He grew up quite poor in São Paulo. His father, my grandfather, actually came out to this country ahead of the rest of the family. He was here several years before he could afford to bring them over. Meanwhile, back in Brazil my father got polio and was hospitalized."

"Was he left with permanent disabilities from the polio?"

"No. He was lucky. But it was all very stressful. When he was twelve he finally came to this country with his mother and brothers and sisters. I think they might have been delayed a year while he was recuperating. I'm not sure.

"Anyway, he came here for high school and then went to college at Ohio State. He majored in physics and went on to medical school. He had just started that when my grandfather had a heart attack and my father had to come home to run the business."

"Oh."

"Yeah. I think that must have been hard."

"You think he's resentful?"

"He might have been, but he's since gotten over it. I think the early part of his life was difficult, with his father leaving and the polio. When he finally got established in this country, he had to give up medical school. Still, he and my mother have had a good life. He says that all the time. Family is what matters most to him. But maybe it had something to do with his anxieties."

"Does he like the restaurant?"

"He expanded by franchising the restaurant. That he enjoys. And he's done well."

"Would he like you to work in the family business?"

"No. Perhaps because of his history, my father wants us to feel free to do whatever we like."

"Do you feel guilty about having the freedom he didn't have?"

"No. I mean, yes, a little. But it's not a problem. My father's very encouraging of me. The one thing they're not happy about is my interest in an international career, because that will mean living abroad for a while, and as I say, they're big on having family around, nearby."

"Are they upset enough to make you conflicted about it?"

"I really don't think so. They're cool. They've accepted it. I'll be back by the time I'm ready to raise a family. It's just something I need to get out of my system."

Roberto was quite convincing. There was no trace of a serious conflict with his family. So we looked elsewhere for what might be the problem.

In one session, Roberto said he himself had reservations about living in Manhattan and traveling all the time for a large consulting firm. "The lifestyle looks attractive," said Roberto, "but it's a rat race. When you're working eighty hours a week, where do you find the time to do anything else? Sometimes I picture the Manhattan skyline with all those skyscrapers lit up all night . . . because people are working in them! I think, 'Do I really want to do that?'"

I feel strongly about psychotherapy not just propping people up to do things they fundamentally do not want to do. "That's what skyscrapers symbolize to you?"

"In a way, yes."

"It's because of interviewing for these jobs that you've come to see me. You've said express elevators in skyscrapers are the hardest."

"Yes."

"Do you think you don't want to be able to do this? Do express elevators symbolize the fast track, which you have mixed feelings about?"

"I definitely have mixed feelings but I know I want to do it. Hey, I'm here, right?"

"That's true. But you can still be very ambivalent."

"I have reservations but I know what I want to do."

"Okay."

In yet another conversation Roberto mentioned that his best friends and girlfriends had always known about his problem. "It's embarrassing but I've been very open about it," he said. "They think it's a joke at first. They think it's ridiculous but they accept it."

"How does it make you feel?"

"I feel like a big baby not being able to ride an elevator. Anyone can do it. People think of me as the together, strong one. I'm usually the person people come to for advice if they're upset. I'm the oldest kid in my family, so I got used to that. It's ridiculous that I can't ride an elevator."

I commented that Roberto had a boyish quality, and he agreed. Was his elevator phobia symbolic of an immature part of him? If he was so responsible in every other way, was this a way of protesting just a little? Of drawing attention to himself and saying, "Here's one thing I can't do"?

"There might be a little of that," Roberto responded. "I don't really want to graduate next spring. I don't really want to leave college and all my friends. But I know I have to."

While intriguing, these feelings did not adequately explain Roberto's phobia. Most people have mixed feelings about graduating from college and moving on into the adult world. Perhaps there were no major issues behind Roberto's phobia. Maybe he just learned it from his father, plain and simple.

The one thing we did turn up were control issues, but these are almost always present in phobias and other forms of anxiety. Roberto repeatedly said he felt "trapped" in elevators. "It's not so much that I'm worried about the elevator cable snapping and falling to the basement. I don't think that's likely to happen. You know what I worry about?"

"What?"

"That the elevator will get stuck and I'll be hours waiting for somebody to get me out."

"But if you'll ultimately be safe, what's the problem?"

"It's that I'm not in control of fixing the problem."

"Fixing the problem?"

"Yeah. If the elevator's stopped, something's wrong, but I don't necessarily trust the people who'll come to fix it."

"Trust?"

Roberto had to struggle to clarify and articulate his feelings. "I'm embarrassed to say this but . . . I work very hard to solve problems, fast. But will someone else, someone who's responsible for my fate?"

"So the problem is thinking you would do it better."

Roberto laughed, embarrassed. "I'm not just making this up."

"Meaning?"

"I remember a couple of years ago I was studying in the Hilles Library up in the Quad and someone got stuck in the elevator."

"Really?"

"I was sitting nearby. I remember the alarm going off, the maintenance men coming and shutting it off. They were talking to the girl in the elevator while they were trying to fix it."

"They were?"

"Yes. Man, I felt so bad for the girl. Anyway, the maintenance men were incredibly slow. I heard them looking for tools they couldn't find and saying they didn't know what they were doing."

"Oh, great."

"I know. And this is what really worries me if I get stuck. That someone's going to take their sweet time or, worse, not really know what they're doing. This girl was stuck in the elevator for hours. I think one of the maintenance men went to lunch and came back. I would never do that."

"It's not optimal, but ultimately, if the girl in the elevator was safe . . ."

"She lost three hours of her life."

"That's not the worst thing in the world."

"What if I had something I needed to do?"

"Look, you can't always account for every minute. And you have to have some degree of trust in people in order to go about living. Every time you step into the street you trust that the driver of the oncoming car will see you and stop."

"It's all in my head."

"It's purely psychological."

"I know. Elevators are just where it hits me. Anyway, I'm working on it."

Roberto made steady progress with the exposure. Periodically he stalled, missing a few days of practice because he was afraid of moving up the ladder of difficulty. Each time, I played the coach, insisting Roberto push himself to new limits.

After mastering the glass elevators, Roberto dragged his feet moving on to enclosed ones. "This is the hardest part for me," he said anxiously.

"Because of the trapped feeling?"

"They're so much more confining."

Working with Roberto, I had actually become a little more conscious of the risks of riding elevators. Although I did not develop problems taking them, I wondered, "Should any of us be riding in these things? Maybe Roberto is sane and society is crazy." This is an occupational hazard of working closely with people with so many kinds of problems. Talking with the Harvard maintenance man in my building one day, I asked him what one would do if an elevator got stuck. He pointed out something I had never noticed: Most elevators have a small trap door in the ceiling big enough for a person to hoist themselves through. I mentioned this to

Roberto in the period when he was delaying moving on to enclosed elevators and it actually helped.

"You're right," he said the following week, somewhat surprised. "I know it's irrational, but it makes me feel better to think I could climb out if I wanted to."

A friend of Roberto's recommended he get a cellular phone to take with him on elevators.

"Do you think that would help?" I asked.

"I do."

"Well, then it's a good idea."

Roberto managed to find a good deal on a cellular phone. "I got the one with the lowest monthly rate," he said. "It would cost me a fortune to actually make a call but I figure I'm never going to use it. If I get stuck in an elevator, I'll be happy to pay for the call."

Finally, Roberto began riding enclosed elevators, taking it a step at a time, gradually increasing the distances he rode. "I'm getting to know every elevator in Harvard Square," he said jokingly one day. "A friend and I were at the Charles Hotel the other day. The bellhop started looking at us strangely after he kept meeting us coming and going on elevators."

Roberto never took any medication to help overcome the elevator phobia. People often find that their anxiety is reduced simply by carrying a small bottle of a Valium-type drug with them as a sort of security blanket, even if they do not use it. I offered this to Roberto, but he declined. Because of the example of his father and brother, he was worried about becoming dependent on drugs. He wanted to overcome the phobia on his own if at all possible. I supported this.

Roberto went home to New Jersey over the Christmas break. I encouraged him to ride elevators there, and possibly even take a train into Manhattan to confront the skyscrapers themselves, but he chose not to. Returning to Cambridge, he resumed the exposure program.

In January and February, Roberto's on-campus job interviews began. He did well and began to get call-backs in New York. With just two weeks to go, now comfortably riding ten-to-twenty-story elevators in Cambridge, he stalled at the final step, going into Boston to ride express elevators.

"I can't do it," Roberto said. He had lost his confidence.

"Of course you can."

"You think so?"

"Of course you can. You've done the hardest part. This is just icing on the cake."

"Maybe I'll just wait and see in New York."

"What do you mean?"

"If I have to, I can always ask to be let into the stairwell."

"No you cannot," I said a little impatiently.

"I can't?"

"No. You know very well that could ruin a job prospect. You have to be able to ride elevators by the summer in order to do the job. So you need to do it now."

"Okay."

The next week Roberto thanked me for "the kick in the pants." He had gone into Boston several times to ride express elevators. Part of getting results with people is pushing at the right junctures, when they still might be inclined to hold back. At some point, most people need to be confronted about how they are contributing to their own problem or reneging on their desire to change. This is not the equivalent of telling a person in pain to "suck it up," or to just use willpower to overcome a longstanding debilitation. On the contrary, Roberto received considerable support and attention to his emotions as he tried to deal with his phobia. In this case, that "kick in the pants" for Roberto was a gentle push at a critical moment.

When Roberto finally went off for his first New York interview, it felt as if he were going to a World Cup competition. Would he make it? Or would the pressure of the job interviews raise his anxiety level so high that his recently established ability to ride elevators would evaporate? "Wish me luck," he said on his way out.

When Roberto came back the next week he happily reported that all had gone well. At the last minute he had thought to take the cell phone with him "just in case." Weeks before, he had gotten out of the habit of taking it with him, but for the final challenge he decided to take it along. The first few times he rode elevators to go to lunch with people who were interviewing him, he was apprehensive, but everything went fine. After that, he had no trouble. Just a few months after beginning treatment, Roberto was able to ride elevators.

While Roberto overcame his elevator phobia without drugs, his father and brother remained on serotonin boosters. His brother also took Valium three times a day. In the last decade, I have often seen patients overcome their difficulties with little or no medication while a number of their family members are on multiple medications, often still symptomatic, and sometimes even deteriorating.

Karen: A Case of Severe Anxiety

Karen was in her third week of an intensive computer programming course when she developed severe anxiety. "I don't know what's happened to me," said Karen, tearfully clutching a fistful of tissues at our first appointment. "For the first time in my life I'm so anxious I can't function."

Karen was referred by the employee assistance program at her company, a Cambridge-based high-technology firm. I was familiar with the intensive, four-month course she was in, having seen other people who became symptomatic while undertaking it. The company periodically offered the course to fill vacancies in their expanding software division. The course allowed qualified individuals to enhance their career opportunities. Since graduating from the University of Massachusetts two years earlier, Karen had worked for the company as a technical support person to computer programmers. Now she had the chance to become a programmer herself.

The immersion course met for eight to ten hours a day, five days a week. Mornings were devoted to four hours of grueling lectures. Afternoons and evenings were spent working in a computer lab doing hands-on programming projects. At night, participants were expected to read long homework assignments in preparation for the next day. During the lectures, they were called upon to answer questions based on the reading. This was what Karen feared most: "I'm petrified of being called on in class. We're being asked questions on material we haven't been taught yet. Some people seem to have more background than I do. If I'm called on and don't know the answer, I feel humiliated."

"Humiliated?"

"I feel so stupid in front of everyone."

"But it's a challenging course, moving at a fast pace. You can't know everything."

"That's just it. I'm a wreck because, for once, I don't."

"What do you mean 'for once'?"

"In college and high school I always overlearned everything. There wasn't anything I didn't know when called on. I can't cope with this."

"How do you feel sitting in class?"

"Like something terrible is going to happen to me that I can't control. My stomach's churning. My mouth gets so dry I have trouble talking. I have a sense of dread and the urge to flee."

"To flee?"

"I'm afraid I'm going to get up and run out of the room. I haven't done it yet. I don't want to call that kind of attention to myself. But I feel like doing it all the time."

In addition to her upset stomach and parched mouth, Karen had episodes in which she experienced a racing heart, pins and needles in her fingertips, the sensation of being unable to catch a full breath, feeling like she might faint, and rapid, shallow breathing. These severe anxiety attacks lasted five minutes or more.

"What brings them to a stop?" I asked.

"Nothing in particular. I grit my teeth until they pass. I'm left exhausted and still pretty anxious but not feeling quite as bad."

"How often are the severe attacks happening?"

"Three or four times a day."

"And what happens when you're actually called on in class?"

"I freeze."

"You freeze?"

"Like a deer in the headlights. Even when I do know the answer, I'm not able to express myself well because I'm so scared. It's terrible. Afternoons in the computer lab are a little easier than the big, morning classes. In the lab we work in small groups. There's more personalized attention. You're not so much on the spot."

Unfortunately, at night Karen's anxiety rose again: "I become obsessed with the reading. I go over and over anything I don't understand, getting more and more anxious. I compulsively make notes and underline things in three different colors of pens. When I try to go to bed I can't get the reading out of my head. I feel wired and can't fall asleep. Especially if I haven't understood everything, I lie in bed obsessing about being called on in class." In a vicious cycle, the insomnia only made Karen more exhausted, more worn down, and more vulnerable to anxiety.

"Has anything like this ever happened to you before?"

"I've always been an anxious person, but nothing like this. I'm a perfectionist. I've always been compulsive about my work."

"But you've never been this symptomatic before."

Karen thought a moment, then recalled, "It happened once before in college. I took an economics course and found myself in over my head. I had the same panicky feelings, like I couldn't cope. That professor, too, called on people cold. I didn't always know the answer and couldn't stand it."

"What happened?"

"I dropped the course."

"Are you afraid of that happening again?"

"That's why I'm here," said Karen tearfully. "I don't want to have to drop out this time. Am I going crazy?"

"No," I said. I explained to Karen that she was experiencing severe anxiety. All her symptoms—panic, insomnia, obsessions, and compulsiveness—were manifestations of the anxiety.

"Can I overcome it?" she asked, plaintively.

"Yes," I reassured her. I explained that we would use a combination of approaches—psychotherapy, relaxation techniques, diet, exercise, and other lifestyle changes. Because her anxiety was severe, we would use a small amount of medication for a limited period of time while waiting for the natural alternatives to take effect.

I referred Karen to a brief course in relaxation training, much like the one I had suggested to Roberto. Karen's class consisted of relaxation tapes, biofeedback, breathing exercises, time-management skills, and cognitive therapy exercises.

Karen learned the techniques quickly and within weeks found them helpful for managing her in-class anxiety. As part of their cognitive-behavioral work, the behavior therapist encouraged Karen to put banners up in her apartment with slogans like "I'm going to make it," "Everything will be all right," and "Just take it a day at a time." Joining in the spirit of these affirmations, I suggested Karen come up with a mantra, a short phrase she could use to reassure herself when she felt panic coming on. Karen's mantra was "I'm free to leave." When I asked what this meant, she said, "It's very important for me to see myself as not being trapped. I keep telling myself I'm taking this course of my own free will and I'm free to leave. Knowing that somehow helps me to stay."

Lifestyle Changes: Diet, Exercise, Sleep, and Work Habits

A remarkable number of anxious people drink strong coffee or other forms of caffeine throughout the day. Many of them complain that their anxiety causes them to lie awake in bed at night, unable to fall asleep. Poorly rested, the next day they resort to coffee to keep themselves awake, which only aggravates their anxiety in a vicious circle. One of the most common scenarios seen in campus health services is that students use strong coffee, over-the-counter stimulants like NoDoz, or prescription stimulants like Ritalin to keep themselves up all night to study for exams or finish papers to meet deadlines. After several days of this, they come in with complaints of anxiety, not aware of the cycle they are caught in. Many people do not realize how much caffeine amplifies anxiety. People experiencing anxiety should eliminate all caffeine from their diet.

Although Karen felt the need for strong coffee to stay alert during her long morning classes, she agreed to taper it off. This has to be done slowly to avoid severe withdrawal headaches. Like many people, Karen was surprised to find herself calmer and more energetic after weaning herself off the caffeine.

Aerobic exercise is as effective for anxiety and insomnia as it is for depression. Karen was "not big on exercise" and resisted the idea of joining a gym, but she began walking briskly twenty minutes to and from her commuter rail station instead of driving. Even this modest amount of regular, aerobic exercise can make a big difference with anxiety and insomnia.

Together, Karen and I went over the guidelines for good sleep habits. Karen's classes prevented her from oversleeping in the morning or taking daytime naps, even though she was often tired after a poor night's sleep. In order to break the cycle of lying in bed ruminating about her reading, I encouraged Karen to stop studying about a half hour before she wanted to go to bed and instead do something relaxing. After considering watching TV, knitting, or reading mysteries, Karen decided on listening to the relaxation tapes from her biofeedback class. Through a catalogue, she bought several more tapes in order to vary them.

On my suggestion, Karen also tried the herbs kava and valerian. Valerian worked well for her insomnia. Although kava works well for many people with mild to moderate daytime anxiety, it was not potent enough to abort Karen's severe anxiety attacks, so I gave her a prescription for a small amount of a Valium-type medication, which she used temporarily in the early weeks of treatment with good results.

Herbal Remedies: Kava and Valerian

In recent years, a number of herbal remedies have become increasingly popular alternatives to more potent, prescription drugs for anxiety and insomnia. Kava is an ancient ceremonial and medicinal herb of the South Sea islands: Tahiti, Fiji, the Marshall and Solomon Islands, Vanuatu, Tonga, and Samoa. Kava's Latin name is *Piper methysticum,* meaning "intoxicating pepper."[2] In the South Pacific, kava is served as a drink in coconut shell bowls. Kava has a mellowing effect, inducing a state of contentment and well-being. During social and ceremonial occasions, kava improves conviviality by relaxing people.

The first Western accounts of kava date to Captain James Cook's eighteenth-century voyage to the South Seas.[3] As recently as 1950, kava was listed in the U.S. Dispensary under the name Neurocardin as a treatment for nervous disorders.[4] In Europe—particularly Germany, Switzerland, and France—kava is a leading antianxiety agent.[5] Kava is also used as a pain reliever and muscle relaxant.

As with St. John's wort, most of the clinical research on herbal antianxiety agents has been carried out in Germany. Clinical studies have demonstrated kava's efficacy in treating anxiety disorders. These studies are similar to those used to win approval of synthetic antianxiety agents and sleeping pills. One of the largest and most recent was a double-blind, placebo-controlled study of 101 patients with a variety of conditions, including agoraphobia, social phobia, and generalized anxiety disorder. Conducted by H. P. Volz at the University of Jena, the study was published in *Pharmacopsychiatry* in 1997.[6] Kava outperformed the placebo and decreased the gamut of physical symptoms of anxiety, from a racing heart to shortness of breath, chest pain, stomach upset, and feeling faint. Other double-blind, placebo-controlled studies of kava's efficacy have obtained similar results.[7] Reviewing the published research, Michael T. Murray concludes in his 1995 book, *Stress, Anxiety, and Insomnia,* "European countries have approved kava preparations on the basis of detailed pharmacological data and favorable clinical studies."[8]

Kava has been compared directly with Valium-type sedatives. A group led by Dr. H. Woelk at the University of Giessen compared kava with Serax and another European Valium-type drug in 164 patients with anxiety symptoms.[9] Kava was comparable with the two synthetic drugs at improving anxiety in the report published in 1993 in the German medical journal *Zeitscrift für Allgemeinmedizin.*

Kava has few side effects when taken at recommended doses. Some patients report mild upset stomach after taking doses of kava. This can usually be remedied by taking the herb with meals. Excessive doses taken over prolonged periods of time can cause yellowing of the skin and a scaly rash known as kava dermopathy. The condition clears when the herb is stopped and does not occur at moderate, recommended doses.

The German formulary recommends kava not be taken for more than three months at a time. Hyla Cass, a psychiatrist at the UCLA School of Medicine, writes in her 1998 book, *Kava: Nature's Answer to Stress, Anxiety, and Insomnia,* "The rationale in Germany for a three-month limit is . . . a general sense that you shouldn't depend on an outside substance on a daily basis. In dealing with anxiety, kava should be regarded as temporary help while finding ways of healing on a deeper level."[10]

The active ingredients in kava are thought to be a group of compounds known as kavalactones. Kava preparations are standardized according to their kavalactone content. When used for daytime anxiety, the recommended dose is 70 milligrams of kavalactones taken one to three times a day. When taken at night for sleep, the recommended dose is 70 to 210 milligrams an hour before bedtime. In my experience, patients find kava more effective for daytime anxiety because it is calming without being sedating.

Valerian grows wild in fields and mountainsides all over Europe. The valerian root has been used medicinally for centuries, dating back to the time of the ancient Greeks. Valerian was used as a decongestant by Galen, one of the foremost Greek physicians whose written works have come down to us.[11] By the nineteenth century, valerian was widely used as a sedative, especially for anxiety associated with gastrointestinal distress. Valerian was officially listed in the *U.S. Pharmacopoeia* until 1936 and in the *National Formulary* as recently as 1950.[12] In this country, herbal remedies were abandoned in the middle of this century with the rise of more powerful pharmaceutical agents. By contrast, in Europe these centuries-old medicines continue to be prescribed.

Today valerian is enjoying a surge in popularity as an herbal sleeping pill. Dr. Andrew Weil describes valerian as a "strong enough sedative to be used for insomnia" in his 1995 best-seller *Spontaneous Healing.*[13] Valerian produces deep, restful sleep, usually without causing a "hangover" the next morning, as is more likely to happen with potent, synthetic drugs.

A number of clinical studies have documented valerian's effects. A group of Swiss doctors headed by Peter Leathwood tested valerian in a short, nine-day placebo-controlled study involving 128 people, which was published in the July 1982 issue of *Pharmacology, Biochemistry, and Behavior.*[14] Valerian shortened the time required to fall asleep and improved the quality of sleep without causing oversedation the next day.

A team of German doctors led by E. Vorbach studied 121 patients with insomnia in a double-blind, placebo-controlled study of valerian.[15] The patients were assessed at two weeks and one month. Valerian was significantly better than placebo at improving sleep and overall mood. In this study, valerian's effects were seen in the latter half of the month, indicating that the herb's benefits may slowly accrue over time.

A team of German doctors led by H. Dressing compared a mixture of valerian and lemon balm to the Valium-type sleeping pill Halcion. The study was published in the German medical journal *Therapiewoch* in 1992.[16] The valerian–lemon balm combination was as effective as Halcion for inducing sleep. Reviewing the studies of valerian in *Psychosomatic Medicine* in 1999, Dr. Jerry Cott—an authority on natural products at the National Institute of

Mental Health—describes the herb as a "popular European botanical medicine used for its mild sedative and tranquilizing properties."[17]

The recommended dose of valerian varies depending on the preparation. Many other sedating herbs are available in health food stores. Some of the most popular preparations contain combinations of herbs: mixtures of valerian, kava, passionflower, skullcap, and hops. For people suffering both anxiety and depression, mixtures of these herbs and St. John's wort are available.

Balancing Medication with Natural Alternatives

Nowadays, many patients like Karen are automatically put on a serotonin booster for years. This should not be done until all other options have been exhausted. These powerful drugs should only be considered in the most debilitating cases of anxiety.

When using serotonin boosters for anxiety, psychopharmacologists advise, "Start low and go slow." That is, one starts with low doses, usually half those typically used in depression, and slowly increase. The more gradual dosing is necessary to avoid worsening anxiety, since the drugs are so stimulating. So long as one allows the nervous system time to gradually adapt, the serotonin booster's energizing, concentration-enhancing, and mood-elevating properties ultimately have a calming effect.

As described in Chapter 4, on suicide and violence, prescribing serotonin boosters to anxious patients is more dangerous than prescribing them for patients who are just depressed. For this reason, a Valium-type sedative may be prescribed simultaneously to "cover" the anxiety short-term. Once the serotonin booster is working, the antianxiety agent can be removed, usually within a month or two. Too often, the sedative is not removed and patients remain on it indefinitely.

Instead of using serotonin boosters with patients who are experiencing high-grade symptoms of anxiety, I prefer short-term use of a Valium-type drug on its own. Even with patients whose anxiety is as severe as Karen's, drugs are best used on an as-needed basis, when they feel panic coming on. Only if the patient's anxiety is debilitating should drugs be used on a regular basis, two or three times a day. In either case, medication should only be used for short periods of time while waiting for the natural alternatives to work.

There are many drugs in the Valium class including Ativan, Xanax, Klonopin, Librium, Serax, Dalmane, Restoril, and Halcion. Some are used primarily for daytime anxiety while others are used primarily as sleeping pills. The main differences among them are how rapidly the drugs take effect and how slowly they wear off.

Valium-type drugs have effects on brain receptors that are similar to the effects of alcohol. With regular, long-term use, patients can develop tolerance, dependence, and addiction, but these can be avoided when the drugs are used sparingly, on an as-needed basis for short periods of time. Used in this way, the risks of Valium-type drugs seem to be minimal by comparison with the long-term use of serotonin boosters.

I gave Karen a prescription for a low dose of a Valium-type antianxiety agent. I instructed her to take between a half and two pills, depending on how much she required to stop incipient panic. This gave her a range within which to find an optimal dose, although even two of the pills was still a small amount. The goal was to cut the edge off Karen's anxiety sufficiently to maintain her ability to function while avoiding taking so much that sedation interfered with her functioning.

After the frightening experience of a few panic attacks, many people develop "anticipatory anxiety." In a vicious cycle of escalating anxiety, they become anxious about becoming anxious. Anticipatory anxiety is often triggered by specific cues in stressful settings. Karen's anticipatory anxiety improved dramatically with the knowledge that she had an effective medication in her possession. In the first month of treatment, Karen used the medication judiciously, once or twice a day on an as-needed basis, three out of four days a week, to control her panic. The point of skipping days is so the nervous system does not become habituated to the drug. In the early weeks of treatment, the medication was invaluable in making it possible for Karen to relax in classes. Thereafter, as other parts of her treatment began to work, she was able to minimize her use of the drug. Still, the small bottle of pills served as a "security blanket" that helped to reduce Karen's anticipatory anxiety even when she no longer needed to use it.

Psychotherapy

All the interventions described so far helped Karen to manage her anxiety. Simultaneously in therapy we were looking for its causes. Karen grew up in Worcester, Massachusetts, an industrial city an hour west of Boston. Her father was a machinist who worked at a factory. Her mother was a billing clerk. Karen had one brother five years younger than she.

Early on, Karen told me her father was psychologically and physically abusive when she was young. Karen seemed reluctant to discuss the abuse in any detail and I did not press her. She said her father had "mellowed" with age. He had not hit her in years, since she was in her early teens. Perhaps this was why she preferred not to talk about the abuse, to leave it in the past. Or perhaps she was too anxious already with the stress of her class to delve into upsetting material.

From an early age, Karen was a diligent student. In retrospect, she recognized this as a bid for attention from teachers to make up for a lack of attention at home. In addition to being a good student, she became involved in numerous extracurricular activities that kept her at school until six or seven o'clock in the evening. "As a kid, I was an overachiever," said Karen. "I overlearned every detail. It made me incredibly anxious not to know something. I had to get perfect grades, because my teachers' attention depended on it. And I wanted to go to college. I knew I needed a full scholarship. My father would never have paid for it."

Was this history the reason Karen felt so anxious in the computer programming class? The fast pace of the class, which inundated students with material, challenged the way Karen had always functioned in school. By making it impossible for her to know everything, to be the perfect student, did it threaten her academic performance, the jewel in her crown? Even though Karen was older, two years out of college, and independent, going back into a classroom setting naturally triggered these issues. Was this the full explanation for the severity of Karen's anxiety? Or was there something deeper?

Karen's relationship with her family was still strained. Since college she had been living with her boyfriend, a situation her parents did not approve of. "They're pretty opinionated," said Karen. "They're not very tolerant."

As the numerous psychosocial interventions—relaxation techniques, aerobic exercise, valerian for sleep, giving up coffee, and sparing use of the prescription medication to abort panic—began to work, Karen became a little more relaxed. "I'm still anxious," she said, "but I feel like I have tools to deal with it." As she relaxed somewhat, in therapy Karen gradually became more open about the abuse by her father.

Karen's father had worked the morning shift at his job. In the midafternoon, when Karen and her brother came home from school, her father would just be getting back from work. Typically, he would be irritable and bad-tempered. Often he would ask Karen to prepare him some food. Even when she went to some trouble, her father would usually find fault with what Karen made for him: the food was too hot or too cold, undercooked or overcooked, too little or too much. "I look back on it now," said Karen, upset, "and realize I couldn't win." She never had the right answer, I thought, beginning to hear the themes of her abuse overlap with her problems in her class. "He was just looking for someone to take out his frustration on. He was always criticizing me, telling me I was stupid, ugly, and useless." Being stupid was precisely Karen's fear in class, I thought. Often when people feel out of control in one area of their lives, they try to exert overcontrol in another, to compensate. In addition, because she was being told she was so awful at home, doing well at school was a way for Karen to try to redeem herself. "Frequently, when I was young, he would haul off, slapping, punching, and kicking me. My younger brother got much better treatment. Watching what was happening to me, he stayed out of my father's way. And as a boy, he wasn't expected to wait on him." I refrained from making the direct connection between the abuse and the classroom, feeling Karen might not be ready for that yet. Karen sometimes took refuge in a neighbor's house when her father assaulted her. "The family next door was wonderful. When I could, I ran over there." Here was the powerful urge to flee Karen often felt in class.

"Remember I told you I joined all kinds of after-school activities as soon as I was old enough?" asked Karen one day.

"Yes."

"That's the reason why. I stayed out until I knew my mother would be home from work and he could no longer hit me."

"Did she know he was hitting you?"

"Yes. My mother never felt she could leave him. He made more money than she did and controlled the purse strings. He's mellowed a lot but their marriage is pretty empty. I tell her all the time to leave him, but she won't."

"How has your brother fared?"

"I used to think he did much better than I, because he wasn't much of a target of my father's. But he's actually done quite poorly. I at least got out of the house, did well, and went to college. I developed a whole life outside the family. My brother didn't. He never went to college, lives at home, and works a menial job. I worry a lot about him."

A few weeks later, Karen's unconscious connected the abuse and the class in a vivid nightmare that woke her in the middle of the night. "I was back in a classroom in grade school," said Karen, upset the next day. "But the teacher was one of the instructors from my computer course. You know the way things can be like that in dreams?"

"Yes. Dreams can cut across time and space."

"This teacher paces in the classroom. He gets very excited when he's moving at a fast clip. My father used to pace just before he hit me."

"Oh, really."

"Yes. In the dream I'm getting more and more anxious sitting there. The teacher starts to look menacing. He goes up to people and is in their face. And ..." Tears started streaming down Karen's face.

"What did the teacher do?" I asked gently.

"Suddenly he came up and punched me."

"He punched you?"

"In the dream."

"What for?"

"I don't know. Nothing. I didn't know the answer? For nothing. Does there have to be a reason? For being there."

"Just like your father."

"Yeah ... ," said Karen, choking on her tears.

In the wake of the dream, Karen's anxiety became worse before it got better. By now she had stopped using the medication, and I encouraged her not to return to it unless she absolutely had to. This was the emotion, the connection between the classroom and her father's abuse, which she needed to work through.

As she untangled the connections, Karen became aware of actually being afraid in the classroom of being hit by an instructor. "You asked me earlier," she said, "if I was more prone to panic in any particular class and I said no. But I've thought about it and noticed a pattern. There is one instructor whose class I'm more likely to panic in. He's the one who really paces. I think that's the trigger, the pacing and his impatience."

"That's what comes closest to your father when he was in a rage?"

"Yes."

Karen was literally afraid of being punched in class to a degree that surprised me. Her fear was a transference reaction: Karen was transferring the abusive childhood scene with her father onto the stressful classroom and the impatient teacher in particular. I went over with her repeatedly that she was, in fact, safe in the class. No matter how excited they might get, these instructors were not going to hit her.

Until now, Karen had warded off this anxiety. She kept a tight lid on it by only taking courses where she could feel in control. The one other insurmountable challenge was the economics course in college, which she had quickly dropped. Now, because she was unable to control things in the fast-paced computer programming course, the anxiety had flooded through again.

Often, as in Karen's case, there is a kernel of truth to transference reactions. Certainly, the course was fast-paced. The way in which it hammered people with material and questions may have bordered on being abusive. Over the years, I had heard from others who became symptomatic in the course that the particular instructor who made Karen the most anxious was, in fact, quite impatient, even nasty at times.

Karen's current circumstances had acted as a trigger around which her long-repressed anxieties crystallized. In chemistry, crystals form in supersaturated solutions. Often such solutions can sit indefinitely without crystallizing until some small solid object, a nidus, is dropped into them. Just a grain of sand will do to start the process. But once the crystal begins to form around the nidus, the reaction is unstoppable; the crystal rapidly spreads throughout the solution. Karen's long-repressed emotions were like a supersaturated solution. The pressurized course and the impatient teacher in particular were the nidus around which her seeming overreaction crystallized.

As Karen worked through these buried emotions, her anxiety subsided. Nevertheless, she stayed in therapy for two months after the course was over to help make the difficult transition into her first computer programming job.

Clinical Research on Treating Anxiety with Therapy Versus Drugs

Extensive clinical research on anxiety has shown psychological treatment is superior in the long run to medication. As in depression, research on the effectiveness of psychological interventions has focused on structured, reproducible cognitive-behavioral treatments. Therapists at different research centers can be trained in cognitive-behavioral techniques using standardized procedure manuals. Patients can be given instructional workbooks with "homework" to follow.

In the last two decades, numerous studies have documented the effectiveness of the psychological treatment of anxiety. Typically, a high percentage of patients (two-thirds to three-quarters) respond within just a few months, as did Karen and Roberto. This has been true for a variety of types of anxiety, including agoraphobia, panic attacks, specific phobias, and obsessive-compulsive rituals. Perhaps most important, once treatment is complete, the gains endure long-term. Studies following patients for nearly ten years after psychological treatment have documented this long-term effect.

One of the pioneers in this research is psychiatrist Isaac Marks, professor of experimental psychopathology at the Institute of Psychiatry and the

Bethlem-Maudsley Hospital in London. Marks is one of the world's lead-ing authorities on research comparing behavioral and drug treatment for a variety of psychiatric conditions. In a typical study, Marks and his col-leagues studied 154 patients with panic attacks and agoraphobia in London and Toronto, Canada. Patients were treated with exposure therapy, such as that used to treat Roberto's elevator phobia, or Xanax (a Valium-type seda-tive) either alone or in combination. Patients received two months of treat-ment. Those on Xanax were then tapered off the drug over the course of two months. After treatment was complete, the patients were followed for an additional six months to monitor whether or not they relapsed.

Writing in the *British Journal of Psychiatry* in 1993, Marks and his group reported that patients treated with Xanax improved but only while they re-mained on the drug.[18] When the drug was stopped, the improvement evap-orated: "After Xanax withdrawal, the Xanax effect disappeared on every measure." Indeed, on a number of measures of anxiety, patients were *worse* off than patients who had been given a placebo. Apparently, being taken off the medication they felt dependent on made them more anxious than peo-ple who were never medicated.

Exposure was more effective than the drug, and its effects were sus-tained after treatment stopped. "Long-term outcome is a key issue for pa-tients with chronic disorders," wrote Marks. In many studies, patients with panic disorder have suffered from the condition for five to ten years. "It is, therefore, not only legitimate but essential to examine outcome long after both Xanax and exposure were discontinued. Xanax is like insulin," which a diabetic has to "continue indefinitely to maintain its effect." This would be true of other medications as well. By contrast, exposure "is more like chemotherapy for neoplasia [cancer]. Once patients have improved with exposure, no further treatment is needed unless relapse threatens, in which case brief booster self-exposure is helpful."

When exposure was combined with Xanax, the drug added no signifi-cant benefit during treatment. Still worse, after treatment, patients lost the gains they had made and quickly relapsed. In other words, the presence of medication undermined the psychological treatment's lasting effects! Writ-ing in the *British Journal of Psychiatry* in 1992, Marks said, While "expo-sure is certainly no panacea and is hard work for the sufferers, its superiority to Xanax in yielding lasting improvement is ... now clear."[19] The same result would be expected with other, similar drugs. But, said Marks, "With no major industry to advertise its superiority, exposure may take a long time to become widely used."

Numerous other studies have demonstrated the negative impact of drugs on treatment outcome. Doctors Tom Roth and Frank Wilhelm at the Stanford University School of Medicine studied twenty-eight people with airplane flying phobias. On an initial plane flight, all of the patients were treated with exposure. Half of them also received Xanax. On retest, in a second flight one week later, those who had been given Xanax had a worsening of their anxiety while those treated only with exposure had an improvement. Writing in *Behavior Research and Therapy* in 1997, Roth and Wilhelm reported medication "hinders [the] therapeutic effects of exposure in flying phobia."[20]

One of the most ambitious clinical studies to date was funded by the National Institute of Mental Health (NIMH) in the early 1990s.[21] Completed in 1997, the study was headed by David Barlow, professor of psychology at Boston University; Jack Gorman, professor of psychiatry at Columbia Medical School; Scott Woods, professor of psychiatry at Yale Medical School; and Katherine Shear, professor of psychiatry at the Western Psychiatric Institute and Clinic, University of Pittsburgh School of Medicine. Over three hundred patients with severe anxiety (panic attacks) were enrolled in the study. Patients received either cognitive-behavioral therapy, antidepressant drugs, or a combination of both for twelve weeks. After treatment stopped, they were evaluated monthly for six months of follow-up to monitor relapse rates.

The national, collaborative project reached the same conclusion as earlier studies: Psychotherapy is superior to medication in the long run. During active treatment, psychotherapy was as effective as drugs: By the end of three months, roughly two-thirds of patients had responded to either treatment. The combination of medication and psychotherapy was no more effective than psychotherapy alone. Once active treatment stopped, patients who had been medicated relapsed quickly. Indeed, within six months, they were doing no better than patients who only received placebo pills. By contrast, the gains made by patients treated psychologically were sustained over time. Sponsored by the NIMH and involving researchers at prestigious institutions, the study is a landmark in the treatment of anxiety, like the NIMH-sponsored study of depression in the mid-1980s.

Many researchers have speculated on why drugs interfere with overcoming anxiety long-term. The central principle of psychological approaches is to remove anxiety one step at a time, in increasingly stressful situations. But this process requires experiencing the anxiety in tolerable, incremental doses.[22] Drugs that numb feelings prevent people from experiencing anxiety and thereby block its wearing off. Once the drug is withdrawn, the suppressed anxiety returns.

Moreover, medicated patients tend to attribute their progress to the drugs rather than their own efforts.[23] Withdrawing a drug that they feel dependent on may make them even more anxious than they were at the start. What patients ascribe their progress to may be a critical variable.

Why do patients in studies fail to overcome anxiety long-term if given medication when someone like Karen was able to balance medication and the alternatives? In research studies medication is taken regularly at doses that substantially suppress anxiety. In contrast, Karen used medication only in low doses on an as-needed basis, which does not suppress anxiety so profoundly as to impair the patients' ability to learn from their own efforts to overcome the problem. Used in this way, medication plays only a minor role in the early weeks of treatment before the natural alternatives start to work. The focus is on psychotherapy, relaxation techniques, exposure, stopping caffeine, exercising, and other lifestyle changes.

One might expect that while mild anxiety responds to psychological treatment, severe conditions do not, but research has shown otherwise. A team of British behavior therapists—Gary McNamee, Geraldine O'Sullivan, and Isaac Marks—used exposure techniques to treat severe agoraphobics, some of whom had been housebound for decades. The patients' agoraphobia was so severe that they could not come to the doctor's office to be treated. Treatment had to be conducted over the phone. The patients were mailed audiotape instructions on relaxation techniques and workbooks with detailed instructions in exposure treatment. Patients were encouraged to enlist a family member as a "cotherapist" to read the material and work with them in person. Telephone contact monitoring their progress was weekly for two months and then tapered off to every other week for an additional month. Many of the patients had been on high doses of medication for years, even decades. To participate in the study, they were required to reduce the medication drastically.

Even though their conditions were severe, patients who completed exposure treatment improved significantly. Reporting the results in the journal *Behavior Therapy*, McNamee, O'Sullivan, and Marks described the case of a fifty-six-year-old widow who had been "virtually housebound for eighteen [years]. . . . She lived with her daughter who carried out all tasks outside the home."[24] For twenty years she had been on high doses of barbiturates and Valium (up to 80 milligrams a day). Before entering treatment, she eliminated the barbiturates and reduced the Valium to one-twentieth the dose, just 4 milligrams a day. Within just four weeks with telephone-guided exposure treatment, the patient "was shopping in large supermarkets and using public transportation." Seven months after the brief treatment ended, she flew on an overseas vacation to Italy.

Long-term follow-up studies have shown the gains made with psychological treatment are enduring. British psychiatrist Isaac Marks and his colleagues evaluated thirty-one patients three and a half years after being treated for panic attacks and agoraphobia with exposure or Xanax. Writing in the July 1997 issue of *Psychotherapy and Psychosomatics,* Marks's group reported that, overall, patients treated with exposure "maintained their gains over the 3.5 years."[25] By contrast, those treated with Xanax showed "no difference on clinical measures" from those who had been given a placebo. Marks's group commented, "This was to be expected given the relapse of patients as soon as they stopped their medication."

Even longer follow-up was available in another study, led by Dr. Giovanni Fava in Italy.[26] Eighty-one patients with panic attacks and agoraphobia who were panic-free after just twelve half-hour sessions of psychotherapy and exposure homework were evaluated yearly for two to nine years. An estimated 96% of patients remained panic-free for two years and 77.5% for five years. For the minority of patients who relapsed at some point during follow-up, 87% became panic-free again after a short course of booster therapy. Writing in the *British Journal of Psychiatry* in 1995, Fava's group concluded that "exposure treatment can provide lasting relief for the majority of patients. . . . The powerful effects of a total of six hours of individual behavioral psychotherapy per patient were certainly impressive. If compared with the very high frequency of relapse upon medication discontinuation in patients with panic disorder, the results lend support to the striking superiority of exposure alone against drug treatment. . . . These findings challenge the view that long-term drug treatment is the most appropriate therapy for patients with panic disorder and agoraphobia."

Why do more doctors not prescribe psychosocial interventions for anxiety instead of prescribing pills? Most doctors are unaware how powerful and conclusive the clinical research is. Part of the problem is that in this country the mental health field is divided among psychiatrists, psychologists, and social workers, each with their own turf. Behavioral treatments that are effective for anxiety (such as relaxation techniques and exposure) are the province of psychologists rather than medical doctors. Primary-care clinicians and psychiatrists rarely receive training in these methodologies. Instead, they are taught to prescribe pills. The majority of patients with anxiety are treated by their primary-care doctor. In the primary-care setting, serotonin boosters or Valium-type drugs provide a quick fix even if they can be detrimental in the long run to people's overcoming their fears.

Like serotonin boosters, long-term use of the Valium group entails significant risks. Because their effects on brain receptors are similar to those of alcohol, they can cause tolerance, dependence, and withdrawal. Valium-type drugs can cause morning hangovers, memory problems, drowsiness, and a host of other side effects. Some patients have seizures while trying to withdraw from them. For these reasons, use of Valium-type medications on a regular basis for prolonged periods of time should be avoided.

Jason: A Case of Mild Anxiety

Not all anxious patients have symptoms as severe as Karen's and Roberto's. Jason was a sixteen-year-old sophomore in high school when he sought help because of mild to moderate anxiety. Jason was a tall, lanky track star at a local high school. A popular actor in the school's drama society and a writer for the student newspaper, in the fall of his sophomore year Jason surprised his parents and teachers when he suddenly became anxious and withdrawn. When his first-quarter grades dropped, his parents became concerned. Jason's mother thought she saw signs of obsessive-compulsive behavior: Jason was taking many more showers than usual, washing his hands excessively, and checking to be sure faucets were completely turned off. When Jason announced he might drop the track team, of which he was one of the stars, the school telephoned his parents. The conversation led to their seeking a psychiatric evaluation for him.

I found Jason to be a likable teenager, more articulate and comfortable with adults than most. Jason's turmoil had been growing since the summer, he said. He felt anxious, "like the ground was falling out from underneath" him, edgy, and alienated much of the time. He was not having full-blown panic attacks (racing heart, shortness of breath, flushing, sweating, etc.). Instead, Jason was preoccupied with obsessive thoughts, which made it difficult for him to concentrate on his studies.

"What are you preoccupied with?" I asked.

"That I'm going to embarrass myself or already have. That it's going to be found out and I'll be exposed."

"Embarrass yourself how?"

"Every day it's something different. The other day I was convinced I had plagiarized on a paper."

"Plagiarized?"

"Part of me knew I hadn't. I've never plagiarized. You know how you read things and are influenced by them. . . . I became obsessed that I'd put something in a history paper, not a direct quote but an idea, and forgot to cite the source. The concern became a runaway fear in my head. Every time

I saw my history teacher I was convinced he was looking at me funny, like I'd done something wrong. I was afraid he'd already gone to the principal and the administration had begun the process of expelling me. When this happens I can't think about anything else. I can't read. Can't study. Can't even exercise. I just get totally preoccupied with the idea that my life is ruined."

In another common scenario, Jason would become convinced he had "done something inappropriate like shouting a profanity or injuring someone." Said Jason, "One day last week I was bored in my biology class. I was daydreaming and became fixated on this guy sitting across from me. He had on an earring, a hoop, kind of a big one, I thought, for a guy. It looked big enough to put a finger through. So I imagined starting to tug on it. The next thing I knew, I was pulling really hard and he was howling. Everyone else in the class and the teacher started yelling at me, aghast. When I came out of the daydream, the class was ending. People were standing up and leaving. I felt shaken. It seemed like my friends all brushed past me. I became concerned that maybe I'd really done it."

"Yanked on the guy's earring?"

"I knew I hadn't. But I got preoccupied with the thought that maybe I had.... What if I did do it? I know it's irrational but I can't get the thought out of my head. And again, I think my whole life is ruined ... I'm disgraced ... I'm going to be expelled. This may sound ridiculous but at lunch I actually sought the guy out to talk to...."

"The guy with the earring?"

Jason nodded. "Just to be sure he was friendly, that nothing had happened."

"Do you ever become convinced, even for a minute, that something actually has happened?"

"No. I always know the thoughts are irrational but I can't stop them. And I do become concerned, at the time."

We discussed the compulsive rituals Jason had developed since the summer. He acknowledged taking showers and washing his hands more frequently. Sometimes when he turned the stove off, locked a door, or shut off a faucet, he would go back repeatedly, two or three times, to be sure it was secured. He worried about the stove "blowing up" his parents' house, an intruder "breaking in," or a faucet dripping.

"For some reason, faucets are the worst," said Jason.

"You worry that you've left a faucet dripping?"

"Not just dripping ... the house is flooded."

"Flooded?"

"I imagine I've left the faucet running and the drain doesn't work. Both the drain at the bottom of the bowl and the backup drain at the top are blocked. As the sink fills up, water runs over the edge onto the floor. The bathroom fills with water, which starts leaking down to the first floor. Soon there's a foot of water, the furniture is floating, and the house is ruined."

"No wonder you're distracted if you have all these fears."

"They're all-consuming," said Jason, becoming upset. "Am I losing my mind?"

"No. You're not losing your mind," I reassured him.

"Why are you so sure?"

"Because you told me you never actually lose touch with reality. At some level you always know it isn't true, it's an irrational fear."

"That makes a difference?"

"A big difference. If you lost touch with reality then you'd be psychotic and, yes, this would be a lot more serious."

"That's a relief," said Jason, looking visibly eased.

"What you're experiencing are intrusive thoughts."

"Intrusive thoughts?"

"The fear that you've embarrassed yourself and ruined your life."

"Other people have them, too?"

"They're not uncommon. You don't even have that bad a case. This is mild to moderate. You're not checking the faucet twenty times. You just check once or twice and not every time."

"That's true. But why am I doing it at all? What's going on?"

I explained to Jason that as upsetting as they are, obsessive thoughts are often a way of avoiding thinking about something even more troubling. By filling one's mental space, the thoughts block out even more disturbing concerns. Similarly, compulsively securing stoves, locks, and faucets can be a way of trying to keep a lid on larger anxieties one feels unable to control. Was there anything deeper that was bothering him, which these obsessive-compulsive symptoms might be symptomatic of?

Initially, Jason said he could not think of anything. He had a good relationship with both his parents. His father was an engineer; his mother worked part-time as a nurse. His family were churchgoing Catholics. Jason was the second of four boys. He said there was "the usual sibling rivalry, especially among so many boys," but that, in general, the four got along "surprisingly well."

When Jason reported nothing in the family, I asked about school: Was there anything about high school, tenth grade in particular, or looking ahead to college that was upsetting him? Jason was "as surprised as everyone else" that his grades went down "just when they started to count" for college. He did not feel under any more pressure than his peers. "School has always come easy to me," he said. "I don't know what's happened."

Pursuing another line of inquiry, I asked Jason what he had been doing in the summer when these symptoms began. He had had a summer job working in the warehouse of a large chain of department stores. The job consisted of moving merchandise in the warehouse, loading and unloading trucks, lifting boxes by hand or moving them with a forklift.

So far, we were turning up nothing. Then, as we talked about a range of topics, Jason told me a vignette that caught my attention. One day in the early fall, Jason and his coach took a cab to practice because they were running late and the coach was without his car. Relating the incident, Jason said, "It was another one of those situations where I thought I had done something wrong."

"Like what?"

"I hailed the cab down. As we got in, I thought, 'Was I rude to the driver? Did I say something inappropriate?' I was uncomfortable sitting in the back seat with the coach. It seemed to me he moved away a little, like I was sitting too close. Was my knee too close to his? Should I turn away, cross my legs . . . I don't know. This is making me very uncomfortable."

"To talk about?"

"Yes."

"Do you know why?"

"No," said Jason quickly, as though something was on his mind but he was hesitant to voice it.

Men who are uncomfortable in close quarters with other men are often consciously or unconsciously struggling with fears of homosexuality. They fear doing something inappropriate. Or they project the fear, expecting some overture or advance. Were doubts about his sexual identity bothering Jason? Was this what he was trying to ward off with his obsessive thoughts and rituals?

"What about relationships?" I asked Jason. "Are you dating anyone?"

"No."

"Have you in the past?"

"I had a girlfriend last year. There's no one I'm interested in right now."

"Was it a sexual relationship?"

"Yes." Jason looked surprised by my directness. Introducing the subject of sexuality, I was gradually building up to the more sensitive question.

"Is there anything sexual bothering you?"

"Not really. . . ."

"The extra showers you take and the hand washing, are they after you've masturbated?"

Jason looked away, guiltily.

Phrasing the question tactfully, I said, "Sometimes people your age become symptomatic because doubts about their sexual identity are weighing on them."

For the first time, Jason's face reddened. His eyes welled up. He pursed his lips as though trying to decide whether or not to speak. His gaze remained averted.

At first, Jason's head movements were imperceptible. Slowly, they turned into definite nodding. Recognizing he was too choked up to speak, I said gently, "It's okay. Take your time. There's no rush."

After Jason had a good cry, he said he first became concerned about his sexual identity over the summer, while working in the warehouse. He described the warehouse as an all-male, macho environment. He was surprised by the ribald humor among the young men who worked in the warehouse full-time. Their crude banter created a sexualized atmosphere. Many of the men wore Timberlane boots, even though it was summer, tight jeans, and tank tops. Bending and stretching to lift boxes side-by-side with other men, Jason became aware he was attracted to some of them. Shocked by his inability to control his desire, he became concerned that he might not be able to check his behavior.

"Did anything happen?" I asked.

"No. It didn't. But working there became excruciating. I took a lot of days off sick. Nobody knew why."

At almost the same time, Jason was "weirded out" by three coincidences in which characters in his favorite TV shows or books turned out to be gay. The first was a character in the novel *The Big Nowhere,* by James Elroy, the author of *L. A. Confidential.* Jason described the book as a "twisted, hard-boiled cop story." Said Jason, "One of the main characters was a cop who suddenly realizes at the end that he's gay. I was really shocked. There was no build-up to it. I didn't think the reader could see it coming at all.

"Then, about a week later I was watching this TV show *South Park* on Comedy Central and this guy's dog turned out to be gay."

"His dog?" I expressed surprise as Jason and I both laughed at the humor and timing of this. The laughter broke the ice on the distress Jason had been feeling, crying just a few minutes before.

On the heels of these two incidents, yet a third one happened: "This time I was watching the TV show *Homicide.* It's about the Baltimore police department. I like cop stories. In this episode, the police were investigating a rash of gay murders in Baltimore. As part of the investigation, they inter-view the owner of a gay restaurant. Afterwards, one of the cops decides he's gay and asks the owner out on a date. Again, there was no build-up. I was blown away."

Humorous as these coincidences were, there was a more ominous side. "What happened to these people once they realized they were gay?" I asked.

"The cop in *The Big Nowhere* killed himself."

"He suicided?"

"He was scheduled to have a psychiatric evaluation for his job and they were going to give him truth serum. Rather than face that, he killed him-self."

"Good grief," I said. In fact, this was a topic I planned to touch on with Jason. The suicide rate among gay teenagers is significantly higher than the adolescent average. "I know you've been distressed about this all fall," I said. "Have you been at all suicidal?"

"No," said Jason definitely. "I couldn't do that."

Jason and I talked about the parallels between his obsessions and his un-derlying anxiety. His fears in many different areas of "embarrassing" him-self, doing something "inappropriate," and "ruining" his life were symbolic representations of his sexual concerns. His showers and hand washing were attempts to rid himself of the idea that he was gay. His doubts about his sex-ual identity were the "intruder" he wanted to bolt the door against or the explosion in the stove he wanted to prevent from "blowing up" his parents' house. Jason's compulsive rituals were attempts to manage an uncontrol-lable sexual force.

Jason said his family's Catholicism posed a particular problem when he thought that he might be gay. Because his mother was a nurse, he thought she had "seen more of life" than his father and was "a little less conserva-tive." Still, he was fearful of what their response might be.

I reassured Jason that he was not the only teenager struggling with these issues. Jason was baffled by his difficulties because the sexual relationship with his girlfriend the year before had gone well, he thought. Like the book and TV characters, he "didn't know where this was coming from." I told Jason it would take time to sort out his sexual identity. He needed to try to have an open mind and sort out his feelings. In fact, Jason had not had a ho-mosexual experience to date. I cautioned him that he needed to practice safe sex in any sexual relationship in this day and age. He agreed wholeheart-edly. I commented that the current atmosphere on many high school and college campuses is much more open and helpful in these matters than in the past. If Jason was unsure of his sexual orientation, he should not feel pushed in either direction. In some instances nowadays, the pendulum has swung to the opposite extreme: People come under more pressure from their gay and lesbian friends than from their straight ones to declare themselves. What Jason needed was support and encouragement to find himself, free of any pressure.

Jason came back the next week saying he was feeling much better. "Telling someone what was on my mind was a huge relief," he said. Following our meeting, Jason confided in his mother, who "took it much better" than he expected. He was not yet ready to discuss the issue with his father. Jason also approached a classmate who was active in the gay-and-lesbian student club at school. This was someone he felt he could trust to keep his confidence. Talking with a peer who had struggled with similar issues was extremely helpful.

Jason said his obsessive thoughts and rituals had improved dramatically. "They're not completely gone," he said, "but now I understand them. If I start to obsess about having offended someone I say to myself, 'You're not really worried about this. What's really bothering you?' Sometimes I can figure it out. Like I was attracted to someone for a fleeting moment and tried to put it out of mind. Other times I can't connect it to something that just happened. But that's all right."

Jason did not feel the need to be in long-term psychotherapy. "This is something I need to figure out for myself," he said. Since he was feeling much better, I agreed. With patients like Jason, their symptoms can improve dramatically if one manages to quickly go to the heart of a secret that is bottled up and festering and needing to be aired. A year later I bumped into Jason in Harvard Square. His improvement was sustained; his grades had rebounded. He was co-captain of his high school track team and a state medalist. He was "still sorting out" his sexual identity.

What if Jason and I had not gotten to what was really bothering him? When I met him he was a scared teenager, not about to volunteer the source of his pain. He needed someone to listen and watch for the subtle signals of what was eating away at him.

Unfortunately, nowadays patients like Jason are often medicated without any exploration of psychological issues. To justify medicating him, Jason would have been diagnosed with "obsessive-compulsive disorder," or OCD. Since serotonin boosters have been approved for OCD, it has become another of the trendy diagnoses of the past decade. Merely medicating Jason would have left him further isolated with his sexual confusion. Moreover, the severe sexual side effects of a serotonin booster could have further complicated his problems. What if his interest in sex suddenly died? What if he found he could only orgasm with excruciating effort? As is often the case, what if he was not told about the sexual side effects of the drugs and ascribed the difficulties to his confusion? This could well have worsened his predicament. As always, medicating with drugs should be undertaken with great caution.

As Roberto's, Karen's, and Jason's cases illustrate, the role of medication in the comprehensive, balanced treatment of anxiety is the same as its role in depression: Medication is reserved for moderate to severe cases where it is used short-term to effect symptomatic relief while the patient is waiting for the natural alternatives to begin to work. Used in this way, prescription drugs can be helpful for controlling severe anxiety, making it possible for a patient to continue to function. However, overmedicating—completely suppressing anxiety—is counterproductive, interfering with a patient's ability to unlearn anxiety through alternative approaches like exposure, relaxation techniques, and psychotherapy. In some cases, anxiety is not rooted in deep, traumatic psychological events as in Roberto's elevator phobia, which he simply learned from his father's having served as a role model for this anxious reflex. In these cases, treatment consists of unlearning the anxiety through behavioral techniques. In other instances, like Karen's panic attacks or Jason's obsessions, symptoms of anxiety are symbolic representations of deeper psychological issues that need to be resolved in order for the patient to be truly freed from the problem.

8

Conquering Addictions
Substance Abuse, Sexual Addictions, and Eating Disorders

Addictions to alcohol, cocaine, amphetamines, marijuana, and narcotics all involve the use of drugs to create highs and to numb feelings. Sexual addictions are remarkably similar to drug abuse. Here, sexual excess becomes a drug-like escape. In bulimia or compulsive overeating, food becomes a drug most often used as an escape, to comfort oneself, to quell psychic distress.

As with depression and anxiety, the treatment of addictions is twofold. First, the short-term management of symptoms, in this case the addictive behavior, is tackled. Second, the more profound and lasting treatment seeks to resolve any underlying psychological issues. Since their introduction, serotonin boosters have been widely used to suppress all kinds of addictive behavior. Unfortunately, while they do suppress addictive behavior, they do not touch the underlying problem, which cannot be resolved unless approached in a more humanistic way.

As a practical method of controlling addictive behavior, twelve-step groups and behaviorally oriented psychotherapy groups are far preferable to serotonin boosters. These natural alternatives entail none of the risks of potent, synthetic drugs. In addition to their side effects, prescription drugs numb feelings just as the addictive behavior once did. In the process, they rob people of the very emotions they need to deal with in order to successfully overcome their compulsive urges.

Seth: A Case of Sexual Addiction

I first met Seth when he called, distraught, and requested that I speak with him on an urgent basis because he was in the midst of a personal crisis. He had read my earlier book, *Sexual Mysteries: Tales of Psychotherapy,* and wanted to consult with me. As it happened, I had a cancellation that afternoon and was able to fit him in.

Seth arrived half an hour early for the appointment, another indication of his acute distress. As we sat down, Seth told me he had recently been discovered viewing pornography over the Internet on his computer at work.

"What do you mean 'discovered'?" I asked, imagining a coworker had come upon Seth in his office. In fact, his predicament was much more dramatic.

"A newspaper reporter called me yesterday to say he had a list of everyone at my work who's looked at pornography on the company computers."

"A newspaper reporter?"

"He's writing an article about pornography on the Internet. He wants to make the point that viewing it at work is much more common than people might think. He knew exactly when I'd been on the computer the day before and what I was looking at. He said he has detailed logs on everyone at my company and several other companies."

"How did he get the logs?"

"He said something about a computer hacker breaking into the company's databases. I had no idea anybody could come by the information. If a hacker can get it, then people inside the company must be able to. I'm a wreck."

"He said he's writing an article?"

"He wanted to know if I would like to make a statement."

"He wanted to quote you?"

"Exactly. He's writing about First Amendment rights, freedom of speech, on the Internet."

"What did you say?"

"I said no way. I was really upset."

"Is that the end of it?"

"No. My name may appear in the article along with a lot of other people's."

"When is the article being published?"

"I don't know. Sometime in the next few days."

"Good grief!"

Seth's company was a large defense contractor headquartered in the

Boston area. "The fact that we work on government contracts I presume will make the revelations more sensational," said Seth.

After he received the phone call, Seth felt so ill he went home from work early. "My wife is pregnant and I made the excuse that she needed me to come home."

"Your wife is pregnant?"

"The timing couldn't be worse for this to happen. She's due to deliver next month."

"Did you tell her?"

"Yes. I was afraid my name might be in the paper today!"

"She must have been upset."

"Terribly. I felt sick having to tell her at a time like this. Of course, she was shocked. She didn't think I would do something like this, looking at pornography for hours every day."

"Hours?"

"Some days. Not every day. I don't know what's happened in the last few months. I'm just completely hooked. I have to use the computer every day for work so I can't avoid the temptation."

"You've been doing this for the last few months?"

"I had a problem looking at pornographic magazines in high school," said Seth. "But I outgrew that. I haven't looked at pornography in years. I don't know why, but the whole thing came back in the last six months."

"When you say 'the whole thing,' are you buying magazines or videotapes in addition to looking on the Internet?"

"No. Just the computer. It started with me being curious to find this stuff on the Internet you hear about all the time. I had no idea I'd get hooked."

Seth's focus was on how to deal with the prospect of the upcoming newspaper article. If he was named, as he feared, this would be extremely stressful for him and his wife, especially with the impending birth of their baby and their already having a four-year-old daughter. I felt particularly bad for his wife in the last month of her pregnancy. Might I be able to persuade the reporter not to name Seth, I wondered? Contemplating the idea, I was relieved he had told his wife about the problem. Having divulged it to her, he would not be able to just sweep it under the carpet even if he was spared the embarrassment of being named publicly. Otherwise, I might have had more mixed feelings about interceding, fearing that if I was successful I might unwittingly enable his addiction.

Seth jumped at the idea of my contacting the reporter. I cautioned him that my calling would compromise his privacy further and that I might not succeed in altering the reporter's course. Seth thought the risk worth taking. "I'm desperate," he said. "I'd try anything."

After Seth left, I called the reporter several times, always getting his voice mail. Finally, I left a message asking him to telephone me at home in the evening. I wondered, Would he call me back? Had the story already gone to press? Would I be trying to help Seth deal with the headlines later in the week? What if I did speak with the reporter and failed in my mission? How disappointed would Seth be? Could this jeopardize a nascent therapeutic relationship?

Such were the thoughts running through my head that evening as the hours passed by. Finally, the reporter telephoned, apologizing for calling so late. He was surprised and intrigued to have heard from me. After establishing the article was not yet in press, I proceeded to discuss Seth's situation.

Initially, the reporter was resistant to the idea of withholding the names in his piece, although he said the final decision whether to publish them had not yet been made. As we talked, he seemed to grow more concerned about the consequences for individuals like Seth, who would be identified publicly. Although he remained noncommittal, in the end he thanked me for calling.

When Seth and I met a week later, the article had still not appeared. He had been monitoring the paper vigilantly, and his feelings were still running high. During the week, Seth had abstained from viewing pornography on the computer. He readily acknowledged this was easy to do for the moment because the pull of pornography was temporarily "spoiled" by the acute scare. But what would he do long-term to curb his behavior?

I suggested Seth join a program like Sex and Love Addicts Anonymous (SLAA), or Sexaholics Anonymous (SA). Modeled on Alcoholics Anonymous, these are twelve-step programs for people with sexual addictions. In recent decades the programs have grown nationwide. In any twelve-step program, the first nine steps are a prescribed sequence of exercises for establishing control over one's addictive behavior. The three final steps are the maintenance phase of sobriety. Sobriety, or abstinence, is achieved "one day at a time." Early in sobriety, this keeps the task small enough to be manageable. Later on, it guards against overconfidence and relapse.

The strength of twelve-step programs is their commonsense approach and their utterly practical, behavioral emphasis: The focus is on eradicating addictive behavior. Twelve-step groups provide a forum of peers to support abstinence and confront addictive behavior. Those with established sobriety act as role models for fledgling members.

A few days after our second meeting, Seth called to express relief that the newspaper article finally appeared without naming any individuals. His wife, too, was enormously relieved.

At our next meeting, Seth talked about his positive experience at the SLAA meetings he had attended. Sitting with so many people who were all struggling with problems similar to his own helped reduce his sense of shame and isolation. "It helps to see I'm not the only one who's succumbed to using sex as a drug," said Seth. "I was surprised to see so many 'normal-looking' people in the room. Meeting them in any other context, I'd never guess they had such a problem. I guess the same is true for me. Having to admit my difficulty openly to the group was powerful."

One day Seth reported an incident in an SLAA meeting that highlighted for me the relationship between twelve-step groups and individual psychotherapy. A woman in the group described how her childhood sexual abuse led to promiscuity in her early teens. Sitting across from her in the circle, Seth identified with this intelligent, articulate woman. When it came his turn to speak, Seth addressed her directly, commenting on her experience and the articulate, moving way in which she was able to describe it. After he spoke, another member of the group "reprimanded" Seth for "cross-talking."

"What's cross-talking?" I asked.

Seth said he had not known before this incident. He then explained that in twelve-step groups, cross-talking is directly addressing what someone else said. In order to avoid these two-way conversations, people are instead encouraged to comment obliquely. They can relate their own experiences but are not supposed to tie their comments directly to what someone else has said. This prevents deepening, one-on-one conversation, which can quickly exclude other members of the group. The emphasis stays on group dynamics and behavioral change—that is, sobriety. This is the strength of twelve-step programs. Complementing this, psychotherapy's strength is emotional intimacy, one-on-one depth.

Indeed, in his psychotherapy, Seth and I continued to try to understand the source of his compulsion. The type of pornographic images a person looks at can be an important clue to what is going on psychologically. This is a kind of projective test, like a Rorschach, in which the particular images a person is drawn to and the themes one sees in them are reflections of the individual's own issues. Whether consciously or unconsciously, a personal element is always present, some identification with the images that makes them particularly appealing to the individual.

Seth talked about his preferences in pornography only reluctantly, because he was so embarrassed by his compulsion. He said he was interested in "more than just women on display." He preferred pictures depicting a man and a woman having sex.

"What kind of sex?" I asked.

"Oral sex."

"More so than intercourse?"

"Yes."

"Do you have any idea why?"

Seth had to think a moment before answering: "It seems like the woman is very focused on the man."

"Focused?"

"Like she's acting on the man as opposed to the other way around."

"Any other thoughts?"

"I like when it appears that the woman is the aggressor."

"Really."

"When the man looks almost reluctant or . . ."

"Can you complete the sentence?"

". . . a little overwhelmed."

"With pleasure?"

"No. Like he was a little hesitant and is overwhelmed by the whole thing."

"Do you have any other associations?"

"Associations?"

"You know the term 'free-associate'?"

"Vaguely. I'm not sure what it really means."

"If you stay with this image of a woman performing oral sex on a man and he's a little reluctant, perhaps even overwhelmed, does anything else come to mind?"

Seth looked at me blankly.

"Even something seemingly far-fetched?" I asked. "Anything at all?"

"No. Nothing."

Was this because we had reached the end of a cul-de-sac with nothing more to be learned from the particular images in which Seth was interested? Or was it because he was blocked, because associating to the images any further would stir up emotions that would be too uncomfortable? Finishing the discussion, Seth said he had no interest in hard-core pornography, group scenes, or gay and lesbian images.

Regarding the question of why the problem had flared now, Seth thought boredom with his job might be responsible. A designer and engineer, he worked for the division of his company manufacturing products for NASA. Until just a year before, his work had been quite hands-on, designing new products for NASA, helping them to meet the technical challenges of the space program. Then, Seth had advanced to his first administrative position. Initially, he found the oversight role, frequent meetings, number crunching, flowcharting, and monitoring the work of others intriguing. But the novelty quickly wore off. Seth missed the satisfaction of tackling and solving real design problems. He was surprised by how much politics entered into administration. Although bored with the work, he liked the increase in his pay and felt "guilty" about wanting to go back to "real work" instead of climbing farther up the corporate ladder. Was there any association between this boredom and how he felt in high school when he bought pornographic magazines? Had Seth been bored then?

"No," he said. "Not at all. That was a tumultuous time."

Our discussions of Seth's work were interrupted one week by his announcement that his wife, Emily, had delivered a baby boy, Andrew. All had gone well and she was already home with the infant. In fact, everyone was already feeling tired from being up at night. Seth said his four-year-old daughter was as "besotted" as his wife with the new baby.

"And what about you?" I asked.

"I feel much better now that Andrew's here."

"What do you mean?"

"I knew all along we would have a boy. I had a lot of apprehension about having a son."

"You knew from an ultrasound?"

"Exactly."

"And that made you apprehensive?"

"Oh, yes."

I had been mindful that Seth's pornography addiction had flared during Emily's pregnancy. The idea that he was apprehensive over having a son introduced a new element.

"What is it you were afraid of about having a son?"

Initially, Seth had a difficult time articulating an inchoate "dread." Slowly, over several meetings, a clearer picture of his fears emerged. Ultimately, Seth said, he had a difficult relationship with both his parents. His father was a successful insurance broker who was arrogant and distant from Seth and the rest of the family. He described his mother as an attractive, "highly sexual" woman.

"What do you mean by 'highly sexual'?"

"She always wore heavy makeup, low necklines, and tight-fitting, revealing clothes. She exuded sexuality . . . deliberately."

Seth said his mother was also an alcoholic. Looking increasingly un-comfortable, he said, "Sometimes her drinking made her sloppy."

"Sloppy?"

Seth looked away, staring at the floor. Was he embarrassed or ashamed? "What are you feeling?" I asked.

After a long silence, Seth said, "Sometimes when she was drunk she was ... inappropriate with my brother and me."

"Inappropriate?"

Seth grew flush in the neck and face. His skin grew raw looking with the red blotches. What was making him so anxious? His gaze still averted, he said, "When she was drunk, she would kiss us and you know ... tongue us."

"Oh," I said sympathetically. After a long silence I asked, "Is that all she did?"

"She used to give us baths," said Seth, welling up with tears. "I have ..." Seth shook his head, as though trying to shake off the memories.

"It's okay. Take your time."

Eventually he blurted out, "I have a few memories of her fondling me in the bathtub. My brother has a lot more. He's much more messed-up than I am. He's a drug addict. He's a very sweet guy ... with a lot of problems."

I felt great sympathy for Seth and his brother over these experiences. Men who have been violated as children feel just as embarrassed and ashamed as women do about abuse. Seth said the only other person he had ever told was Emily. Part of the reason he told her was that he never wanted his mother to be left alone with his children. What a sad state of affairs, I said, while completely supporting Seth's need to protect his children. After we had discussed his mother's inappropriate behavior over several sessions, one day Seth asked, "Remember the conversation we had about what kinds of pornography I like?"

"Yes."

"Do you think that has any more meaning now?"

"Do you?"

"Well, I was thinking about liking pictures, or imagining into pictures that the man was overwhelmed. In a way, isn't that what happened to me?"

"Exactly."

"What I don't understand is why would I want to look at scenes where a woman overwhelms a man if that was traumatic for me?"

"Because that's where you were stuck. It's like revisiting the scene of a crime, trying to solve it."

I told Seth about a monograph called "A Male Grief: Notes on Pornog-raphy and Addiction," by the poet David Mura, a short-story-like piece describing how childhood sexual abuse can lead to a fixation with pornography. Seth found the poetic monograph deeply moving. Says Mura, "At the essence of pornography is the image of flesh used as a drug, a way of numbing psychic pain. . . . For the addict the rush is more than an attraction. He is helpless before it. Completely out of control. . . . The addiction to pornography is not fun. Underneath all the assertions of liberty and 'healthy fun' lie the desperation and anxiety, the shame and fear, the loneliness and sadness, that fuels the endless consumption" of pornographic images.[1]

Seth now thought his interest in pornography surfaced in high school because adolescent sexuality was bursting on the scene. "By college," said Seth, "I was involved in satisfying relationships with women. Once that happened, I think the trauma with my mother receded."

He now felt that the pending birth of his son, much more so than boredom on his job, precipitated a return of the problem: "I've thought about it. I've been bored many times before and this didn't happen."

The one possible connection between the job and family issues was a fear that being bored at work made him more flat, less engaged, and potentially more like his father: "I know it was an overreaction. I'm fundamentally not like him. But I was afraid of becoming more remote just as I was about to have a son. I feel more strongly than ever about changing my situation at work. I can't be bored with what I do. I used to love my work."

Trying to cope with his anxieties now that he understood them better, Seth reassured himself on several points: "Emily and I have a very different kind of relationship than my parents'. I'm not arrogant and distant like my father. Emily's not alcoholic or inappropriate like my mother. What happened to me is not going to happen to Andrew."

Emily actually came to meet with me once. I did not see her and Seth as a couple. They preferred to have Emily just come on her own. In fact, she brought Andrew, who was still a small baby. I found Emily incredibly warm and down-to-earth. She confirmed Seth's descriptions of his family.

For many people, sexual addictions, particularly those like addictions to pornography, are difficult to understand and sympathize with. Most people would find it hard to believe a couple as "normal" and wholesome looking as Seth and Emily could be struggling with such a problem. Yet society does not benefit any more than individuals do from denying the existence of these conditions. Recognizing that traumas like Seth's can underlie sexual compulsions helps us better understand and deal with the problem.

With the help of psychotherapy and Sex and Love Addicts Anonymous,

Seth did not return to viewing pornography. Had he not entered treatment, his brush with embarrassing publicity might well have only brought about a temporary stay in his addiction.

Dan: A Case of Alcoholism

I first met Dan when he returned to the business school at the Massachusetts Institute of Technology (MIT) after a six-year leave of absence because of severe alcoholism. During the first four years he was away, his drinking only worsened. Eventually he "hit bottom," losing his job, his apartment, and most of his friends. At this point, he finally joined Alcoholics Anonymous, AA, which he described as "life-saving." Now he was back in business school after being sober two years.

"During the whole six years I was on leave, business school loomed in the back of my mind as unfinished business," said Dan. "I'm picking my life up where I left off. I want to finish the degree but I don't know whether or not I want to work in a large company. I'm trying to take it 'one day at a time,' as they say in AA."

Dan came to see me because in addition to being back in school, he wanted to be in psychotherapy. There were many painful incidents in his childhood and the years he was drinking that he wished to revisit. Since becoming sober, he had often considered getting into therapy. He thought now would be a good time.

For someone whose drinking had been as severe as Dan's, psychotherapy entails risks, stirring up the very emotions that once drove the individual to drink. Was Dan's sobriety firmly enough established to make embarking on such a journey safe? Surely coming back to business school was already a challenge. Was this the best time to take on therapy as well? The last thing I wanted was for therapy to drive him once again to drink, to a possible second withdrawal from business school.

I suggested to Dan that we proceed slowly. Initially, I thought, our focus should be on his transition back to school and staying sober. Once he finished a semester, if he felt ready, he could begin delving into older, more painful material.

In retrospect, Dan must have been eager to address the issues from his past, because after just a few weeks he launched headlong into them. This made me apprehensive, but I felt that it was important to respect Dan's energy and courage. In order not to accelerate Dan's already fast pace, however, I exercised restraint in my responses. I stayed with the material as he presented it, refraining from asking too many probing questions when he was already elaborating his story at a fast clip.

Dan's parents married when they were quite young, in their early twenties. His father was a "ruthless" businessman who eventually made a small fortune. He was also an alcoholic, quite handsome, and a womanizer. Dan had vivid memories of his father coming home drunk in the morning to shave and dress for work after spending nights with other women. His parents' fights would escalate to screaming matches and throwing things. After seven years of marriage, they divorced. Dan's mother took Dan to live with her parents.

He described the years after his parents' divorce as extremely painful. His grandparents were severely disapproving of his mother on account of her failed marriage. "We lived as second-class citizens in a downstairs apartment in their house in Pittsburgh," he said. Although still young and pretty, his mother avoided dating and socializing. She took a job in a meat-packing plant, which she "hated." Throughout this period Dan was his mother's confidant, listening endlessly to her anger at his father and her parents.

Relations with Dan's father were always strained. He was perpetually late with child support payments. While Dan lived a "meager, blue-collar existence" with his mother, his father lived in a large house with his new wife.

Dan's visits with his father in the summer were especially stressful. His father was a "gun nut" who collected pistols and rifles. Although violence was never threatened overtly, Dan often felt unsafe. "I used to have to sit on his bed with him and admire his guns and watches," he said. "Once when I was nine years old, I had just handed him back a Colt .45. Sitting two feet away from me, he aimed it at a closet door just a little to the left of my head. I thought he was joking, aiming it with an exaggerated, macho air. But when he pulled the trigger, it went off! The explosion threw me to the ground. The room reeked of gunpowder. His new wife, whom I had just met, came screaming into the bedroom. I was petrified. My father looked shocked. He said he hadn't known the gun was loaded but I've always wondered. The year before, he'd been suicidally depressed. He shot a revolver in his car, putting a bullet through the windshield. It was downplayed as an accident but I just never felt safe with him again."

Vivid scenes like this brought back feelings of immense helplessness, anger, and sadness from Dan's childhood. Ultimately, these were the buried emotions he needed to deal with. They had once fueled his drinking. Periodically, I would ask Dan if there was any risk of that now. Was he going to all his business school classes? Was he keeping up with the reading? Was he feeling at all like drinking? Dan said he always felt "close to the edge of drinking," but that he took sobriety one day at a time, which did not exactly reassure me. As the semester progressed, Dan decided to forgo on-campus interviews with companies recruiting students for jobs after graduation, because he felt he already had a lot on his plate. These kinds of interviews had been his "downfall," he said, the last time around. He did not feel ready for them. He would "take his chances" finding a job on his own later in the academic year.

Meanwhile, Dan launched forward with his history. When he was ten, his mother abruptly remarried after dating her new husband for just a month. She met him while he was vacationing in Pennsylvania near where they lived. After the wedding, she moved to Connecticut with him, transferring Dan abruptly in the middle of the school year. When they got to Connecticut they discovered that Dan's new stepfather lived with his father, who was a "nasty, abusive old" man. "Unfortunately," said Dan, "he owned the house, so we were all trapped there with him." Still worse, after just a few days in Connecticut, it became apparent that Dan's new stepfather was psychotic. "He went three days in a row with no sleep and drinking heavily. He became irritable and threatening. Finally, he became psychotic. He thought the wallpaper was talking to him. He believed the house was bugged by the CIA. He insisted that my mother had married his brother, not him, as part of a plot. The police had to come and take him away to be locked up in a hospital.

"Once again, my mother turned to me. I remember like it happened yesterday her sitting me down on the living room couch and saying, 'Dan, Mr. Barton is crazy. What should we do?' How the hell was I supposed to know? I was ten. She was the one who had just married him after only knowing him a month.

"While he was in the hospital, his family told my mother that he was manic-depressive and an alcoholic. He'd gone off his medication and disappeared—to Pennsylvania, as it turned out, where he met my mother. The whole romance with her was part of his escalation into a manic break. In spite of everything, she stood by him. I think she couldn't face going back to her parents again after another unsuccessful marriage. He went off his medication and was hospitalized many more times while I was in junior high and high school. Once when we didn't know he was getting psychotic, he tried to poison us. He served us soup with Drano in it. Fortunately, my mother saw the Drano bottle on the counter just before we were about to drink it."

Dan began drinking alcohol heavily in high school. Most of the drinking was with his buddies on the football team. Dan played a defensive linesman on the football squad. "I used to love to go out there and smash into people," he said. "It was a great outlet for my frustration and anger."

Dan said it was a "relief" at seventeen to go to Connecticut College and escape the family scene. But during his freshman year, while he was home over Christmas vacation, his stepfather committed suicide. In fact, Dan was the one who discovered his stepfather hanging in the basement.

Again, I stopped Dan to check on how the steady stream of emotional images were affecting him. Were these memories making him feel at all like drinking? In fact, said Dan, our discussions were making him feel much better: "Ever since becoming sober, I've been aware of a monolithic pain, which I'm finally beginning to feel is breaking up."

"A monolithic pain?"

"I think it was the cumulative emotion. . . . I called it monolithic because I thought it would never go away."

Dan finished the semester successfully, which was a relief. I cautioned him that many people are vigilant their first semester back in school but get into trouble in the second semester because they relax, thinking they are home free. As the academic year progressed, he continued with his story and psychotherapy.

In spite of his drinking, Dan had done well at Connecticut College. After college he worked for a few years and then was accepted to the business school at MIT. Here, too, he did extremely well academically. On the basis of his grades, Dan received invitations to interview at some of the most prestigious consulting firms in New York, but he had found dressing up for the interviews in dark suits and going into the august firms unbearably stressful. In one incident, he had gone into a New York firm that had scheduled lunch and six interviews. After checking in with the secretary, Dan found himself too anxious to go through with the meetings. Excusing himself to allegedly go the bathroom, he disappeared, exiting the building and standing up the bewildered interviewers. He finished his exams at the end of the first year and withdrew from business school.

"I think I understand better now why those interviews did me in," said Dan one day.

"Oh?"

Reflecting on his life, Dan thought the constant upheavals and threats as a child had left him with a profound sense of instability and unreliability. "'Mayhem' is the word that keeps coming to mind," he said. "My life was mayhem: My parents' violent arguments when I was a young kid. My grandparents' harsh disapproval after the divorce. My father nearly blowing my head off with a gun. My stepfather getting psychotic and my mother asking me what to do. His trying to poison us. My later finding him hanging from a rope. These are just a few of the high points, you know. It was mayhem, on a daily basis.

"I think when I dressed up to go in to those consulting firms, part of me was like a four-year-old kid sitting down in the middle of the street, bawling, 'I can't go on. I've had enough.' It must have felt like another incomprehensible leap . . . into adulthood or the establishment . . . I don't know what, but I wasn't ready for it."

During his first years after leaving business school, Dan's drinking escalated. He moved to New York, worked on construction sites in Manhattan, and lived with a girlfriend who was also an alcoholic. "The construction sites were teeming with a whole other life in the heart of the city but at the same time entirely separate from it," said Dan. "I found it incredibly colorful. I developed this romantic idea of myself as a writer. Since college and especially business school, there had been this question in my mind of whether I was an establishment figure or an outsider. If I could succeed as a writer, I could be both."

Dan began writing poetry and actually finished a three-act play about the characters he was meeting at work. Unfortunately, he was also drinking daily in tough blue-collar bars. Always robust and physically fit, during this period Dan got into numerous barroom brawls, in which he sometimes sustained serious injuries. Eventually, the drinking caught up with him. He stopped writing. He couldn't work and was laid off from his job. Unemployment lasted only for a year. When it ran out, he was evicted from his apartment.

Alcoholics Anonymous uses the terms "bottoming out," or "hitting bottom," for an alcoholic's suffering enough losses in life that he is finally willing to actively engage in treatment. Destitute, he checked into an alcohol rehabilitation center.

During the month-long inpatient detoxification program, Dan became actively involved in AA. When discharged from the hospital, he moved into a halfway house for recovering alcoholics and continued in AA. After being sober several months, he took a job in a lumberyard. "Obviously, I'd fallen far from my days at MIT or as an aspiring playwright," said Dan sadly. "I spent my days driving a forklift moving lumber from one end of the yard to another. I needed a mindless job to keep my life simple and focus on sobriety. I was petrified of going back to drinking."

Taking his recovery slowly, Dan lived at the halfway house for six months before moving into a small apartment of his own. He lived in the apartment and worked at the lumberyard for another year before moving back to Boston. "Returning to Boston was the first step in returning to school," said Dan. In Boston, he established the same simple lifestyle: living on his own, working a blue-collar job, attending AA meetings several times a week, working out at a gym, and depending on a small group of friends, most of whom he met in AA.

In the summer before I met him, Dan got up the "courage" to write to the business school inquiring whether or not he could return after such a long absence. Like most schools, MIT was happy to have a student return from leave. Dan was surprised by the warm reception he received.

As the second semester progressed, one day in mid-April Dan commented on how much better he was feeling: "Last week I was jogging with a buddy in my neighborhood. The day was unusually warm. It felt as if spring was coming. As we jogged, I found myself looking into people's backyards and noticing picnic tables and barbecues. I thought, 'This is good. Families live in these houses. Nice things happen here.' You have to realize how unusual it was for me to have thoughts like that because they were so positive. Usually my thoughts are much more cynical. It's a really refreshing change."

Later in the month, when he came to see me, Dan announced he had accepted a job at a start-up Internet company in Boston: "After I understood a little better why interviewing had been so difficult the last time around, I felt I could face it. Writing to companies and going in to see them wasn't easy. It brought back a lot of memories. But it was okay. I think I'll be fine working after graduation."

As business school came to a close, Dan said of the relationship between AA and psychotherapy, "In AA, I learned to abstain from alcohol and get on with my life, to keep trucking, like a foot soldier. But I often experienced a black mood, which would descend on me for days. Many of my friends in AA experience the same thing. We called it 'being in the tank,' submerged in a gloomy darkness. I think it was the closest I came to feeling the monolithic pain. But in AA's foot-soldier culture, I couldn't have indulged the emotions that have come up in here. Only now that the pain is breaking up am I aware how strong a presence it's been all these years."

I have found that twelve-step programs and individual psychotherapy complement each other in just this way. Twelve-step programs seem to have intuitively hit on a cognitive-behavioral approach to controlling addictive behavior. Peer groups reduce an addict's sense of shame and isolation. For those who become actively involved, they provide a new social life revolving around abstinence to replace one that revolved around alcohol, cocaine, narcotics, or other drugs.

While AA's strength is group dynamics and a behavioral emphasis, psychotherapy's is one-on-one emotional depth. Dan's story is typical of people who enter therapy after firmly establishing sobriety. At the time that he bottomed out, Dan's drinking was so severe he never could have done psychotherapy. A strict emphasis on sobriety had to be the focus. Yet this left many emotions on hold. Later, psychotherapy provided an opportunity to work through them. Dan and I were able to do the emotional work we did because he could rely—we both could rely—on AA to keep him sober.

Amanda: A Case of Bulimia

"I hate myself," Amanda sobbed. An attractive Harvard undergraduate with an olive complexion, watery green eyes, and a cascade of curly black hair, Amanda pulled her legs up in the chair and wrapped her slender arms around them. Tears streaming down her cheeks, she said, "I've been eating all week. I can't stop myself. I went to the gym this morning hoping to break the cycle. That anorexic girl was there. She's always there on the treadmill, the exercise bike, or the StairMaster. She's so thin it's unhealthy. You can see every bone in her body. She looks like she could fall off the bike she's so frail."

"Really," I said gravely, wanting to reinforce Amanda's concern for the girl and her implicit rejection of anorexia. For Amanda herself had been anorexic in high school.

"But part of me is jealous of her." Amanda's reddened, tear-stained face convulsed in a cry.

"Oh dear." My concern for Amanda rose.

"I envy her determination. The fact that she's so thin. Where's my willpower gone? The worst mistake was weighing myself before I left the gym. I weigh one hundred thirty-two pounds! I can't believe I'm in the hundred-and-thirties!" Amanda tore at the slim flesh on her upper arms. "I'm so fat. I feel so ugly."

In addition to bingeing, Amanda had been purging, vomiting up the food she ate hoping to minimize the calories she absorbed. In painful detail, she described going to the local convenience store to buy bags of junk food. In the middle of the night, when it was too late to go out, she would descend into the basement of her dormitory to a small room lined with vending machines. In the fluorescent-lit, linoleum-tiled room she would furtively drop her quarters into the steely machines and yank on their plungers to get bags of potato chips or chocolate chip cookies.

"I always meet one or two other girls," said Amanda, "either at the machines or going down to them. We barely acknowledge one another with a guilty look of 'I know what you're doing.'"

The trek to the store or the vending machines is always suspenseful, an adrenalinized mixture of anticipation and fear. From a psychological point of view, this procurement ritual is remarkably like an alcoholic's trip to the liquor store, a drug addict's rendezvous with his pusher, or a sex addict's pursuit of a thrill. If the vending machines were already empty, Amanda would raid her dormitory's small communal kitchen. Women stealing their roommates' food to fuel binges is quite a serious problem on college campuses.

Back in her room, Amanda hastily consumed bags of cheese twists, boxes of vanilla wafers, cartons of Häagen-Dazs ice cream, or whatever the high-carbohydrate food happened to be. Some women describe eating whole loaves of white bread because that was all they could find in the cupboard.

Amanda ate until her stomach was so full it was distended. She knew she could not indulge this bloated feeling for long if she wanted to avoid the consequences. She would have to vomit before she absorbed much of the food, with its high caloric content.

Although it may seem nauseating to the uninitiated and has distasteful elements even for the most jaded bulimic, vomiting after a binge is a convulsive, cleansing experience. Purging oneself of the bloated feeling is the climax of the bulimic ritual. After this high, one is left exhausted, sated, at least temporarily. Of course, after a quiescent period, the call of the addictive cycle inevitably returns.

"Why am I stuffing my face when I'm full and don't want to eat?" implored Amanda.

Sitting opposite Amanda, her face flush with tears, I was struck by the incongruity of a beautiful young woman feeling so ugly and worthless. Hers was a peculiarly upper-middle-class problem, one I had seen before. I felt sympathetic toward her because I did not take what she said literally. Rather, I heard her talk about food metaphorically: as symbolic of her feeling empty, bereft, confused, plagued by doubt and self-loathing.

Amanda had been in treatment with me for two months. In the previous few weeks, she had been doing better, avoiding bingeing and keeping to a reasonable exercise schedule. What caused her to fall off the wagon?

"I went home over the weekend," said Amanda.

"You did?" I said surprised, since Amanda's family were in Manhattan.

"My father called to say, 'Why don't you fly down? It's Becca's birthday.' So I went." Rebecca was Amanda's younger sister.

"How was it?"

"Awful."

"What happened?"

"Becca and I had a big fight with my mother."

"Over what?"

"My aunt gave Becca an ankle bracelet. It was really pretty. Eighteen-carat gold. From Tiffany's. Becca was sporting the ankle bracelet quite proudly until my mother said, dripping with mock sympathy, 'Oh, Becca, you have ankles just like mine.' All our childhood, my mother complained bitterly that her calves and ankles were too thick, that she could never find shoes she looked good in. She gets special tailor-made pants to come down just right and cover her ankles. She was always saying, 'My ankles are so ugly.' So for her to say Becca's ankles were like hers was to say, 'They're ugly. You have to cover them up. You can't wear ankle bracelets. Don't get a big head.' It was as though Becca had lead feet; she could never be light and graceful and feminine. Hell, her ankles are fine. They're just not as thin as my mother thinks they should be. What can Becca do about that? I felt so bad for her."

"Did you say anything?"

"Becca did. The next day. She was incredibly tactful. She simply said, 'You know, Mom, I wish you wouldn't make comments like that about my body. I've asked you not to many times before. It makes me feel very self-conscious.'"

"How did your mother respond?"

"She denied saying it."

"Denied it?"

"It was less than twenty-four hours later, and she adamantly denied she'd made any comment about Becca's ankles."

"Did Becca challenge her?"

"Yes. Not only did Mom continue to deny what she'd said, she insisted she never complained about her own ankles! That's when I chimed in."

"With?"

"'Come on, Mom. We've heard you complain our whole lives about your ankles. Whenever you go shopping for shoes. Whenever you're getting dressed up. Whenever you're packing for a trip. It's a constant refrain.'"

"What happened?"

"She wouldn't budge. She got all tearful. She took to her bed. She wouldn't get up to say goodbye when my father was taking me to the airport. I heard him go in and ask her to but she refused."

"Why would she have denied it?"

"When Becca repeated it, Mom knew that wasn't a nice thing to have said. Obviously, it was very insensitive. So she denied it."

Even before leaving her parents' house to go back to school, Amanda had started "eating everything in sight."

"Why?"

"I wish I knew."

"You have no idea?"

"None," she said, baffled.

"Do you remember how you felt right after the fight, before you started to eat?"

Amanda looked at me blankly and shook her head.

In previous sessions, Amanda had described both her parents as growing up in lower-middle-class circumstances. Amanda's father was now a partner in a large Manhattan law firm. His position and income gave them entrée into social circles they were "desperate to join." Amanda said her father was a "workaholic," who kept long hours at the office and "had no real involvement with the family."

For Amanda's mother, life revolved around "doing the socially correct thing": designer labels, prestigious clubs, and brand-name schools. Highly self-conscious, she placed inordinate emphasis on superficial appearances and achievement. Amanda said her mother's love was conditional, contingent on one's performance: "I was loved *so long as* I didn't wear jeans to the country club party, so long as my scarf matched my shoes, so long as I wore my hair down because my mother thought when I wore it up I looked 'pluggy' . . . so long as I was thin, so long as my boyfriend was Jewish, so long as I got into Harvard."

Her mother first put Amanda on a diet when she was ten years old. By fifth grade Amanda was already counting calories and knew the fat content of most foods. Amanda's mother, too, was perpetually gaining and losing weight.

Amanda was naturally slimmer and prettier than her sister Rebecca and often felt guilty about it. A competitive atmosphere existed between the three women in the household, driven by her mother's constant, intrusive comments about their bodies. Amanda's mother noticed whenever anyone lost or gained a pound in their face, stomach, or thighs.

In this atmosphere, Amanda "almost naturally" became anorexic in high school. When her weight dropped to a hundred pounds, her parents "panicked." After meeting with a psychiatrist who specialized in eating disorders, Amanda refused to enter therapy. Instead, Amanda's weight was monitored by her primary-care doctor. Over the course of a year, she slowly regained fifteen pounds under threat of being forced into treatment, potentially including force-feeding. Her weight remained stable until she left home to come to Harvard.

Given this background, it might seem surprising that Amanda had no idea why she began eating in the wake of the family fight. What mixture of feelings might have been stirred up by her sister's birthday, her mother's insensitivity, and her father's remoteness from the scene? Of course, the feelings would not have been limited to this particular argument but rather would have tapped into a long history of similar ones.

This bingeing episode precipitated a crisis in Amanda's treatment. "What am I going to do to stop eating?" she demanded. We discussed the possibility of Prozac to suppress her appetite. But this would only be temporary. Over the longer haul, the drug could increase her appetite and weight, a risk Amanda was unwilling to take, to say nothing of its other side effects. When she first came to therapy, I suggested Amanda consider an eating-disorders group as an adjunct to our work. At the time she scoffed at the idea. Now she expressed more interest.

Eating-disorders groups include the twelve-step program Overeaters Anonymous and psychotherapy groups with a cognitive-behavioral emphasis. Members are educated about the medical dangers of vomiting, being overweight, or anorexic. The groups are focused on learning appropriate behavior around food: recognizing when one is full, eating for nutritional instead of emotional reasons, taking responsibility for what one eats by refraining from purging, following reasonable diet and exercise regimens rather than draconian ones, and checking one's weight on a weekly or monthly basis, rather than on a more obsessive daily basis. Members are encouraged to keep a food diary, a log of what they eat and their mood at the time. Unlike Overeaters Anonymous, most eating-disorders groups meet for limited periods of time, ten to sixteen weeks.

Because she felt "desperate," Amanda joined a group in Boston specifically for college students with bulimia. Initially overwhelmed by other people's stories, after just a few weeks she began to enjoy the camaraderie of others struggling with the same problem. In their stories Amanda heard themes echoing her own. The group helped break down Amanda's sense of isolation and shame. Because they shared the same problem, her peers could quickly confront Amanda's distorted thinking about her body and food.

Meanwhile, in psychotherapy, Amanda and I revisited the "ankle incident," trying to retrieve how she felt about it. She expressed sadness and guilt over Rebecca's birthday celebration having been ruined. Why guilt, when she had not made the offensive comment and she had defended her sister when her mother denied it? "When your whole self-worth is based on how you look, even if you're the 'winner' you feel like you don't deserve it. Why did I get thinner ankles than Becca? Wouldn't she feel better if I put on weight? At times my mother has given me clothes and explicitly said, 'Don't wear this around Becca. She'll be jealous.' It makes me feel awful. I feel like saying, 'Then don't give it to me. What have I done to deserve it?'"

"Have you ever said that to her?"

"Yes. It made her apeshit. I was rejecting her generosity."

"You were just rejecting the intrigue."

"Try to tell her that!"

Amanda had mixed feelings toward her father. On the one hand, she thought him dull, uninteresting, dependent on her mother for friends and a social life. Distant and unpsychological, he was unable to mitigate her relationship with her mother. Like her mother, he most valued status, prestige, and appearances. Yet at times he could be thoughtful, as in suggesting Amanda fly home for her sister's birthday. "I feel like he peeks into my life but is not really there," said Amanda sadly. "He ducks away the minute the going gets rough. Ultimately, I think of him as weak."

Amanda's struggle with her parents—over her worth, her appearance, and above all, control in her life—was at the center of her difficulties, as it is for so many eating-disordered women. "My mother was so adamant that she hadn't commented on Becca's ankles that I begin to wonder . . . ," said Amanda one day. "Anytime I was upset about something she did, that's what would happen. Whenever I tried to address an incident, she would become belligerent. 'I don't know what you're talking about,' she would say. 'That never happened.' She claimed I made things up. That I was impossible. I was ungrateful after all she did for me. I'd get so confused. . . . This ankle incident is actually rare, where I can hold on to what really happened. If Becca hadn't been there as a witness, I would doubt my own perceptions. My mother's so forceful, she's so adamant, and I was so dependent on her."

All kinds of interactions with family, friends, teachers, or even strangers could cause Amanda to want to eat. We had to go over dozens of incidents before she began to recognize the pattern in which she used bingeing and purging to distract herself from overwhelming feelings. "I've realized," she said one day, "if I'm feeling sad, angry, disappointed, vulnerable, confused—whatever the feelings are—eating totally distracts me, bingeing completely derails the feelings. By the time I've found food, found a place where I can eat it, and thrown up, I've forgotten the feelings. I've switched the channel. I've gotten on another track, at least temporarily."

This is the nub of the problem: Like other forms of substance abuse, eating disorders are driven by emotional short circuits; affective overload triggers the addictive behavior as a way of coping with overwhelming, inchoate feelings. Gradually, Amanda became better able to recognize her feelings in the moment, in the very midst of her interactions with people. This was literally a process of coming to know herself emotionally, being able to articulate feelings and deal with them rather than eating them away. In the process, Amanda had to become comfortable with strong emotions like anger, sadness, and disappointment. She had to learn how to assert herself, how to confront people and work through differences, instead of consoling herself with food.

This central struggle to know oneself emotionally is well described in Kim Chernin's feminist interpretation of eating disorders, *The Hungry Self*. Says Chernin, "We cannot indeed even begin to think about self-healing until we stop using words like 'eating disorder' to hide from ourselves the formidable struggle for a self in which every woman suffering in her relationship to food is secretly engaged. . . . This is the hunger knot, in which identity, the mother-separation struggle, love, rage, food, and the female body are all entangled. It is this we must unravel, patiently, meticulously, strand by strand, until we know ourselves."[2]

As Amanda made steady progress in psychotherapy and the eating-disorders group, one day I asked her to articulate how the group helped. Said Amanda, "I don't feel alone anymore. Bulimia entails so much shame. I don't feel like this weird pig demon who does all this crazy stuff when I sit in a room full of other women driven to do the same thing.

"When you're bulimic, you can't really share that with the people you love, your family and friends. They don't want to hear it. They can't understand. But the isolation is part of the problem. Having a place to talk about it, to bring it out in the open, makes it so much less powerful."

How do psychotherapy and the group relate? I asked.

"Therapy is much more focused on me. It's more probing. If I don't want to speak in group one week, I don't have to. I can just listen. There isn't the same kind of building from week to week on what I've been talking about and where I'm going. In therapy I'm held more accountable for digging into the past, pushing myself to get in touch with feelings, and trying to understand my behavior. Group is very practical. Therapy is delving down deep."

Amanda was in the group for four months, until the end of the academic year. She stayed in therapy an additional year, solidifying the progress she had made. As with any addiction, the goal was not to completely eradicate any urge to binge and purge. This would be unrealistic. "Once a vulnerability, always a vulnerability," I tell patients. Under sufficient duress, the old temptation will raise its head. In the throes of bulimia, many women binge and purge on a daily basis. The goal instead is that when they feel the urge a few times a year they are able to resist it.

As Seth's, Dan's, and Amanda's cases illustrate, different though they may seem at first glance, sexual compulsions, substance abuse, and eating disorders have much in common: They are all forms of addictive behavior in which excessive sex, drugs, or food are used to numb painful emotions. As an alternative to prescription medication, group psychotherapy or twelve-step programs are far preferable for curbing the addictive behavior. In severe cases, like Dan's alcoholism, the initial focus of treatment needs to be exclusively on mastering sobriety. As in Dan's case, this may take years. Only after sobriety is established is it safe to proceed with addressing the underlying emotions that fueled the addictive behavior in the first place. In other instances, as in Seth's and Amanda's cases, where the addictive behavior is not totally disruptive or life-threatening, learning to curb the behavior through a group program and exploring the underlying emotions in psychotherapy can proceed simultaneously.

Effecting Personal Change

Often, only as one finishes up a therapy is it clear why it was undertaken in the first place; the real, underlying issues become most evident in hindsight. The same may be said of writing a book: Only as I approached the end did I realize how much this book was born out of my and my patients' attempts to understand a cultural phenomenon in which we have all been swept up.

A decade ago, Prozac burst onto the scene like an armed intruder demanding my attention and that of my patients. Before long the Prozac group included Zoloft, Paxil, and more. What were these drugs? What confluence of forces brought about their stunning success? What benefits did they offer? What risks did they entail?

The search for answers to these questions brought many surprises. Little did I know that in trying to understand withdrawal, dependence, and the drugs' wearing off, I would discover neurotoxicity research on related medications that would raise profoundly disturbing questions. And in attempting to understand Prozac's relationship to suicide and violence, I did not expect to come upon a secret settlement in the test case that went to trial, conflicts of interest in the FDA committee that investigated the issue, and ongoing research that had quietly shed new light on this side effect.

As I was completing the manuscript, an article entitled "The Antidepressant Web" in the *International Journal of Risk & Safety in Medicine* came to my attention.[1] The article was on withdrawal side effects and dependency on the Prozac group. In an accompanying commentary, the editor of the *Journal* said the article's author "is worried, and many with him. Concerned because we seem to be facing here a phenomenon which is capable of expanding exponentially—a headlong rush into the unknown, propelled by forces on which society as a whole has little grip."[2] Yes, I thought, and that is exactly why I set out to write this book. Now, as I finish it, I hope we understand a little better the forces we have been swept up in.

Similar concerns were the motivation for many of the people who helped me in my research for the book. As they generously gave of their time and energy, many were remarkably candid about their own experiences. Said one researcher whose work I was quoting, "I was unhappy with my job a number of years ago. I went to a psychiatrist who offered me Prozac. I was horrified. What I needed was a career change, which I made after talking to another psychiatrist for a few months. I've felt better ever since."

A journalist who helped me find original sources commented, "What I don't understand is why doctors offer patients pills for normal emotions. I had a stillbirth a few years ago. My doctor immediately said I was a 'candidate' for Paxil. Aren't we allowed to have normal grief anymore?"

Still another person observed, "A few years ago I felt under pressure to go on Zoloft because so many of my coworkers were on it to feel 'better than normal' and to be more productive. I felt pressure to keep up with them. I didn't want to be at a pharmacologic disadvantage. Fortunately, my girlfriend brought me to my senses." From wanting to be left in peace with normal emotions to feeling pressured to keep up with the Joneses pharmacologically, the Prozac phenomenon has touched all our lives.

A few people have reacted more cautiously to some of the book's topics. "Do you realize what you're asking?" said one researcher when I mentioned Prozac in a discussion on neurotoxicity, as though the question touched forbidden territory. "You mustn't scare patients," commented a psychiatrist. "You must be careful not to alarm them."

In both instances, the comments were made by older men in their late sixties. I think they reflect a conservative, paternalistic, perhaps even chauvinistic attitude toward patients. They reflect the stance "We doctors know best. Concerns like tic disorders, brain damage, and neurotoxicity should stay within the profession until the evidence is unequivocal. Patients are already fragile enough. We shouldn't worry them. Instead, we should reassure them until and unless it becomes impossible to do so."

In my estimation and that of many of my colleagues, this approach is outdated. Patients want and have a right to know all of the concerns in order to factor them into their decisions. I have discussed these issues with patients for some time now. One reason I wrote the book is that it is impossible in brief weekly or monthly meetings to relate every detail and construct all the arguments in the depth that I have been able to here. Many of my patients have chosen to stay on the drugs in spite of these concerns.

Others have chosen not to begin taking drugs or to go off them as soon as possible. In any case, patients have been grateful to be fully informed. No one has run distraught from the office. No one has been too "fragile," too "scared," or too "alarmed" to deal with information presented in a balanced, straightforward way.

Anyone who would invoke such an alleged need to protect patients might better have led an outcry against the exaggerated claims made on behalf of these drugs for the past decade. Throughout this book, I have been careful to note where I speculate beyond what is definitely known regarding issues that desperately need further research. My speculations are tempered and cautious, rooted well within the known evidence, small steps dwarfed by the wild leaps that have been made by others in the efforts to promote these drugs.

Prozac-type drugs are by no means harmless candy, although in some settings they are currently being prescribed almost as though they were. These and other antidepressants should be reserved for moderate to severe symptoms that interfere with one's ability to function. Serotonin boosters have serious side effects and many unanswered questions about their long-term safety.

Certainly antidepressants can have an important place in balanced, comprehensive psychiatric treatment. For patients with moderate to severe symptoms, judicious use of medication can be invaluable, even life-saving. But in making the decision to use drugs, patients need to be fully informed of both the potential benefits and the risks.

If one's symptoms are severe enough to warrant medication, it should not be the only form of treatment. Medication merely provides symptomatic relief; it is never a cure. One or more of the many alternatives should simultaneously be undertaken to effect genuine personal change, ultimately reducing or eliminating one's dependence on drugs.

Treating psychiatric symptoms with the Prozac group is analogous to using aspirin to relieve a fever caused by an infection. Aspirin merely reduces the fever and makes the patient more comfortable. Patients need diagnostic tests such as chest X-rays, blood cultures, sputum cultures, and spinal taps, depending on the particular type of infection suspected. Once the infection is identified, appropriate antibiotic treatment is continued until the infection has cleared. Like aspirin, Prozac relieves symptoms and makes patients more comfortable. But other treatments—like psychotherapy, cognitive-behavioral techniques, and twelve-step programs—may be required to address the underlying problem. In no other branch of medicine would we tolerate treating symptoms without investigating and treat-

ing the underlying problem. Can one imagine patients with pneumonia being put on aspirin indefinitely and not receiving any other treatment? Why
should we tolerate this kind of "treatment" for psychiatric conditions?

Obviously we are in need of several research initiatives and reforms. A
few deserve particular note:

We need immediate research on the potential neurotoxicity of antidepressant drugs. Animal research—such as the studies on cocaine, amphetamines, and the diet pill Redux—should be done on the Prozac group and
other antidepressants that are so widely prescribed. Even though these
drugs are still covered by their patent, pharmaceutical companies should
not be able to force researchers to sign agreements giving the pharmaceutical companies the right to veto publication of this critically important research. Related clinical studies following patients are needed to assess
whether or not antidepressants worsen the long-term course of depression
by sensitizing brain tissue, which can create a vicious cycle in which patients who have been on the drugs a long time cannot get off them without
causing a relapse.

We do know, from documented clinical experience and research, that
these drugs have led to suicidal and violent urges in some patients. We desperately need warnings for patients and doctors, together with information
on prevention and coping with suicidal and violent impulses when they occur. Additional research to help us understand the phenomenon is desirable
but should not be merely a ploy to delay such warnings and preventive
steps.

The widespread prescribing of these drugs to children also needs careful scrutiny. With their developing nervous systems, children are a special
case. They cannot protect themselves, so families and society bear an additional responsibility to help them.

We need new curbs on excesses in the way the drugs are promoted.
There is no established biochemical imbalance for depression. There is no
established gene for depression. Prescription antidepressants should not be
promoted as though these hypothetical models were established. Psychiatric diagnoses should not be expanded and marketed as part of the efforts
to market the drugs. Medical ethics, not business standards, need to prevail
in health care.

Given the public health issues involved, we need a national database in
which health care professionals are required to report any financial ties to
pharmaceutical companies. The database should be readily accessible on
the Internet, so journalists and the public can easily use the information to
put in perspective comments made on behalf of drugs by seemingly independent spokespeople. The information would not just be a list of affilia-

tions with pharmaceutical companies. Rather, the full dollar amounts should be disclosed so that the public is informed of the huge sums of money often involved. The argument that this would be an invasion of the individuals' privacy is more than overridden by the public safety issues at stake. Academic institutions have a long tradition of neutrality. The purpose of tenured academic faculty is to have independent researchers, clinicians, educators, and thinkers who are unencumbered by commercial self-interest. Independent academics can perform a critical role in society, safeguarding the public interest and the pursuit of scientific truth. A few individuals with serious behind-the-scenes conflicts of interest should not be allowed to spoil this rich tradition.

We now have enough experience with drugs that boost neurotransmitters like serotonin, dopamine, and adrenaline to know that all of them will inevitably precipitate a backlash in which the brain seeks to counteract the effects of the drugs.[3] This backlash is responsible for most of the serious, long-term side effects of psychiatric drugs.

Because of the limited clinical testing that drugs receive before being marketed, in the early decades in which they are prescribed to patients every new psychiatric drug is an ongoing human experiment. As the more serious side effects of the Prozac group are more widely recognized, no doubt new drugs will emerge and be promoted as "safer." Indeed, a new, "improved" Prozac has already been announced.[4] Chemicals like Prozac have two mirror-image forms—called right-Prozac and left-Prozac. The original version contains a mixture of the two. But as the patent on Prozac expires, its right and left forms can each be separately patented and marketed as "new" drugs. The new, "improved" version of Prozac already announced is right-Prozac, scheduled for release at about the time that the patent on the original mixture expires. Unfortunately, especially given the timing, one is left to question whether the marketing of the new, "improved" drug is little more than an effort to prolong a patentable product.

The new, "improved" Prozac is already being promoted as having fewer side effects. But is there any real substance to this claim? Are the chances not far more likely that the new drug—like virtually every other major psychiatric drug—will prove to have serious side effects and dangers once large numbers of people begin taking it for months or years? Like any new drug, it too will be an ongoing experiment. In fact, we have a recent analogy that is not reassuring. Like the new Prozac, the diet pill Redux was the right half of the right and left forms of its parent compound.[5] Redux was marketed as a new, breakthrough drug. Of course, Redux did not prove any safer than the parent drug.

The many stories of patients in this book are examples of effecting personal change that is truly liberating, leaving them substantially less vulnerable to depression, anxiety, obsessions, compulsions, addictions, eating disorders, and other psychiatric syndromes. Roberto overcame his elevator phobia through perseverance in behavioral therapy without the use of any drugs. After Tanya developed Paxil withdrawal symptoms—electric shock–like sensations that made her think she was being electrocuted while swimming in a pool—she was determined to slowly wean herself off a drug to which she felt held "hostage." She and her boyfriend, Richard, then worked together to sort out the issues in their relationship that had precipitated her anxiety. They are now happily married, pursuing challenging careers, and planning a family. At the opposite end of the life cycle, when Dora retired from teaching her Holocaust memories came back to haunt her. After a year of being given only Prozac at her HMO, she sought more balanced, comprehensive treatment. In just six months of psychotherapy, she worked through the Holocaust memories and moved on with her life drug-free. Sunita became psychotic and suicidal shortly after starting Prozac. Once the Prozac was stopped, Sunita's suicidality waned over several weeks, but her psychosis took months to clear. She declined antipsychotic medication "after what happened on Prozac." Sunita put an enormous effort into psychotherapy, resolving her grief over her mother's death and her relationship with her demanding, alcoholic father. No longer depressed, Sunita went on to graduate school and an academic career. All of these patients, and the many others described in this book, worked hard to overcome their difficulties. All of them feel the hard work was well worth the results.

In my experience, 75% or more of people who are currently being prescribed Prozac-type antidepressants can dramatically lower their dose or eliminate the medication altogether. Drugs can serve a purpose when they are used judiciously and with a recognition of their limitations. But most people can overcome the obstacles to leading satisfying lives through the help of more natural alternatives that treat our whole selves—psychological, physical, intellectual, and emotional.

NOTES

In academic and professional journals, the chemical rather than the commercial names for drugs are typically used. For example, Prozac is referred to as fluoxetine. When these journals are quoted in the text, for readability the well-recognized commercial names of the drugs have been substituted for their chemical names.

INTRODUCTION
The Prozac Phenomenon

1. R. J. Leo, "Movement Disorders Associated with the Serotonin Selective Reuptake Inhibitors [serotonin boosters]," *Journal of Clinical Psychiatry* 57 (1996) 449–54; R. Pies, "Serotonergic Agents [serotonin boosters] and Extrapyramidal [neurological] Side Effects," *Psychiatric Times*, January 1999, pp. 20–22.

2. The percentage of patients with withdrawal effects varies widely among the drugs, depending upon how quickly they wash out of the body. Withdrawal symptoms are rare with Prozac. At the other end of the spectrum, they are estimated to occur in 86% of patients stopping Luvox and 50% of patients stopping Paxil. These are estimates based on small-scale studies, since systematic studies have not been done. See L. C. Barr, W. K. Goodman, and L. H. Price, "Physical Symptoms Associated with Paroxetine [Paxil] Discontinuation [withdrawal], *American Journal of Psychiatry* 151 (1994): 289; D. W. Black, R. Wesner, and J. Gabel, "The Abrupt Discontinuation [withdrawal] of Fluvoxamine [Luvox] in Patients with Panic Disorder," *Journal of Clinical Psychiatry* 54 (1993): 146–49.

3. A. L. Montejo-González, G. Llorca, J. A. Izquierdo, A. Ledesma, M. Bousono, A. Calcedo, J. L. Carrasco, J. Ciudad, E. Daniel, J. De la Gandara, J. Derecho, M. Franco, M. J. Gomez, J. A. Macias, T. Martin, V. Perez, J. M. Sanchez, S. Sanchez, and E. Vicens, "SSRI-Induced Sexual Dysfunction: Fluoxetine [Prozac], Paroxetine [Paxil], Sertraline [Zoloft], and Fluvoxamine [Luvox] in a Prospective, Multicenter, and Descriptive Clinical Study of 344 Patients," *Journal of Sex and Marital Therapy* 23 (1997): 176–94.

4. L. Slater, *Prozac Diary* (New York: Random House, 1998), pp. 179–85; D. Abramson, "Hooked: Antidepressants Can Take Away as Much of You as They Give Back," *Boston Phoenix*, April 17, 1998, p. 7.

5. An example is the recently withdrawn diet pill Redux, which targets serotonin. See M. E. Molliver, U. V. Berger, L. A. Mamounas, D. C. Molliver, E. O'Hearn, and M. A. Wilson, "Neurotoxicity of MDMA [Ecstasy] and Related Compounds [including discussion of Redux]: Anatomic Studies," *Annals of the New York Academy of Science* 600 (1990): 640–64. For a study that compared the effects of Prozac to a lobotomy, see R. Hoehn-Saric, G. Harris, G. Pearlson, C. Cox, S. Machlin, and E. Calmargo, "A Fluoxetine [Prozac]-Induced Frontal Lobe Syndrome [apathy and indifference] in an Obsessive Compulsive Patient," *Journal of Clinical Psychiatry* 52 (1991): 131–33.

6. M. Fava, S. M. Rappe, J. A. Pava, A. A. Nierenberg, J. E. Alpert, and J. F. Rosenbaum, "Relapse in Patients on Long-Term Fluoxetine [Prozac] Treatment: Response to Increased Fluoxetine [Prozac] Dose," *Journal of Clinical Psychiatry* 56 (1995): 52–55.

7. J. Cornwell, *The Power to Harm: Mind, Medicine, and Murder on Trial* (New York: Viking, 1996).

8. American Psychiatric Association, *Diagnostic and Statistical Manual of Mental Disorders (DSM)*, 4th edition (Washington, D.C.: American Psychiatric Association, 1994),

p. 748. While the tics are permanent in less than 50% of young patients, they are permanent in 60–95% of elderly patients. Because tics associated with Prozac-type medications have not been thoroughly investigated, we do not have an estimate of what percentage may be permanent.

9. I use the term "involuntary motor system" to refer to the extrapyramidal motor system in the brain.

10. R. Pies, "Must We Now Consider SRIs [serotonin boosters] Neuroleptics [major tranquilizers]?," *Journal of Clinical Psychopharmacology* 17 (1997): 443–45.

11. A. Weil, "The New Politics of Coca," *New Yorker,* May 15, 1995, pp. 70–80.

12. G. Cowley, "The Promise of Prozac," cover story, *Newsweek,* March 26, 1990, p. 38.

13. Both *New York* magazine and the *National Enquirer* are cited in G. Cowley, "The Promise of Prozac," cover story, *Newsweek,* March 26, 1990, p. 38.

14. P. Kramer, *Listening to Prozac* (New York: Viking, 1993).

15. Ibid., pp. xvi–xix.

16. Ibid., p. 15.

17. S. Begley, "Beyond Prozac: How Science Will Let You Change Your Personality with a Pill," cover story, *Newsweek,* February 7, 1994, pp. 36–43.

18. J. Solomon, "Breaking the Silence: From Congress to Hollywood, Prominent Americans Are Trying to Erase the Lingering Shame of Mental Illness," *Newsweek,* May 20, 1996, pp. 20–24.

19. M. J. Grinfeld, "Protecting Prozac," *California Lawyer,* December 1998, pp. 36–40, 79. See also E. J. Pollock, "Managed Care's Focus on Psychiatric Drugs Alarms Many Doctors," *Wall Street Journal,* December 1, 1995, p. 1.

20. M. J. Grinfeld, "New Weight Loss Controversy Flares: Lilly Tries to Stop Nutri/Systems Marketing [Prozac as a diet pill] as Experts Assess Consumer Health Risks," *Psychiatric Times,* November 1997, pp. 1, 10–12.

21. T. Copeland, Interviewed on National Public Radio's "Morning Edition," October 10, 1997, in a segment called "Overtime at Boeing." Copeland is a psychologist who treats Boeing employees.

22. Review of *Listening to Prozac* in the *New Yorker,* August 16, 1993, p. 95.

23. *New Yorker,* September 27, 1993, p. 67.

24. *New Yorker,* November 8, 1993, p. 92.

25. L. Menand, "Listening to Bourbon," *New Yorker,* April 18, 1994, p. 108.

26. D. X. Freedman, "On Beyond Wellness," review of *Listening to Prozac,* in the *New York Times Book Review,* August 8, 1993, p. 6.

27. D. Rothman, "That Prozac Moment! Shiny Happy People," review of *Listening to Prozac,* in the *New Republic,* cover story, February 14, 1994, pp. 34–38.

28. S. Nuland, "The Pill of Pills," review of *Listening to Prozac,* in the *New York Review of Books,* June 9, 1994, pp. 4–8.

29. The data pharmaceutical companies release on the sales of their drugs are in dollar amounts and numbers of prescriptions, so that only rough estimates are available for the numbers of patients exposed to the drugs.

30. M. Leonard, "Children Are the Hot New Market for Antidepressants. But Is This How to Make Them Feel Better?," *Boston Sunday Globe,* May 25, 1997, pp. D1, D5; B. Strauch, "Use of Antidepression Medicine for Young Patients Has Soared," *New York Times,* August 10, 1997, p. 1.

31. R. L. Fisher and S. Fisher, "Antidepressants for Children: Is Scientific Support Necessary?," *Journal of Nervous and Mental Disease* 184 (1996): 99–102; L. Eisenberg, "Commentary: What Should Doctors Do in the Face of Negative Evidence?," *Journal of Nervous and Mental Disease* 184 (1996): 103–5; E. D. Pellegrino, "Commentary: Clinical Judgment, Scientific Data, and Ethics: Antidepressant Therapy in Adolescents and Children," *Journal of Nervous and Mental Disease* 184 (1996): 106–8.

32. P. Kramer, *Listening to Prozac,* (New York: Viking, 1993), p. 10.

33. In the text, I use the word "adrenaline" for both adrenaline and the closely related noradrenaline (also called epinephrine and norepinephrine, respectively), because "adrenaline" is the term well known to a nontechnical audience. Noradrenaline—or norepinephrine—is the form found in the brain.

34. W. Douglas, "Histamine and 5-Hydroxytryptamine [serotonin] and Their Antagonists,"

in A. G. Gilman, L. S. Goodman, and A. Gilman, eds., *The Pharmacological Basis of Therapeutics,* 6th edition (New York: Macmillan, 1980), p. 635.

35. E. Sanders-Bush and S. E. Mayer, "5-Hydroxytryptamine (Serotonin) Receptor Agonists and Antagonists," in J. G. Hardman and L. E. Limbird, eds., *Goodman and Gilman's The Pharmacological Basis of Therapeutics,* 9th edition (New York: McGraw-Hill, 1996), pp. 249–63.

36. G. Frajese, R. Lazzari, A. Magnani, C. Moretti, V. Sforza, and D. Nerozzi, "Neurotransmitter, Opiodergic System, Steroid-Hormone Interaction and Involvement in the Replacement Therapy of Sexual Disorders," *Journal of Steroid Biochemistry and Molecular Biology* 37 (1990): 411–19; G. L. Gessa and A. Tagliamonte, "Role of Brain Monoamines in Male Sexual Behavior," *Life Sciences* 14 (1974): 425–36.

37. E. C. Azmitia and P. M. Whitaker-Azmitia, "Awakening the Sleeping Giant: Anatomy and Plasticity of the Brain Serotonergic System," *Journal of Clinical Psychiatry* 52 (1991) [12, suppl.]: 4–16.

38. B. L. Jacobs, "Serotonin and Behavior: Emphasis on Motor Control," *Journal of Clinical Psychiatry* 52 (1991) [12, suppl.]: 17–23.

39. S. E. Hyman and E. J. Nestler, "Initiation and Adaptation: A Paradigm for Understanding Psychotropic Drug Action," *American Journal of Psychiatry* 153 (1996): 151–62.

40. J. Ichikawa and H. Y. Meltzer, "Effect of Antidepressants on Striatal [involuntary motor system] and Accumbens [another region of the brain] Extracellular Dopamine Levels," *European Journal of Pharmacology* 281 (1995): 225–61. S. L. Dewey, G. S. Smith, J. Logan, D. Alexoff, Y.-S. Ding, P. King, N. Pappas, J. D. Brodie, and C. R. Ashby, "Serotonergic Modulation of Striatal [involuntary motor system] Dopamine Measured with Positron Emission Tomography (PET) and In Vivo Microdialysis," *Journal of Neuroscience* 15 (1995): 821–29. A. Di Rocco, T. Brannan, A. Prikhojan, and M. D. Yahr, "Sertraline [Zoloft] Induced Parkinsonism. A Case Report and an In Vivo Study of the Effect of Sertraline [Zoloft] on Dopamine Metabolism," *Journal of Neural Transmission* 105 (1998): 247–51.

41. The official, or medical, name for the Prozac group is "selective serotonin reuptake inhibitors," or SSRIs. Sometimes the term "serotonin reuptake inhibitors," SRIs, is used because the drugs are, in fact, not so selective. I use terms like "Prozac group," "Prozac-type antidepressants," and "serotonin boosters" for this class of agents.

42. R. Baldessarini, Keynote Address, "Psychopharmacology: Where Have We Been; Where Are We; Where Are We Going?," Massachusetts General Hospital/Harvard Medical School Conference on Psychopharmacology, October 16, 1998.

43. T. Moore, *Prescription for Disaster* (New York: Simon & Schuster, 1998), p. 115.

44. D. A. Kessler, "Introducing MedWatch," *Journal of the American Medical Association* 269 (1993): 2765–68.

45. T. Moore, *Prescription for Disaster* (New York: Simon & Schuster, 1998), pp. 172–74.

46. Ibid., p. 115.

47. Ibid, pp. 117, 53.

48. *Physicians' Desk Reference (PDR)* (Montvale, N.J.: Medical Economics, 1999). See Table 1 on p. 926. Most authors report 1–2% for Lilly's official figure for sexual side effects in depressed patients on Prozac. See A. L. Montejo-González, G. Llorca, J. A. Izquierdo, A. Ledesma, M. Bousono, A. Calcedo, J. L. Carrasco, J. Ciudad, E. Daniel, J. De la Gandara, J. Derecho, M. Franco, M. J. Gomez, J. A. Macias, T. Martin, V. Perez, J. M. Sanchez, S. Sanchez, and E. Vicens, "SSRI-Induced Sexual Dysfunction: Fluoxetine [Prozac], Paroxetine [Paxil], Sertraline [Zoloft], and Fluvoxamine [Luvox] in a Prospective, Multicenter, and Descriptive Clinical Study of 344 Patients," *Journal of Sex and Marital Therapy* 23 (1997): 176–94 (see page 182); M. J. Gitlin, "Psychotropic Medications and Their Effects on Sexual Function: Diagnosis, Biology, and Treatment Approaches," *Journal of Clinical Psychiatry* 55 (1994): 406–13 (see page 410). I have used the 2–5% figure because in Lilly's Table 1 on page 926 of the *PDR,* in addition to 2% of depressed patients on the drug having impotence, the figure of 3% is also listed for decreased libido. It is impossible to tell from Lilly's table whether or not these two groups overlap. The 5% figure therefore represents the maximum percent possible based on Lilly's figures. These figures are based on Lilly's original prerelease studies of the drug for depression. Later studies by other researchers in which patients were asked directly about sexual dysfunction have found rates

as high as 75% of patients. One of the earliest studies of 60 patients found this high rate. See W. M. Patterson, "Fluoxetine [Prozac]-Induced Sexual Dysfunction," *Journal of Clinical Psychiatry* 54 (1993): 71. Later, large-scale studies include that of Modell, who found rates of sexual side effects of 73% for Prozac, 67% for Zoloft, and 86% for Paxil. See J. G. Modell, C. R. Katholi, J. D. Modell, and R. L. DePalma, "Comparative Sexual Side Effects of Bupropion [Wellbutrin], Fluoxetine [Prozac], Paroxetine [Paxil], and Sertraline [Zoloft]," *Clinical Pharmacology and Therapeutics* 61 (1997): 476–87. The most comprehensive study was that of the Montejo-González group, who found an overall rate of 58% of patients on Prozac, Zoloft, Paxil, or Luvox reporting sexual side effects. See A. L. Montejo-González, G. Llorca, J. A. Izquierdo, A. Ledesma, M. Bousono, A. Calcedo, J. L. Carrasco, J. Ciudad, E. Daniel, J. De la Gandara, J. Derecho, M. Franco, M. J. Gomez, J. A. Macias, T. Martin, V. Perez, J. M. Sanchez, S. Sanchez, and E. Vicens, "SSRI-Induced Sexual Dysfunction: Fluoxetine [Prozac], Paroxetine [Paxil], Sertraline [Zoloft], and Fluvoxamine [Luvox} in a Prospective, Multicenter, and Descriptive Clinical Study of 344 Patients," *Journal of Sex and Marital Therapy* 23 (1997): 176–94.

49. A. F. Schatzberg, "Introduction: Antidepressant Discontinuation [withdrawal] Syndrome: An Update on Serotonin Reuptake Inhibitors [Prozac-type drugs]," *Journal of Clinical Psychiatry* 58 (1997) [suppl. 7]: 3–4; A. F. Schatzberg, P. Haddad, E. M. Kaplan, M. Lejoyeux, J. F. Rosenbaum, A. H. Young, and J. Zajecka, "Serotonin Reuptake Inhibitor [Prozac-type drug] Discontinuation [withdrawal] Syndrome: A Hypothetical Definition," *Journal of Clinical Psychiatry* 58 (1997) [suppl. 7]: 5–10; M. Lejoyeux and J. Adès, "Antidepressant Discontinuation [withdrawal]: A Review of the Literature," *Journal of Clinical Psychiatry* 58 (1997) [suppl. 7]: 11–16; P. Haddad, "Newer Antidepressants and the Discontinuation [withdrawal] Syndrome," *Journal of Clinical Psychiatry* 58 (1997) [suppl. 7]: 17–22; A. F. Schatzberg, P. Haddad, E. M. Kaplan, M. Lejoyeux, J. F. Rosenbaum, A. H. Young, and J. Zajecka, "Possible Biological Mechanisms of the Serotonin Reuptake Inhibitor [Prozac-type drug] Discontinuation [withdrawal] Syndrome," *Journal of Clinical Psychiatry* 58 (1997) [suppl. 7]: 23–27; A. H. Young and A. Currie, "Physicians' Knowledge of Antidepressant Withdrawal Effects: A Survey," *Journal of Clinical Psychiatry* 58 (1997) [suppl. 7]: 28–30; E. M. Kaplan, "Antidepressant Noncompliance as a Factor in the Discontinuation [withdrawal] Syndrome," *Journal of Clinical Psychiatry* 58 (1997) [suppl. 7]: 31–36; J. F. Rosenbaum and J. Zajecka, "Clinical Management of Antidepressant Discontinuation [withdrawal]," *Journal of Clinical Psychiatry* 58 (1997) [suppl. 7]: 37–40.

50. N. Varchaver, "Lilly's Phantom Verdict," *American Lawyer,* September 1995, pp. 74–83.

51. Ibid.

52. Ibid.

53. J. Cornwell, *The Power to Harm: Mind, Medicine, and Murder on Trial* (New York: Viking, 1996) p. 271.

54. Court's Motion Pursuant to Civil Rule 60.01 and Notice, *Joyce Fentress, et al. v. Shea Communications, et al.* [the official name of the Wesbecker trial], Jefferson Circuit Court, Division 1. No 90CI-6033.

55. *Potter v. Eli Lilly and Company,* Supreme Court of Kentucky No. 926 S.W.2d 449. Opinion of the Court by Justice Wintersheimer, May 23, 1996.

56. Report of the Friend of the Court [the Office of the Attorney General of Kentucky] in *Joyce Fentress, et al. v. Shea Communications, et al.* [the official name of the Wesbecker trial], March 4, 1997.

57. Corrected Judgment, *Joyce Fentress, et al. v. Shea Communications, et al.* [the official name of the Wesbecker trial] March 24, 1997. Jefferson Circuit Court, Div 5. No. 90-CI-6033.

58. Report of the Friend of the Court [the Office of the Attorney General of Kentucky] in *Joyce Fentress et al, v Shea Communications, et al.* [the official name of the Wesbecker trial], March 4, 1997.

59. American Psychiatric Association, *Diagnostic and Statistical Manual of Mental Disorders (DSM),* 4th edition (Washington, D.C.: American Psychiatric Association, 1994), pp. 735–51. The category Medication-Induced Movement Disorder Not Otherwise Specified on page 751 was added for involuntary movement disorders caused by drugs such as the Prozac-type antidepressants. See R. J. Leo, "Movement Disorders Associated

with the Serotonin Selective Reuptake Inhibitors [the Prozac group]," *Journal of Clinical Psychiatry* 57 (1996): 449–54.

60. D. Abramson, "Hooked: Antidepressants Can Take Away as Much of You as They Give Back," *Boston Phoenix*, April 17, 1998, p. 7.
61. E. Wurtzel, *Prozac Nation: Young and Depressed in America* (Boston: Houghton Mifflin, 1994), pp. 16, 8.
62. Ibid, pp. 16–17.
63. K. Linde, G. Ramirez, C. D. Mulrow, A. Pauls, W. Weidenhammer, and D. Melchart, "St. John's Wort for Depression—An Overview and Meta-Analysis of Randomised Clinical Trials," *British Medical Journal* 313 (1996): 253–58.

1
The Awakened Giant's Wrath:
Risking Brain Damage

1. The medical term for these tics and twitches is "tardive dyskinesia," meaning late-appearing abnormal movements. In addition to jerking movements, some patients have more rhythmic, sinuous, or writhing movements. "Late-appearing" is defined as after at least one month of treatment in the elderly or at least three months in patients less than sixty years old. The term "dyskinesia" is used for similar tics that appear even earlier. Early-onset cases are more likely to occur in patients with histories of prior exposure to drugs that cause the tics or medical conditions that predispose to them, or in the elderly who are more vulnerable because of the loss of brain cells that accompanies aging.
2. *Physicians' Desk Reference (PDR)* (Montvale, N.J.: Medical Economics, 1999), p. 927.
3. The medical term for this neurologically driven agitation is "akathisia."
4. The medical term for these muscle spasms is "acute dystonic reactions."
5. Because these side effects have not been systematically studied, we do not know what their relative frequencies are with the different serotonin boosters. The majority of published reports are associated with Prozac, the most commonly prescribed serotonin booster, but reports of these neurological side effects have been published with all four serotonin boosters.
6. I use the term "involuntary motor system" for the extrapyramidal motor system. "Extrapyramidal syndromes" is the medical term for the group of related conditions that I am calling the "neurological side effects" of the Prozac group.
7. D. A. Fishbain, M. Dominguez, M. Goldberg, E. Olsen, and H. Rosomoff, "Dyskinesia [tics] Associated with Fluoxetine [Prozac] Use," *Neuropsychiatry, Neuropsychology, and Behavioral Neurology* 5 (1992): 97–100.
8. C. L. Budman and R. D. Bruun, "Persistent Dyskinesia [tics] in a Patient Receiving Fluoxetine [Prozac]," *American Journal of Psychiatry* 148 (1991): 1403.
9. D. K. Arya and E. Szabadi, "Dyskinesia [tics] Associated with Fluvoxamine [Luvox]," *Journal of Clinical Psychopharmacology* 13 (1993): 365–66.
10. N. H. Sandler, "Tardive Dyskinesia [tics] Associated with Fluoxetine [Prozac]," *Journal of Clinical Psychiatry* 57 (1996): 91. When academic and professional journals are quoted in the text, for readability the well-recognized commercial names of drugs have been substituted for their chemical names.
11. B. A. Fallon and M. R. Liebowitz, "Fluoxetine [Prozac] and Extrapyramidal Symptoms [neurological side effects] in CNS [central nervous system] Lupus," *Journal of Clinical Psychopharmacology* 11 (1991): 147–48.
12. K. J. Bharucha and K. D. Sethi, "Complex Movement Disorders Induced by Fluoxetine [Prozac]," *Movement Disorders* 11 (1996): 324–26. The patient was also on doxepin, an older, tricyclic antidepressant. She had been on doxepin without involuntary movements for four years prior to adding Prozac. While the Prozac was stopped after the tics emerged, the "doxepin was left unchanged." Bharucha and Sethi observed that the patient "had been taking a combination of doxepin and Prozac, but the prompt resolution of movements on withdrawal of Prozac indicates that the latter was the offending agent." In general, when reviewing reported case studies, one finds a range of patients with different circumstances: Some patients have no prior or current exposure to other psychiatric drugs. Others have a history of exposure to drugs that may have caused silent

damage, leaving them more vulnerable to developing the side effect of a serotonin booster. Still other patients have medical conditions thought to predispose them. And the elderly are more vulnerable because of the loss of brain cells that accompanies aging. In the published cases described in the book, even if another of these circumstances was present the reporting doctor felt the serotonin booster was the critical variable because the time course of the side effect coincided with the serotonin booster's being started and stopped. In some instances, the side effect is dose-dependent, meaning it increases and decreases as the dose of the drug is adjusted up and down. And in the case of some side effects, rechallenge studies have been published. In rechallenge studies, after the drug is stopped and the side effect clears, when the patient is readministered the drug (rechallenged with it) the side effect reappears.

13. Some of the patients' abnormal movements that were unlike those seen traditionally with major tranquilizers were described by Bharucha and Sethi as "mycoclonus," shock-like contractions of a muscle or a portion of a muscle.

14. American Psychiatric Association, *Diagnostic and Statistical Manual of Mental Disorders (DSM)*, 4th edition (Washington, D.C.: American Psychiatric Association, 1994), p. 748. While the tics are permanent in less than 50% of young patients, they are permanent in 60–95% of elderly patients.

15. W. M. Glazer, H. Morgenstern, and J. T. Doucette, "Predicting the Long-Term Risk of Tardive Dyskinesia [tics] in Outpatients Maintained on Neuroleptic [major tranquilizer] Medications," *Journal of Clinical Psychiatry* 54 (1993): 133–39.

16. J. M. Kane, M. Woerner, and J. Lieberman, "Tardive Dyskinesia [tics]: Prevalence, Incidence, and Risk Factors," *Journal of Clinical Psychopharmacology* 8 (1988) [suppl. 4]: S52–S56.

17. M. Berk, "Paroxetine [Paxil] Induces Dystonia [muscle spasms] and Parkinsonism in Obsessive Compulsive Disorder," *Human Psychopharmacology* 8 (1993): 444–45.

18. F. J. Jiménez-Jiménez, J. Tejeiro, G. Martinez-Junquera, F. Cabrera-Valdivia, J. Alarcon, and E. Garcia-Albea, "Parkinsonism Exacerbated by Paroxetine [Paxil]," *Neurology* 44 (1994): 2406.

19. J.M.K. Hesselink, "Serotonin, Depression, and Parkinson's Disease," *Neurology* 43 (1993): 1624–25.

20. R. D. Adams and M. Victor, *Principles of Neurology*, 2d ed. (New York: McGraw-Hill, 1981), p. 344.

21. "Early Parkinsonism Vulnerability a Tardive Dyskinesia [tics] Risk Factor," *Clinical Psychiatry News*, June 1990, p. 2.

22. S. A. Chong, "Fluvoxamine [Luvox] and Mandibular [jaw] Dystonia [muscle spasms]," *Canadian Journal of Psychiatry* 40 (1995): 430–31. In published cases such as this, the patient's name is an arbitrary pseudonym for readability.

23. L. Reccoppa, W. A. Welch, and M. R. Ware, "Acute Dystonia [muscle spasm] and Fluoxetine [Prozac]," *Journal of Clinical Psychiatry* 51 (1990): 487.

24. M. Dave, "Fluoxetine [Prozac]-Associated Dystonia [muscle spasms]," *American Journal of Psychiatry* 151 (1994): 149.

25. V. Porro, S. Fiorenzoni, C. Menga, A. de Cristofaro, and A. Bertolino, "Single-Blind Comparison of the Efficacy of Fluvoxamine [Luvox] Versus Placebo in Patients with Depressive Syndrome," *Current Therapeutic Research* 43 (1988): 621–29.

26. H. Y. Meltzer, M. Young, J. Metz, V. S. Fang, P. S. Schyve, and R. C. Arora, "Extrapyramidal [neurological] Side Effects and Increased Serum Prolactin Following Fluoxetine [Prozac], a New Antidepressant," *Journal of Neural Transmission* 45 (1979): 165–75.

27. M. S. Hamilton and L. A. Opler, "Akathisia [agitation], Suicidality, and Fluoxetine [Prozac]," *Journal of Clinical Psychiatry* 53 (1992): 401–6; W. C. Wirshing, T. Van Putten, J. Rosenberg, S. Marder, D. Ames, and T. Hicks-Gray, "Fluoxetine [Prozac] Akathisia [agitation] and Suicidality: Is There a Causal Connection?," *Archives of General Psychiatry* 49 (1992): 580–81; T. Van Putten, L. R. Mutalipassi, and M. D. Malkin, "Phenothiazine [major tranquilizer]-Induced Decompensation," *Archives of General Psychiatry* 30 (1974): 102–5.

28. J. F. Lipinski, Jr., G. Mallya, P. Zimmerman, and H. G. Pope, "Fluoxetine [Prozac]-Induced Akathisia [agitation]: Clinical and Theoretical Implications," *Journal of Clinical Psychiatry* 50 (1989): 339–42.

29. C. M. Beasley, M. E. Sayler, A. M. Weiss, and J. H. Potvin, "Fluoxetine [Prozac]: Acti-

vating and Sedating Effects at Multiple Fixed Doses," *Journal of Clinical Psychopharmacology* 12 (1992): 328–33.

30. O. Sacks, *Awakenings* (New York: Harper Perennial, 1990). Agitation (akathisia) in the postinfectious Parkinson's disease patients is described on page 6. Their muscle spasms (dystonias) and tics are described on pages 16–17.

31. Ibid., pp. 351–65.

32. J. Davies and P. Tongroach, "Neuropharmacological Studies on the Nigro-Striatal [involuntary motor] and Raphe-Striatal [serotonin-dopamine] System in the Rat," *European Journal of Pharmacology* 51 (1978): 91–100; A. Dray, J. Davies, N. R. Oakley, P. Tongroach, and S. Vellucci, "The Dorsal and Medial Raphe [serotonin] Projections to the Substantia Nigra [involuntary motor system] in the Rat: Electrophysiological, Biochemical, and Behavioural Observations," *Brain Research* 151 (1978): 431–42; H. C. Fibiger and J. J. Miller, "An Anatomical and Electrophysiological Investigation of the Serotonergic Projection from the Dorsal Raphe Nucleus to the Substantia Nigra [involuntary motor system] in the Rat," *Neuroscience* 2 (1977): 975–87; A. Dray, "Serotonin in the Basal Ganglia [involuntary motor system]: Functions and Interactions with Other Neuronal Pathways," *Journal of Physiology* (Paris) 77 (1981): 393–403.

33. J. M. K. Hesselink, "Serotonin, Depression, and Parkinson's Disease," *Neurology* 43 (1993): 1624–25.

34. D. K. Arya, "Extrapyramidal Symptoms [neurological side effects] with Selective Serotonin Reuptake Inhibitors [serotonin boosters]," *British Journal of Psychiatry* 165 (1994): 728–33.

35. M. Laruelle, M.-A. Vanisberg, and J.-M. Maloteaux, "Regional and Subcellular Localization in Human Brain of [^{3}H]-Paroxetine [Paxil] Binding, a Marker of Serotonin Uptake Sites," *Biological Psychiatry* 24 (1988): 299–309.

36. J. Ichikawa and H. Y. Meltzer, "Effect of Antidepressants [including Prozac] on Striatal [involuntary motor system] and Accumbens [another region of the brain] Extracellular Dopamine Levels," *European Journal of Pharmacology* 281 (1995): 225–61.

37. S. L. Dewey, G. S. Smith, J. Logan, D. Alexoff, Y.-S. Ding, P. King, N. Pappas, J. D. Brodie, and C. R. Ashby, "Serotonergic Modulation of Striatal [involuntary motor system] Dopamine Measured with Positron Emission Tomography (PET) and In Vivo Microdialysis," *Journal of Neuroscience* 15 (1995): 821–29.

38. A. Di Rocco, T. Brannan, A. Prikhojan, and M. D. Yahr, "Sertraline [Zoloft]-Induced Parkinsonism: A Case Report and an In Vivo Study of the Effect of Sertraline [Zoloft] on Dopamine Metabolism," *Journal of Neural Transmission* 105 (1998): 247–51.

39. S. M. Stahl, "Not So Selective Serotonin Reuptake Inhibitors [serotonin boosters]," *Journal of Clinical Psychiatry* 59 (1998): 343–44; M. Tatsumi, K. Groshan, R. D. Blakely, and E. Richelson, "Pharmacological Profile of Antidepressants and Related Compounds at Human Monoamine Transporters," *European Journal of Pharmacology* 340 (1997): 249–58; E. Richelson, "The Pharmacology of Antidepressants at the Synapse: Focus on Newer Compounds," *Journal of Clinical Psychiatry* 55 (1994) [9, suppl. A]: 34–39; S. L. Dubovsky, "Beyond the Serotonin Reuptake Inhibitors [serotonin boosters]: Rationales for the Development of New Serotonergic Agents," *Journal of Clinical Psychiatry* 55 (1994) [2, suppl.]: 34–44.

40. E. C. Azmitia and P. M. Whitaker-Azmitia, "Awakening the Sleeping Giant: Anatomy and Plasticity of the Brain Serotonergic System," *Journal of Clinical Psychiatry* 52 (1991) [12, suppl.]: 4–16.

41. W. S. Appleton, *Prozac and the New Antidepressants* (New York: Plume, 1997), p. 45.

42. R. D. Adams and M. Victor, *"Principles of Neurology,"* 2d ed. (New York: McGraw-Hill, 1981), p. 778.

43. F. J. Ayd, "Prevention of Recurrence (Maintenance Therapy)," in A. DiMascio and R. I. Shader, eds., *Clinical Handbook of Psychopharmacology* (New York: Science House, 1970), pp. 297–310.

44. G. E. Crane, "Clinical Psychopharmacology in Its 20th Year: Late, Unanticipated Effects of Neuroleptics [major tranquilizers] May Limit Their Use in Psychiatry," *Science* 181 (1973): 124–28.

45. Ibid.

46. D. X. Freedman, Editorial Comment, *Archives of General Psychiatry* 28 (1973): 463–67.

47. G. M. Asnis, M. A. Leopold, R. C. Duvoisin, and A. H. Schwartz, "A Survey of Tardive

Dyskinesia [tics] in Psychiatric Outpatients," *American Journal of Psychiatry* 134 (1977): 1367–70; S. J. Tepper and J. F. Haas, "Prevalence of Tardive Dyskinesia [tics]," *Journal of Clinical Psychiatry* 12 (1979): 508–16.

48. "Neuroleptics [major tranquilizers] to Carry FDA Class Warning," *Psychiatric News,* May 17, 1985, pp. 1, 44.

49. "Early Parkinsonism Vulnerability a Tardive Dyskinesia [tics] Risk Factor," *Clinical Psychiatry News,* June 1990, p. 2.

50. R. Pies, "Must We Now Consider SRIs [serotonin boosters] Neuroleptics [major tranquilizers]?," *Journal of Clinical Psychopharmacology* 17 (1997): 443–45.

51. R. Baldessarini, Keynote Address: "Psychopharmacology: Where Have We Been; Where Are We; Where Are We Going?," Massachusetts General Hospital/Harvard Medical School Conference on Psychopharmacology, October 16, 1998.

52. D. Healy, *The Antidepressant Era* (Cambridge, Mass.: Harvard University Press, 1997), p. 176.

53. L. Slater, *Prozac Diary* (New York: Random House, 1998), pp. 178–79.

54. I. Grant, K. M. Adams, A. S. Carlin, P. M. Rennick, L. L. Judd, and K. Schooff, "The Collaborative Neuropsychological Study of Polydrug Users," *Archives of General Psychiatry* 35 (1978): 1063–74; I. Grant, K. M. Adams, A. S. Carlin, P. M. Rennick, L. L. Judd, K. Schooff, and R. Reed, "Organic Impairment in Polydrug Users: Risk Factors," *American Journal of Psychiatry* 135 (1978): 178–84; P. Breggin, *Toxic Psychiatry* (New York: St. Martin's Press, 1991), pp. 82–84.

55. The exact pathophysiology of these delayed, postinfectious cases has never been fully elucidated. For a detailed discussion of these complex cases, see O. Sacks, *Awakenings* (New York: Harper Perennial, 1990), pp. 12–23. See also R. D. Adams, M. Victor, and A. H. Ropper, *Principles of Neurology,* 6th ed. (New York: McGraw-Hill, 1997), p. 754.

56. P. L. McGeer, E. G. McGeer, and J. S. Suzuki, "Aging and Extrapyramidal [involuntary motor] Function," *Archives of Neurology* 34 (1977): 33–35; B. Pakkenberg, A. Moller, H. J. Gundersen, M. A. Dam, and H. Pakkenberg, "The Absolute Number of Nerve Cells in Substantia Nigra [involuntary motor system] in Normal Subjects and in Patients with Parkinson's Disease Estimated with an Unbiased Stereological Method," *Journal of Neurology, Neurosurgery, and Psychiatry* 54 (1991): 30–33; R. D. Adams, M. Victor, and A. Ropper, *Principles of Neurology,* 6th edition (New York: McGraw-Hill, 1997), p. 1071.

57. R. D. Adams, M. Victor, and A. Ropper, *Principles of Neurology,* 6th ed. (New York: McGraw-Hill, 1997), pp. 423–24.

58. *Physicians' Desk Reference (PDR)* (Montvale, N.J.: Medical Economics, 1999), pp. 823–25.

59. P.C.S. Hoaken, "An Alert to Extrapyramidal [neurological] Side-Effects from SSRIs [serotonin boosters]," *Canadian Journal of Psychiatry* 40 (1995): 51.

60. R. J. Leo, "Movement Disorders Associated with the Serotonin Selective Reuptake Inhibitors [the Prozac group]," *Journal of Clinical Psychiatry* 57 (1996): 449–54.

61. F. J. Ayd, "Biological Psychiatry Update: SSRI [serotonin booster]-Induced Extrapyramidal Syndromes [neurological side effects, including tics]," *Psychiatric Times,* January 1997, p. 28.

62. Committee on Safety of Medicines, Medicine Control Agency, "Dystonia [muscle spasms] and Withdrawal Symptoms with Paroxetine [Paxil]," *Current Problems in Pharmacovigilance* 19 (1993): 1.

63. M. Tatsumi, K. Groshan, R. D. Blakely, and E. Richelson, "Pharmacological Profile of Antidepressants and Related Compounds at Human Monoamine Transporters," *European Journal of Pharmacology* 340 (1997): 249–58.

64. V. Choo, "Paroxetine [Paxil] and Extrapyramidal Reactions [neurological side effects]," *Lancet* 341 (1993): 624.

65. American Psychiatric Association, *Diagnostic and Statistical Manual of Mental Disorders (DSM),* 4th edition (Washington, D.C.: American Psychiatric Association, 1994), pp. 735–51. The category Medication-Induced Movement Disorder Not Otherwise Specified on page 751 was added for involuntary movement disorders caused by drugs such as the Prozac-type antidepressants. See R. J. Leo, "Movement Disorders Associated with the Serotonin Selective Reuptake Inhibitors [the Prozac group]," *Journal of Clinical Psychiatry* 57 (1996): 449–54.

66. R. Pies, "Serotonergic Agents [serotonin boosters] and Extrapyramidal [neurological] Side Effects," *Psychiatric Times*, January 1999, pp. 20–22.

67. M. Leonard, "Children Are the Hot New Market for Antidepressants. But Is This How to Make Them Feel Better?," *Boston Sunday Globe*, May 25, 1997, pp. D1, D5; B. Strauch, "Use of Antidepression Medicine for Young Patients Has Soared," *New York Times*, August 10, 1997, p. 1.

68. R. L. Fisher and S. Fisher, "Antidepressants for Children: Is Scientific Support Necessary?," *Journal of Nervous and Mental Disease* 184 (1996): 99–102; L. Eisenberg, "Commentary: What Should Doctors Do in the Face of Negative Evidence?," *Journal of Nervous and Mental Disease* 184 (1996): 103–5; E. D. Pellegrino, "Commentary: Clinical Judgment, Scientific Data, and Ethics: Antidepressant Therapy in Adolescents and Children," *Journal of Nervous and Mental Disease* 184 (1996): 106–8.

2
Held Hostage:
Withdrawal, Dependence, and Wearing Off

1. L. C. Barr, W. K. Goodman, and L. H. Price, "Physical Symptoms Associated with Paroxetine [Paxil] Discontinuation [withdrawal]," *American Journal of Psychiatry* 151 (1994): 289; L. Pacheco, P. Malo, E. Aragues, and M. Etxebest, "More Cases of Paroxetine [Paxil] Withdrawal Syndrome," *British Journal of Psychiatry* 169 (1996): 384; R. A. Dominguez and P. J. Goodnick, "Adverse Events After the Abrupt Discontinuation [withdrawal] of Paroxetine [Paxil]," *Pharmacotherapy* 15 (1995): 778–80; F. L. Leiter, A. A. Nierenberg, K. M. Sanders, and T. A. Stern, "Discontinuation [withdrawal] Reactions Following Sertraline [Zoloft]," *Biological Psychiatry* 38 (1995): 694–95; L. Frost and S. Lal, "Shock-like Sensations After Discontinuation of Selective Serotonin Reuptake Inhibitors [Prozac-type drugs]," *American Journal of Psychiatry* 152 (1995): 810.

2. N. J. Coupland, C. J. Bell, and J. P. Potokar, "Serotonin Reuptake Inhibitor [Prozac-type drug] Withdrawal," *Journal of Clinical Psychopharmacology* 16 (1996): 356–62.

3. A. F. Schatzberg, P. Haddad, E. M. Kaplan, M. Lejoyeux, J. F. Rosenbaum, A. H. Young, and J. Zajecka, "Serotonin Reuptake Inhibitor [Prozac-type drug] Discontinuation [withdrawal] Syndrome: A Hypothetical Definition," *Journal of Clinical Psychiatry* 58 (1997) [suppl. 7]: 5–10.

4. L. Frost and S. Lal, "Shock-like Sensations After Discontinuation of Selective Serotonin Reuptake Inhibitors [Prozac-type drugs]," *American Journal of Psychiatry* 152 (1995): 810.

5. D. Kasantikul, "Reversible Delirium After Discontinuation of Fluoxetine [Prozac]," *Journal of the Medical Association of Thailand* 78 (1995): 53–54.

6. W. J. Giakas and J. M. Davis, "Intractable Withdrawal from Venlafaxine [Effexor] Treated with Fluoxetine [Prozac]," *Psychiatric Annals* 27 (1997): 85–92.

7. R. E. Pyke, "Paroxetine [Paxil] Withdrawal Syndrome," *American Journal of Psychiatry* 152 (1995): 149–50; A. L. Lazowick, "Potential Withdrawal Syndrome Associated with SSRI [Prozac-type drug] Discontinuation [withdrawal]," *Annals of Pharmacotherapy* 29 (1995): 1284–85.

8. N. J. Keuthen, P. Cyr, J. A. Ricciardi, W. E. Minichiello, M. L. Buttolph, and M. A. Jenike, "Medication Withdrawal Symptoms in Obsessive-Compulsive Disorder Patients Treated with Paroxetine [Paxil]," *Journal of Clinical Psychopharmacology* 14 (1994): 206–7.

9. M. Lejoyeux and J. Adès, "Antidepressant Discontinuation [withdrawal]: A Literature Review," *Journal of Clinical Psychiatry* 58 (1997) [suppl. 7]: 11–16.

10. J. Zajecka, K. A. Tracy, and S. Mitchell, "Discontinuation [withdrawal] Symptoms After Treatment with Serotonin Reuptake Inhibitors [Prozac-type drugs]: A Review of the Literature," *Journal of Clinical Psychiatry* 58 (1997): 291–97.

11. L.S.W. Kent, and J.D.D. Laidlaw, "Suspected Congenital Setraline [Zoloft] Dependence," *British Journal of Psychiatry* 167 (1995): 412–13.

12. N. J. Coupland, C. J. Bell, and J. P. Potokar, "Serotonin Reuptake Inhibitor [Prozac-type drug] Withdrawal," *Journal of Clinical Psychopharmacology* 16 (1996): 356–62.

13. D. W. Black, R. Wesner, and J. Gabel, "The Abrupt Discontinuation [withdrawal] of Fluvoxamine [Luvox] in Patients with Panic Disorder," *Journal of Clinical Psychiatry* 54 (1993): 146–49.

14. L. C. Barr, W. K. Goodman, and L. H. Price, "Physical Symptoms Associated with

Paroxetine [Paxil] Discontinuation [withdrawal]," *American Journal of Psychiatry* 151 (1994): 289.

15. C. S. Berlin, "Fluoxetine [Prozac] Withdrawal Symptoms," *Journal of Clinical Psychiatry* 57 (1996): 93–94.

16. *Physicians' Desk Reference (PDR)* (Montvale, NJ: Medical Economics, 1999). The withdrawal disclaimer for Luvox on page 3124 is quoted. Similar disclaimers for Prozac, Zoloft, and Paxil appear on pages 928, 2247, and 3082, respectively.

17. A. H. Young and A. Currie, "Physicians' Knowledge of Antidepressant Withdrawal Effects: A Survey," *Journal of Clinical Psychiatry* 58 (1997) [suppl. 7]: 28–30.

18. E. Einbinder, "Fluoxetine [Prozac] Withdrawal?," *American Journal of Psychiatry* 152 (1995): 1235.

19. W. J. Giakas, and J. M. Davis, "Intractable Withdrawal from Venlafaxine [Effexor] Treated with Fluoxetine [Prozac]," *Psychiatric Annals* 27 (1997): 85–92.

20. A. Farah and T. E. Lauer, "Possible Venlafaxine [Effexor] Withdrawal Syndrome, *American Journal of Psychiatry* 153 (1996): 576.

21. W. J. Giakas, and J. M. Davis, "Withdrawal from Venlafaxine [Effexor] Treated with Fluoxetine [Prozac]," *Psychiatric Annals* 27 (1997): 85–92.

22. *Journal of Clinical Psychiatry,* 58 (1997) [suppl. 7]: see inside of cover for statement of Lilly sponsorship.

23. A. F. Schatzberg, "Introduction: Antidepressant Discontinuation [withdrawal] Syndrome: An Update on Serotonin Reuptake Inhibitors [Prozac-type drugs]," *Journal of Clinical Psychiatry* 58 (1997) [suppl. 7]: 3–4; A. F. Schatzberg, P. Haddad, E. M. Kaplan, M. Lejoyeux, J. F. Rosenbaum, A. H. Young, and J. Zajecka, "Serotonin Reuptake Inhibitor [Prozac-type drug] Discontinuation [withdrawal] Syndrome: A Hypothetical Definition," *Journal of Clinical Psychiatry* 58 (1997) [suppl. 7]: 5–10; M. Lejoyeux and J. Adès, "Antidepressant Discontinuation [withdrawal]: A Review of the Literature," *Journal of Clinical Psychiatry* 58 (1997) [suppl. 7]: 11–16; P. Haddad, "Newer Antidepressants and the Discontinuation [withdrawal] Syndrome," *Journal of Clinical Psychiatry* 58 (1997) [suppl. 7]: 17–22; A. F. Schatzberg, P. Haddad, E. M. Kaplan, M. Lejoyeux, J. F. Rosenbaum, A. H. Young, and J. Zajecka, "Possible Biological Mechanisms of the Serotonin Reuptake Inhibitor [Prozac-type drug] Discontinuation [withdrawal] Syndrome," *Journal of Clinical Psychiatry* 58 (1997) [suppl. 7]: 23–27; A. H. Young and A. Currie, "Physicians' Knowledge of Antidepressant Withdrawal Effects: A Survey," *Journal of Clinical Psychiatry* 58 (1997) [suppl. 7]: 28–30; E. M. Kaplan, "Antidepressant Noncompliance as a Factor in the Discontinuation [withdrawal] Syndrome," *Journal of Clinical Psychiatry* 58 (1997) [suppl. 7]: 31–36; J. F. Rosenbaum and J. Zajecka, "Clinical Management of Antidepressant Discontinuation [withdrawal]," *Journal of Clinical Psychiatry* 58 (1997) [suppl. 7]: 37–40.

24. J. M. Ferguson and J. P. Feighner, "Fluoxetine [Prozac]-Induced Weight Loss in Overweight Non-depressed Humans," *International Journal of Obesity* 11 (1987): 163–70; J. McGuirk and T. Silverstone, "The Effect of the 5-HT [serotonin] Re-Uptake Inhibitor Fluoxetine [Prozac] on Food Intake and Body Weight in Healthy Male Subjects," *International Journal of Obesity* 14 (1990): 361–72.

25. M. J. Grinfeld, "New Weight Loss Controversy Flares: Lilly Tries to Stop Nutri/Systems Marketing [Prozac as a diet pill] as Experts Assess Consumer Health Risks," *Psychiatric Times,* November 1997, pp. 1, 10–12.

26. Fluoxetine [Prozac] Bulimia Nervosa Collaborative Study Group, "Fluoxetine [Prozac] in the Treatment of Bulimia Nervosa: A Multicenter, Placebo-Controlled, Double-Blind Trial," *Archives of General Psychiatry* 49 (1992): 139–47.

27. Quoted in C. Sherman, "Long-Term Side Effects Surface with SSRIs [Prozac-type drugs]," *Clinical Psychiatry News,* May 1998, pp. 1, 8.

28. B. Knutson, O. Wolkowitz, S. Cole, T. Chan, E. Moore, R. Johnson, J. Terpstra, R. Turner, and V. Reus, "Selective Alteration of Personality and Social Behavior by Serotonergic Intervention [with Paxil]," *American Journal of Psychiatry* 155 (1998): 373–79.

29. J. Zajecka, K. Tracy, and S. Mitchell, "Discontinuation [withdrawal] Symptoms After Treatment with Serotonin Reuptake Inhibitors [Prozac-type drugs]: A Literature Review," *Journal of Clinical Psychiatry* 58 (1997): 291–97.

30. M. Bloch, S. V. Stager, A. R. Braun, and D. R. Rubinow, "Severe Psychiatric Symptoms Associated with Paroxetine [Paxil] Withdrawal," *Lancet* 346 (1995): 57.

31. A. L. Lazowick, "Potential Withdrawal Syndrome Associated with SSRI [Prozac-type drug] Discontinuation [withdrawal]," *Annals of Pharmacotherapy* 29 (1995): 1284–85.
32. P. Kramer, *Listening to Prozac* (New York: Viking, 1993), p. 244.
33. I. Oswald, S. A. Lewis, D.L.F. Dunleavy, V. Brezinova, and M. Briggs, "Drugs of Dependence Though Not of Abuse: Fenfluramine [the parent compound of Redux] and Imipramine [an antidepressant]," *British Medical Journal* 3; 766 (1971): 70–73.
34. S. Rimer, "With Millions Taking Prozac, a Legal Drug Culture Arises," *New York Times,* December 13, 1993, pp. 1, B8.
35. B. Knutson, O. Wolkowitz, S. Cole, T. Chan, E. Moore, R. Johnson, J. Terpstra, R. Turner, and V. Reus, "Selective Alteration of Personality and Social Behavior by Serotonergic Intervention [with Paxil]," *American Journal of Psychiatry* 155 (1998): 373–79.
36. D. Y. Mayer, "Psychotropic Drugs and the 'Antidepressed' Personality," *British Journal of Medical Psychology* 48 (1975): 349–57.
37. D. Abramson, "Hooked: Antidepressants Can Take Away as Much of You as They Give Back," *Boston Phoenix,* April 17, 1998, p. 7
38. G. A. Fava, "Do Antidepressant and Antianxiety Drugs Increase Chronicity in Affective [depressive] Disorders?," *Psychotherapy and Psychosomatics* 61 (1994): 125–31; G. A. Fava, "Holding On: Depression, Sensitization by Antidepressant Drugs, and the Prodigal Experts," *Psychotherapy and Psychosomatics* 64 (1995): 57–61.
39. G. A. Fava and S. Grandi, "Withdrawal Syndromes After Paroxetine [Paxil] and Setraline [Zoloft] Discontinuation," *Journal of Clinical Psychopharmacology* 15 (1995): 374–75.
40. S. B. Levy, *The Antibiotic Paradox: How Miracle Drugs Are Destroying the Miracle* (New York: Plenum, 1992). See also G. A. Fava and E. Tomba, "The Use of Antidepressant Drugs: Some Reasons for Concern," *International Journal of Risk & Safety in Medicine* 11 (1998): 271–74.
41. G. Chouinard, B. D. Jones, and L. Annable, "Neuroleptic [major tranquilizer]-Induced Supersensitivity Psychosis," *American Journal of Psychiatry* 135 (1978): 1409–10; W. Steiner, M. Laporta, and G. Chouinard, "Neuroleptic [major tranquilizer]-Induced Supersensitivity Psychosis in Patients with Bipolar Affective Disorder [manic-depressive illness]," *Acta Psychiatrica Scandinavica* 81 (1990): 437–40.
42. "Editorial Sparks Debate on Effects of Psychoactive Drugs," *Psychiatric News,* May 20, 1994.
43. R. J. Baldessarini, "Risks and Implications of Interrupting Maintenance [long-term] Psychotropic Drug Therapy," *Psychotherapy and Psychosomatics* 63 (1995): 137–41.
44. A. F. Schatzberg, P. Haddad, E. M. Kaplan, M. Lejoyeux, J. F. Rosenbaum, A. H. Young, and J. Zajecka, "Serotonin Reuptake Inhibitor [Prozac-type drug] Discontinuation [withdrawal] Syndrome: A Hypothetical Definition," *Journal of Clinical Psychiatry* 58 (1997) [suppl. 7]: 5–10.
45. R. G. Priest, C. Vize, A. Roberts, M. Roberts, and A. Tylee, "Lay People's Attitudes to Treatment of Depression: Results of Opinion Poll for Defeat Depression Campaign Just Before Its Launch," *British Medical Journal* 313 (1996): 858–59.
46. C. Medawar, "The Antidepressant Web," *International Journal of Risk & Safety in Medicine* 10 (1997): 75–126.
47. C. Medawar, *Power and Dependence, Social Audit on the Safety of Medicines* (London: Social Audit, 1992).
48. *Parade,* September 28, 1997, Prozac advertisement, pp. 20–22.
49. M. Fava, S. M. Rappe, J. A. Pava, A. A. Nierenberg, J. E. Alpert, and J. F. Rosenbaum, "Relapse in Patients on Long-Term Fluoxetine [Prozac] Treatment: Response to Increased Fluoxetine [Prozac] Dose," *Journal of Clinical Psychiatry* 56 (1995): 52–55.
50. E. Wurtzel, *Prozac Nation: Young and Depressed in America* (Boston: Houghton Mifflin, 1994), p. 4.
51. J. Deardorff, "Totally Bummed: Author Elizabeth Wurtzel's Depression May Be Just a Symptom of a Deeper Problem Among Americans of Her Generation," *Chicago Tribune,* February 10, 1995.
52. E. Wurtzel, *Prozac Nation: Young and Depressed in America* (Boston: Houghton Mifflin, 1994) p. 305.
53. A. Solomon, "Anatomy of Melancholy: Personal History," *New Yorker,* January 12, 1998, pp. 46–61.

54. L. Slater, *Prozac Diary* (New York: Random House, 1998), p. 116.
55. K. P. Lesch, C. S. Aulakh, B. L. Wolozin, T. J. Tolliver, J. L. Hill, and D. L. Murphy, "Regional Brain Expression of Serotonin Transporter mRNA [instructions read off DNA] and Its Regulation by Reuptake Inhibiting Antidepressants [including Prozac]," *Molecular Brain Research* 17 (1993): 31–35.
56. S. E. Hyman and E. J. Nestler, "Initiation and Adaptation: A Paradigm for Understanding Psychotropic Drug Action," *American Journal of Psychiatry* 153 (1996): 151–62.
57. L. S. Seiden, "Neurotoxicity of Methamphetamine: Mechanisms of Action and Issues Related to Aging," *National Institute on Drug Abuse Research Monograph Series* 115 (1991): 24–32; G. Ellison, S. Irwin, A. Keys, K. Noguchi, and G. Sulur, "The Neurotoxic Effects of Continuous Cocaine and Amphetamine in Habenula [region of the brain]: Implications for the Substrates of Psychosis," *National Institute on Drug Abuse Research Monograph Series* 163 (1996): 117–45; U. D. McCann, L. S. Seiden, L. J. Rubin, and G. A. Ricaurte, "Brain Serotonin Neurotoxicity and Primary Pulmonary Hypertension from Fenfluramine [Redux's parent compound] and Dexfenfluramine [Redux]: A Systematic Review of the Evidence," *Journal of the American Medical Association* 278 (1997): 666–72; T. D. Steele, U. D. McCann, and G. A. Ricaurte, "3, 4-Methylenedioxymethamphetamine (MDMA, 'Ecstasy'): Pharmacology and Toxicology in Animals and Humans," *Addiction* 89 (1994): 539–51.
58. In the text, I use the word "adrenaline" for both adrenaline and the closely related noradrenaline (also called epinephrine and norepinephrine, respectively), because "adrenaline" is the term well known to a nontechnical audience. Noradrenaline—or norepinephrine—is the form found in the brain.
59. S. Garattini, A. Bizzi, S. Caccia, and T. Mennini, "Progress Report on the Anorectic [appetite-suppressant] Effects of Dexfenfluramine [Redux], Fluoxetine [Prozac], and Sertraline [Zoloft]," *International Journal of Obesity* 16 (1992) [suppl. 3]: S43–S50.
60. B. Caballero, "Brain Serotonin and Carbohydrate Craving in Obesity," *International Journal of Obesity* 11 (1987): 179–83.
61. M. D. Lemonick, "Redux, Fen/Phen, Prozac; How Mood Drugs Work . . . and Fail," *Time,* September 29, 1997, pp. 75–82.
62. Ibid.
63. R. A. Knox and R. Rosenberg, "Major Questions Not Yet Answered in Diet Pill Debacle," *Boston Globe,* September 22, 1997, pp. 1, A6.
64. U. D. McCann, L. S. Seiden, L. J. Rubin, and G. A. Ricaurte, "Brain Serotonin Neurotoxicity and Primary Pulmonary Hypertension from Fenfluramine [Redux's parent compound] and Dexfenfluramine [Redux]: A Systematic Review of the Evidence," *Journal of the American Medical Association* 278 (1997): 666–72.
65. M. E. Molliver, U. V. Berger, L. A. Mamounas, D. C. Molliver, E. O'Hearn, and M. A. Wilson, "Neurotoxicity of MDMA [Ecstasy] and Related Compounds [including discussion of Redux]: Anatomic Studies," *Annals of the New York Academy of Sciences* 600 (1990): 640–64.
66. G. A. Ricaurte, M. E. Molliver, M. B. Martello, J. L. Katz, M. A. Wilson, and A. L. Martello, "Dexfenfluramine [Redux] Neurotoxicity in Brains of Non-human Primates," *Lancet* 338 (1991): 1487–88.
67. U. McCann, G. Hatzidimitriou, A. Ridenour, C. Fischer, J. Yuan, J. Katz, and G. Ricaurte, "Dexfenfluramine [Redux] and Serotonin Neurotoxicity: Further Preclinical Evidence That Clinical Caution Is Indicated," *Journal of Pharmacology and Experimental Therapeutics* 269 (1994): 792–98.
68. J. A. Harvey and S. E. McMaster, "Fenfluramine [Redux's parent compound]: Cumulative Neurotoxicity After Chronic [10 days] Treatment with Low Doses in the Rat," *Communications in Psychopharmacology* 1 (1977): 3–17. See also U. D. McCann, L. S. Seiden, L. J. Rubin, and G. A. Ricaurte, "Brain Serotonin Neurotoxicity and Primary Pulmonary Hypertension from Fenfluramine [Redux's parent compound] and Dexfenfluramine [Redux]: A Systematic Review of the Evidence," *Journal of the American Medical Association* 278 (1997): 666–72.
69. R. I. Westphalen and P. R. Dodd, "The Regeneration of d,l-Fenfluramine [Redux's parent compound]-Destroyed Serotonergic Nerve Terminals," *European Journal of Pharmacology* 238 (1993): 399–402.

70. U. D. McCann, L. S. Seiden, L. J. Rubin, and G. A. Ricaurte, "Brain Serotonin Neurotoxicity and Primary Pulmonary Hypertension from Fenfluramine [Redux's parent compound] and Dexfenfluramine [Redux]: A Systematic Review of the Evidence," *Journal of the American Medical Association* 278 (1997): 666–72.

71. C. Fischer, G. Hatzidimitriou, J. Wlos, J. Katz, and G. Ricaurte, "Reorganization of Ascending 5-HT [serotonin] Axon Projections in Animals Previously Exposed to the Recreational Drug (±3), 4-Methylenedioxymethamphetamine (MDMA, 'Ecstasy')," *Journal of Neuroscience* 15 (1995): 5476–85.

72. G. A. Ricaurte, A. L. Markowska, G. L. Wenk, G. Hatzidimitriou, J. Wlos, and D. S. Olton, "3,4-Methylenedioxymethamphetamine [Ecstasy], Serotonin and Memory," *Journal of Pharmacology and Experiemental Therapeutics* 266 (1993): 1097–1105.

73. D. B. Calne, F. H. Hochberg, B. J. Snow, and T. Nygaard, "Theories of Neurodegeneration," *Annals of the New York Academy of Sciences* 648 (1992): 1–5.

74. M. Z. Wrona, Z. Yang, F. Zhang, and G. Dryhurst, "Potential New Insights into the Molecular Mechanisms of Methamphetamine-Induced Neurodegeneration," *National Institute on Drug Abuse Research Monograph Series* 173 (1997): 146–74. Dopamine is another neurotransmitter that is particularly vulnerable to being oxidized into a neurotoxin. Wellbutrin (Zyban) and Ritalin are two currently widely prescribed drugs that boost dopamine. Note that in the text, I used the word "amphetamine" generically to refer to amphetamine, methamphetamine, and other amphetamine derivatives because this is the term well known to a nontechnical audience.

75. E. Mechcatie, "Despite Drugs' Withdrawal, Fenfluramines' [Redux's parent compound and Redux] Neurotoxicity to Be Studied," *Clinical Psychiatry News,* October 1997, p. 5.

76. U. D. McCann, L. S. Seiden, L. J. Rubin, and G. A. Ricaurte, "Brain Serotonin Neurotoxicity and Primary Pulmonary Hypertension from Fenfluramine [Redux's parent compound] and Dexfenfluramine [Redux]: A Systematic Review of the Evidence," *Journal of the American Medical Association* 278 (1997): 666–72.

77. J. M. Ferguson and J. P. Feighner, "Fluoxetine [Prozac]-Induced Weight Loss in Overweight Non-depressed Humans," *International Journal of Obesity* 11 (1987): 163–70; J. McGuirk and T. Silverstone, "The Effect of the 5-HT [serotonin] Re-uptake Inhibitor Fluoxetine [Prozac] on Food Intake and Body Weight in Healthy Male Subjects," *International Journal of Obesity* 14 (1990): 361–72. Eli Lilly provided funding for McGuirk's study. Lilly considered marketing Prozac as a diet pill under a different name, but after the drug became so successful as an antidepressant, Lilly never did.

78. M. J. Grinfeld, "New Weight Loss Controversy Flares: Lilly Tries to Stop Nutri/Systems Marketing [Prozac as a diet pill] as Experts Assess Consumer Health Risks," *Psychiatric Times,* November 1997, pp. 1, 10–12.

79. M. D. Lemonick, "Redux, Fen/Phen, Prozac: How Mood Drugs Work ... and Fail," *Time,* September 29, 1997, pp. 75–82.

80. I was unable to find any published experiments with photomicrographic studies for Prozac, Zoloft, Paxil, or Luvox in spite of an exhaustive search of databases of medical journals. In addition, I spoke with several leading researchers in the field of neurotoxicity to be sure I had not missed a paper in an obscure journal. The researchers I spoke with were Dr. Lewis Seiden at the University of Chicago, Dr. Mark Molliver at the Johns Hopkins University School of Medicine, Dr. Pavel Hrdina at the University of Ottawa, and Dr. Silvio Garattini at the Institute for Pharmacologic Research Mario Negri in Milan. All of them said they knew of no published photomicrographic studies on the Prozac group.

81. S. Caccia, C. Fracasso, S. Garattini, G. Guiso, and S. Sarati, "Effects of Short [7days]- and Long-Term [21 days] Administration of Fluoxetine [Prozac] on the Monoamine Content of Rat Brain," *Neuropharmacology* 31 (1992): 343–47. The significance of waiting to sacrifice the animals until a week after the last dose is that the longer one waits, the more the evidence suggests a persistent, potentially permanent change. Other studies demonstrating reduced markers that are less conclusive because the animals were sacrificed within a day of the last dose are P. D. Hrdina, "Regulation of High and Low-Affinity [³H] Imipramine Recognition Sites in Rat Brain by Chronic [21 days] Treatment with Antidepressants [including Prozac]," *European Journal of Pharmacology* 138 (1987): 159–68; C. F. Sarkissian, R. J. Wurtman, A. N. Morse, and R. Gleason, "Effects of Flu-

oxetine [Prozac] or d-Fenfluramine [Redux] on Serotonin Release from, and Levels in, Rat Frontal Cortex," *Brain Research* 529 (1990): 294–301; R. W. Fuller, K. W. Perry, and B. B. Molloy, "Effect of an Uptake Inhibitor [Prozac] on Serotonin Metabolism in Rat Brain: Studies with 3-(p-Trifluoromethylphenoxy)-N-Methyl-3-Phenylpropylamine (LY110140)," *Life Sciences* 15 (1974): 1161–71. Note that at the time the paper was published, Fuller, Perry and Molloy were all in-house researchers at Eli Lilly. A study in which the markers are not decreased but the animals were only treated for four to six days is U. D. McCann, J. Yuan, G. Hatzidimitriou, and G. A. Ricaurte, "Selective Serotonin Reuptake Inhibitors [Prozac-type drugs] Dissociate Fenfluramine's [Redux's parent compound] Anorectic and Neurotoxic Effects: Importance of Dose, Species and Drug," *Journal of Pharmacology and Experimental Therapeutics* 281 (1997): 1487–98.

82. M. E. Molliver, U. V. Berger, L. A. Mamounas, D. C. Molliver, E. O'Hearn, and M. A. Wilson, "Neurotoxicity of MDMA [Ecstasy] and Related Compounds [including discussion of Redux]: Anatomic Studies," *Annals of the New York Academy of Sciences* 600 (1990): 640–64.

83. L. S. Seiden and M. S. Kleven, "Lack of Toxic Effects of Cocaine on Dopamine and Serotonin Neurons in the Rat Brain," *National Institute on Drug Abuse Research Monograph Series* 88 (1988): 276–89.

84. G. Ellison, S. Irwin, A. Keys, K. Noguchi, and G. Sulur, "The Neurotoxic Effects of Continuous Cocaine and Amphetamine in Habenula: [region of the brain]: Implications for the Substrates of Psychosis," *National Institute on Drug Abuse Research Monograph Series* 163 (1996): 117–45.

85. G. Ellison, "Stimulant-Induced Psychosis, the Dopamine Theory of Schizophrenia, and the Habenula [region of the brain]," *Brain Research Reviews* 19 (1994): 223–39.

86. G. Ellison, S. Irwin, A. Keys, K. Noguchi, and G. Sulur, "The Neurotoxic Effects of Continuous Cocaine and Amphetamine in Habenula [region of the brain]: Implications for the Substrates of Psychosis," *National Institute on Drug Abuse Research Monograph Series* 163 (1996): 117–45.

87. N. D. Volkow, R. Hitzemann, G. J. Wang, J. S. Fowler, A. P. Wolf, S. L. Dewey, and L. Handlesman, "Long-Term Frontal Brain Metabolic Changes in Cocaine Abusers," *Synapse* 11 (1992): 184–90.

88. R. Hoehn-Saric, J. R. Lipsey, and D. R. McLeod, "Apathy and Indifference in Patients on Fluvoxamine [Luvox] and Fluoxetine [Prozac]," *Journal of Clinical Psychopharmacology* 10 (1990): 343–45.

89. R. Hoehn-Saric, G. Harris, G. Pearlson, C. Cox, S. Machlin, and E. Camargo, "A Fluoxetine [Prozac]-Induced Frontal Lobe Syndrome [apathy and indifference] in an Obsessive Compulsive Patient," *Journal of Clinical Psychiatry* 52 (1991): 131–33.

90. Some monkey studies can be done with the pill form. But monkey studies are very expensive. Moreover, only a few facilities in the country are equipped to study monkeys, so few scientists have access to doing this kind of research.

91. S. Garattini, A. Bizzi, S. Caccia, and T. Mennini, "Progress Report on the Anorectic [appetite suppressant] Effects of Dexfenfluramine [Redux], Fluoxetine [Prozac] and Sertraline [Zoloft]," *International Journal of Obesity* 16 (1992) [suppl. 3]: S43–S50.

92. For a good discussion of the issue of dosage, see U. D. McCann, L. S. Seiden, L. J. Rubin, and G. A. Ricaurte, "Brain Serotonin Neurotoxicity and Primary Pulmonary Hypertension from Fenfluramine [Redux's parent compound] and Dexfenfluramine [Redux]: A Systematic Review of the Evidence," *Journal of the American Medical Association* 278 (1997): 666–72.

93. M. S. Kleven and L. S. Seiden, "Methamphetamine-Induced Neurotoxicity: Structure Activity Relationships," *Annals of the New York Academy of Sciences* 654 (1992): 292–301. See also U. D. McCann, L. S. Seiden, L. J. Rubin, and G. A. Ricaurte, "Brain Serotonin Neurotoxicity and Primary Pulmonary Hypertension from Fenfluramine [Redux's parent compound] and Dexfenfluramine [Redux]: A Systematic Review of the Evidence," *Journal of the American Medical Association* 278 (1997): 666–72.

94. C. N. Karson, J.E.O. Newton, R. Livingston, J. B. Jolly, T. B. Cooper, J. Sprigg, and R. A. Komoroski, "Human Brain Fluoxetine [Prozac] Concentrations," *Journal of Neuropsychiatry and Clinical Neurosciences* 5 (1993): 322–29.

95. G. Hanson, L. Matsuda, and J. Gibb, "Effects of Cocaine on Methamphetamine-

Induced Neurochemical Changes: Characterization of Cocaine as a Monamine Uptake [reuptake] Blocker [inhibitor]," *Journal of Pharmacology and Experimental Therapeutics* 242 (1987): 507–13. See also G. Ellison, "Continuous Amphetamine and Cocaine Have Similar Neurotoxic Effects in Lateral Habenular Nucleus and Fasciculus Retroflexus [regions of the brain]" *Brain Research* 598 (1992): 353–56.

96. "Editorial Sparks Debate on Effects of Psychoactive Drugs," *Psychiatric News*, May 20, 1994.

3
Not Tonight, Dear–I'm on Prozac:
Sexual Dysfunction

1. Studies in which patients on serotonin boosters are directly asked about sexual dysfunction have found rates as high as 75% of patients. One of the earliest systematic studies of 60 patients found this high rate. See W. M. Patterson, "Fluoxetine [Prozac]-Induced Sexual Dysfunction," *Journal of Clinical Psychiatry* 54 (1993): 71. Later, large-scale studies include that of Modell, who found rates of sexual side effects of 73% for Prozac, 67% for Zoloft, and 86% for Paxil. See J. G. Modell, C. R. Katholi, J. D. Modell, and R. L. DePalma, "Comparative Sexual Side Effects of Bupropion [Wellbutrin], Fluoxetine [Prozac], Paroxetine [Paxil], and Sertraline [Zoloft]," *Clinical Pharmacology and Therapeutics* 61 (1997): 476–87; The most comprehensive study was that of the Montejo-González group, who found an overall rate of 58% of patients on Prozac, Zoloft, Paxil, or Luvox reporting sexual side effects. See A. L. Montejo-González, G. Llorca, J. A. Izquierdo, A. Ledesma, M. Bousono, A. Calcedo, J. L. Carrasco, J. Ciudad, E. Daniel, J. De la Gandara, J. Derecho, M. Franco, M. J. Gomez, J. A. Macias, T. Martin, V. Perez, J. M. Sanchez, S. Sanchez, and E. Vicens, "SSRI-Induced Sexual Dysfunction: Fluoxetine [Prozac], Paroxetine [Paxil], Sertraline [Zoloft], and Fluvoxamine [Luvox] in a Prospective, Multicenter, and Descriptive Clinical Study of 344 Patients," *Journal of Sex and Marital Therapy* 23 (1997): 176–94.

2. *Physicians' Desk Reference (PDR)* (Montvale, N.J.: Medical Economics, 1999). See Table 1 on page 926. Most authors report 1–2% for Lilly's official figure for sexual side effects in depressed patients on Prozac. See A. L. Montejo-González, G. Llorca, J. A. Izquierdo, A. Ledesma, M. Bousono, A. Calcedo, J. L. Carrasco, J. Ciudad, E. Daniel, J. De la Gandara, J. Derecho, M. Franco, M. J. Gomez, J. A. Macias, T. Martin, V. Perez, J. M. Sanchez, S. Sanchez, and E. Vicens, "SSRI-Induced Sexual Dysfunction: Fluoxetine [Prozac], Paroxetine [Paxil], Sertraline [Zoloft], and Fluvoxamine [Luvox] in a Prospective Multicenter and Descriptive Clinical Study of 344 Patients," *Journal of Sex and Marital Therapy* 23 (1997): 176–94 (see page 182); M. J. Gitlin, "Psychotropic Medications and Their Effects on Sexual Function: Diagnosis, Biology, and Treatment Approaches," *Journal of Clinical Psychiatry* 55 (1994): 406–13 (see page 410). I have used the 2–5% figure because in Lilly's Table 1 on page 926 of the *PDR*, in addition to 2% of depressed patients on the drug having impotence, the figure of 3% is also listed for decreased libido. It is impossible to tell from Lilly's table whether or not these two groups overlap. The 5% figure therefore represents the maximum percent possible based on Lilly's figures. These figures are based on Lilly's original prerelease studies of the drug for depression.

3. *Physicians' Desk Reference (PDR)* (Montvale, N.J.: Medical Economics, 1999). For Zoloft, see Table 1 on page 2445. For Paxil, see Table 1 on page 3081. For Luvox, see Table 2 on page 3123.

4. For a discussion of pharmaceutical companies' relying on spontaneous reports of sexual dysfunction in their clinical studies of the drugs rather than directly inquiring of patients, see A. L. Montejo-González, G. Llorca, J. A. Izquierdo, A. Ledesma, M. Bousono, A. Calcedo, J. L. Carrasco, J. Ciudad, E. Daniel, J. De la Gandara, J. Derecho, M. Franco, M. J. Gomez, J. A. Macias, T. Martin, V. Perez, J. M. Sanchez, S. Sanchez, and E. Vicens, "SSRI-Induced Sexual Dysfunction: Fluoxetine [Prozac], Paroxetine [Paxil], Sertraline [Zoloft], and Fluvoxamine [Luvox] in a Prospective, Multicenter, and Descriptive Clinical Study of 344 Patients," *Journal of Sex and Marital Therapy* 23 (1997): 176–94 (see p. 182); J. G. Modell, C. R. Katholi, J. D. Modell, and R. L. DePalma, "Com-

parative Sexual Side Effects of Bupropion [Wellbutrin], Fluoxetine [Prozac], Paroxetine [Paxil], and Sertraline [Zoloft]," *Clinical Pharmacology and Therapeutics* 61 (1997): 476–87 (see pp. 482 and 484).

5. V. L. King, Jr., and I. R. Horowitz, "Vaginal Anesthesia Associated with Fluoxetine [Prozac] Use," *American Journal of Psychiatry* 150 (1993): 984–85.

6. J. Glenmullen, *Sexual Mysteries: Tales of Psychotherapy* (Cambridge, Mass.: Orbit Publishing, 1999).

7. J. R. Neill, "Penile Anesthesia Associated with Fluoxetine [Prozac] Use," *American Journal of Psychiatry* 148 (1991): 1603.

8. W. H. Masters and V. E. Johnson, *Human Sexual Inadequacy* (Boston: Little, Brown, 1970), pp. 92–115. See also H. S. Kaplan, *The New Sex Therapy* (New York: Times Books/Random House, 1974), p. 314.

9. Glenmullen, *Sexual Mysteries: Tales of Psychotherapy* (Cambridge, Mass.: Orbit Publishing, 1999).

10. M. D. Waldinger, M. W. Hengeveld, and A. H. Zwinderman, "Paroxetine [Paxil] Treatment of Premature Ejaculation: A Double-Blind, Randomized, Placebo-Controlled Study," *American Journal of Psychiatry* 151 (1994): 1377–79.

11. J. Mendels, "Sertraline [Zoloft] for Premature Ejaculation," *Journal of Clinical Psychiatry* 56 (1995): 591.

12. A. Graziottin, "Prozac in the Treatment of Premature Ejaculation," presented at the 1995 Annual Meeting of the American Urological Association, Las Vegas, 1995. Cited in R. Balon, note 13.

13. R. Balon, "Antidepressants in the Treatment of Premature Ejaculation," *Journal of Sex and Marital Therapy* 22 (1996): 85–96.

14. P. Kramer, *Listening to Prozac* (New York: Viking, 1993), pp. ix–xi.

15. M. P. Kafka, "Successful Antidepressant Treatment of Nonparaphilic Sexual Addictions and Paraphilias in Men," *Journal of Clinical Psychiatry* 52 (1991): 60–65; D. J. Stein, E. Hollander, D. T. Anthony, F. R. Schneier, B. A. Fallon, M. R. Liebowitz, and D. F. Klein, "Serotonergic Medications [Prozac-type antidepressants] for Sexual Obsessions, Sexual Addictions, and Paraphilias," *Journal of Clinical Psychiatry* 53 (1992): 267–71.

16. D. H. Golwyn and C. P. Sevlie, "Adventitious Change in Homosexual Behavior During Treatment of Social Phobia with Phenelzine [Nardil]," *Journal of Clinical Psychiatry* 54 (1993): 39–40. For a report on Prozac's effect on homosexual interests, see L. S. Lorefice, "Fluoxetine [Prozac] Treatment of a Fetish," *Journal of Clinical Psychiatry* 52 (1991): 41.

17. S. E. Althof, "Pharmacologic Treatment of Rapid Ejaculation," *Psychiatric Clinics of North America* 18 (1995): 85–94.

18. R. Balon, "Sexual Obsessions Associated with Fluoxetine [Prozac]," *Journal of Clinical Psychiatry* 55 (1994): 496; J. Garcia-Campayo, C. Sanz-Carrillo, and A. Lobo, "Orgasmic Sexual Experiences as a Side Effect of Fluoxetine [Prozac]: A Case Report," *Acta Psychiatrica Scandinavica* 91 (1995): 69–70.

19. J. G. Modell, "Repeated Observations of Yawning, Clitoral Engorgement, and Orgasm Associated with Fluoxetine [Prozac] Administration," *Journal of Clinical Psychopharmacology* 9 (1989): 63–65.

20. J. M. Ellison, "Exercise-Induced Orgasms Associated with Fluoxetine [Prozac] Treatment of Depression," *Journal of Clinical Psychiatry* 57 (1996): 596–97.

21. C. T. Gualtieri, "Paradoxical Effects of Fluoxetine [Prozac]," *Journal of Clinical Psychopharmacology* 11 (1991): 393–94.

22. Pharmaceutical companies' relying on spontaneous reports of sexual dysfunction rather than directly inquiring of patients during their clinical studies of the drugs is discussed in note 4 above.

23. *Physicians' Desk Reference (PDR)* (Montvale, N.J.: Medical Economics, 1999). For Zoloft, see Table 1 on page 2445. For Paxil, see Table 1 on page 3081. For Luvox, see Table 2 on page 3123.

24. R. B. Lydiard and M. S. George, "Fluoxetine [Prozac]-Related Anorgasmy," *Southern Medical Journal* 82 (1989): 933–34; M. D. Kline, "Fluoxetine [Prozac] and Anorgasmia," *American Journal of Psychiatry* 146 (1989): 804–5; J. S. Musher, "Anorgasmia with the Use of Fluoxetine [Prozac]," *American Journal of Psychiatry* 147 (1990): 948; M. J. Murray and D. Hooberman, "Fluoxetine [Prozac] and Prolonged Erection," *American Jour-*

nal of Psychiatry 150 (1993): 167–68; W. M. Patterson, "Fluoxetine [Prozac]-Induced Sexual Dysfunction," *Journal of Clinical Psychiatry* 54 (1993): 71.

25. M. J. Gitlin, "Psychotropic Medications and Their Effects on Sexual Function: Diagnosis, Biology, and Treatment Approaches," *Journal of Clinical Psychiatry* 55 (1994): 406–13.

26. A. L. Montejo-González, G. Llorca, J. A. Izquierdo, A. Ledesma, M. Bousono, A. Calcedo, J. L. Carrasco, J. Ciudad, E. Daniel, J. De la Gandara, J. Derecho, M. Franco, M. J. Gomez, J. A. Macias, T. Martin, V. Perez, J. M. Sanchez, S. Sanchez, and E. Vicens, "SSRI-Induced Sexual Dysfunction: Fluoxetine [Prozac], Paroxetine [Paxil], Sertraline [Zoloft], and Fluvoxamine [Luvox] in a Prospective, Multicenter, and Descriptive Clinical Study of 344 Patients," *Journal of Sex and Marital Therapy* 23 (1997): 176–94.

27. B. D. Bartlik, P. Kaplan, and H. S. Kaplan, "Psychostimulants Apparently Reverse Sexual Dysfunction Secondary to Selective Serotonin Re-uptake Inhibitors [Prozac-type antidepressants]," *Journal of Sex and Marital Therapy* 21 (1995): 264–71.

28. M. J. Gitlin, "Psychotropic Medications and Their Effects on Sexual Function: Diagnosis, Biology, and Treatment Approaches," *Journal of Clinical Psychiatry* 55 (1994): 406–13.

29. J. G. Modell, C. R. Katholi, J. D. Modell, and R. L. DePalma, "Comparative Sexual Side Effects of Bupropion [Wellbutrin], Fluoxetine [Prozac], Paroxetine [Paxil], and Sertraline [Zoloft]," *Clinical Pharmacology and Therapeutics* 61 (1997): 476–87.

30. G. Frajese, R. Lazzari, A. Magnani, C. Moretti V. Sforza, and D. Nerozzi, "Neurotransmitter, Opiodergic System, Steroid-Hormone Interaction and Involvement in the Replacement Therapy of Sexual Disorders," *Journal of Steroid Biochemistry and Molecular Biology* 37 (1990): 411–19.

31. S. Balogh, S. E. Hendricks, and J. Kang, "Treatment of Fluoxetine [Prozac]-Induced Anorgasmia with Amantadine," *Journal of Clinical Psychiatry* 53 (1992): 212–13.

32. A. L. Montejo-González, G. Llorca, J. A. Izquierdo, A. Ledesma, M. Bousono, A. Calcedo, J. L. Carrasco, J. Ciudad, E. Daniel, J. De la Gandara, J. Derecho, M. Franco, M. J. Gomez, J. A. Macias, T. Martin, V. Perez, J. M. Sanchez, S. Sanchez, and E. Vicens, "SSRI-Induced Sexual Dysfunction: Fluoxetine [Prozac], Paroxetine [Paxil], Sertraline [Zoloft], and Fluvoxamine [Luvox] in a Prospective, Multicenter, and Descriptive Clinical Study of 344 Patients," *Journal of Sex and Marital Therapy* 23 (1997): 176–94.

33. H. Y. Meltzer, M. Young, J. Metz, V. S. Fang, P. S. Schyve, and R. C. Arora, "Extrapyramidal [neurological] Side Effects and Increased Serum Prolactin Following Fluoxetine [Prozac], a New Antidepressant," *Journal of Neural Transmission* 45 (1979): 165–75. Although this study is widely cited in the psychiatric literature as evidence of the serotonin-dopamine connection, it is worth noting that Meltzer only obtained this result with one patient. Given the importance of the subject, further studies are warranted.

34. K. Degen, "Sexual Dysfunction in Women Using Major Tranquilizers," *Psychosomatics* 23 (1982): 959–61; J. E. Mitchell and M. K. Popkin, "Antipsychotic [major tranquilizer] Drug Therapy and Sexual Dysfunction in Men," *American Journal of Psychiatry* 139 (1982): 633–37.

35. J. Kotin, D. Wilbert, D. Verburg, and S. Soldinger, "Thioridazine [Mellaril, a major tranquilizer] and Sexual Dysfunction," *American Journal of Psychiatry* 133 (1976): 82–85; G. Sullivan and D. Lukoff, "Sexual Side Effects of Antipsychotic [major tranquilizer] Medication: Evaluation and Interventions," *Hospital and Community Psychiatry* 41 (1990): 1238–41.

36. H. Singh, "Therapeutic Use of Thioridazine [Mellaril, a major tranquilizer] in Premature Ejaculation," *American Journal of Psychiatry* 119 (1963): 891; D. Bártová and M. Bouchal, "Thioridazine [Mellaril, a major tranquilizer] Treatment of Ejaculatio Praecox [premature ejaculation]," *Activitas Nervosa Superior (Praha)* [Prague] 7 (1965): 244–45.

37. I. Haider, "Thioridazine [Mellaril, a major tranquilizer] and Sexual Dysfunctions," *International Journal of Neuropsychiatry* 2 (1966): 255–67.

38. I. Kamm, "Control of Sexual Hyperactivity with Thioridazine [Mellaril, a major tranquilizer]," *American Journal of Psychiatry* 121 (1965): 922–23.

39. L. Clein, "Thioridazine [Mellaril, a major tranquilizer] and Ejaculation," *British Medical Journal* 2; 5303 (1962): 548–49.

40. K. Witton, "Sexual Dysfunction Secondary to Mellaril [a major tranquilizer]," *Diseases of the Nervous System* 23 (1962): 175.

41. J. Ichikawa and H. Y. Meltzer, "Effect of Antidepressants [including Prozac] on Striatal [involuntary motor system] and Accumbens [another region of the brain] Extracellular Dopamine Levels," *European Journal of Pharmacology* 281 (1995): 225–61.

42. A. J. Rothschild, "Selective Serotonin Reuptake Inhibitor [Prozac-type antidepressant]-Induced Sexual Dysfunction: Efficacy of a Drug Holiday," *American Journal of Psychiatry* 152 (1995): 1514–16.

43. R. T. Segraves, T. L. Thompson, and T. Wise, "Sexual Dysfunction and Antidepressants," *Journal of Clinical Psychiatry* 57 (1996) [12, Intercom, the Experts Converse]: 1–12.

44. J. G. Modell, C. R. Katholi, J. D. Modell, and R. L. DePalma, "Comparative Sexual Side Effects of Bupropion [Wellbutrin], Fluoxetine [Prozac], Paroxetine [Paxil], and Sertraline [Zoloft]," *Clinical Pharmacology and Therapeutics* 61 (1997): 476–87.

45. W. S. Appleton, *Prozac and the New Antidepressants* (New York: Plume, 1997), pp. 131–32.

46. As in previous chapters, I am using the word "adrenaline" for both adrenaline and the closely related noradrenaline (also called epinephrine and norepinephrine, respectively), because "adrenaline" is the term well known to a nontechnical audience. Noradrenaline—or norepinephrine—is the form found in the brain.

47. *Physicians' Desk Reference (PDR)* (Montvale, N.J.: Medical Economics, 1999), pp. 1252–58.

48. More recently, Glaxo Wellcome introduced a longer-acting, sustained-release form of Wellbutrin.

49. J. A. Bodkin, R. A. Lasser, J. D. Wines, D. M. Gardner, and R. J. Baldessarini, "Combining Serotonin Reuptake Inhibitors [Prozac-type antidepressants] and Bupropion [Wellbutrin] in Partial Responders to Antidepressant Monotherapy," *Journal of Clinical Psychiatry* 58 (1997): 137–45. See also T. R. Green, "Bupropion [Wellbutrin] for SSRI [Prozac-type antidepressant]-Induced Fatigue," *Journal of Clinical Psychiatry* 58 (1997): 174.

50. Quoted in B. Hendrick, "Mind and Body: New Depression Drug Leaves Libido Intact," *Atlanta Journal and Constitution*, May 22, 1997, Features section, p. G3.

51. *Physicians' Desk Reference (PDR)* (Montvale, N.J.: Medical Economics, 1999), pp. 1277–82.

52. A. Weil, "The New Politics of Coca," *New Yorker*, May 15, 1995, pp. 70–80.

53. H. S. Kaplan, *The New Sex Therapy* (New York: Times Books/Random House, 1974), p. 91.

54. L. A. Labbate and M. H. Pollack, "Treatment of Fluoxetine [Prozac]-Induced Sexual Dysfunction with Bupropion [Wellbutrin]: A Case Report," *Annals of Clinical Psychiatry* 6 (1994): 13–15.

55. B. D. Bartlik, P. Kaplan, and H. S. Kaplan, "Psychostimulants Apparently Reverse Sexual Dysfunction Secondary to Selective Serotonin Re-Uptake Inhibitors [Prozac-type antidepressants]," *Journal of Sex and Marital Therapy* 21 (1995): 264–71.

56. R. K. Shrivastava, S. Shrivastava, N. Overweg, and M. Schmitt, "Amantadine in the Treatment of Sexual Dysfunction Associated with Selective Serotonin Reuptake Inhibitors [Prozac-type antidepressants]," *Journal of Clinical Psychopharmacology* 15 (1995): 83–84; R. Balon, "Intermittent Amantadine for Fluoxetine [Prozac]-Induced Anorgasmia," *Journal of Sex and Marital Therapy* 22 (1996): 290–92; M. J. Gitlin, "Treatment of Sexual Side Effects with Dopaminergic Agents," *Journal of Clinical Psychiatry* 56 (1995): 124; C. Roeloffs, B. Bartlik, P. M. Kaplan, and J. H. Kocsis, "Methylphenidate [Ritalin] and SSRI [Prozac-type antidepressant]-Induced Sexual Side Effects," *Journal of Clinical Psychiatry* 57 (1996): 548.

57. C. Roeloffs, B. Bartlik, P. M. Kaplan, and J. H. Kocsis, "Methylphenidate [Ritalin] and SSRI [Prozac-type antidepressant]-Induced Sexual Side Effects," *Journal of Clinical Psychiatry* 57 (1996): 548.

58. A. J. Cohen and B. Bartlik, "Ginkgo Biloba for Antidepressant-Induced Sexual Dysfunction," *Journal of Sex and Marital Therapy* 24 (1998): 139–43.

59. G. Frajese, R. Lazzari, A. Magnani, C. Moretti, V. Sforza, and D. Nerozzi, "Neurotransmitter, Opiodergic System, Steroid-Hormone Interaction and Involvement in the Replacement Therapy of Sexual Disorders," *Journal of Steroid Biochemistry and Molec-*

ular Biology 37 (1990): 411–19; G. L. Gessa and A. Tagliamonte, "Role of Brain Monoamines in Male Sexual Behavior," *Life Sciences* 14 (1974): 425–36.

60. R. Pear, "Proposal to Test Drugs in Children Meets Resistance," *New York Times,* November 30, 1997, pp. 1, 28.

61. J. Brody, Personal Health column, *New York Times,* May 15, 1996, Health section, p. C8.

62. P. W. Walker, J. O. Cole, E. A. Gardner, A. R. Hughes, J. A. Johnston, S. R. Batey, and C. G. Lineberry, "Improvement in Fluoxetine [Prozac]-Associated Sexual Dysfunction in Patients Switched to Bupropion [Wellbutrin]," *Journal of Clinical Psychiatry* 54 (1993): 459–65; R. T. Segraves, K. B. Segraves, and C. N. Bubna, "Sexual Function in Patients Taking Bupropion [Wellbutrin] Sustained Release," *Journal of Clinical Psychiatry* 56 (1995): 374.

63. A. Feiger, A. Kiev, R. K. Shrivastava, P. G. Wisselink, and C. S. Wilcox, "Nefazodone [Serzone] Versus Sertraline [Zoloft] in Outpatients with Major Depression: Focus on Efficacy, Tolerability, and Effects on Sexual Function and Satisfaction," *Journal of Clinical Psychiatry* 57 (1996) [suppl. 2]: 53–62.

64. R. Jacobsen, "Bristol Drug Seen Having Fewer Sexual Side Effects," Reuters Financial Service, New York Newsdesk, May 8, 1996.

65. J. Brody, "Wonder Drugs to Brighten Moods Can Dim Libido: But There Are Solutions Available to Those Left Sexually Bereft," *Star Tribune* (Minneapolis), May 19, 1996, Variety section, p. E3.

66. J. Brody, Personal Health column, *New York Times,* May 15, 1996, Health section, p. C8.

67. S. G. Boodman, "Some Antidepressants Put Hex on Sex," *Des Moines Register,* July 22, 1996, Today section, p. 3.

68. S. G. Boodman, "Antidepressants Can Interfere with Sex; Studies Compare Problems of Patients Taking Serzone and Zoloft," *Washington Post,* May 21, 1996.

69. Cited in D. M. Rios, "Women Urged to Talk About Antidepressants' Effects on Sex," *Austin American-Statesman,* November 16, 1997, Lifestyle section, p. D1.

70. J. Brody, "Sexual Side Effects of Antidepressants," *International Herald Tribune,* May 16, 1996, Feature section.

71. J. Dominquez, "Withdrawal Symptoms," *Sunday Times* (London), July 27, 1997, Features section.

72. E. A. Nofzinger, M. E. Thase, C. F. Reynolds, E. Frank, J. R. Jennings, G. L. Garamoni, A. L. Fasiczka, and D. J. Kupfer, "Sexual Function in Depressed Men: Assessment by Self-Report, Behavioral, and Nocturnal Penile Tumescence Measures Before and After Treatment with Cognitive Behavior Therapy," *Archives of General Psychiatry* 50 (1993): 24–30.

73. J. Dominquez, "Withdrawal Symptoms," *Sunday Times* (London), July 27, 1997, Features section.

74. J. T. Neely, "Secret Side Effects: Users of Prozac and Similar Antidepression Drugs May Suffer Unexpected Impacts on Their Sex Lives," *Spokesman-Review* (Spokane, Washington), November 11, 1997, In Life section, p. D3.

75. R. T. Segraves, T. L. Thompson, and T. Wise, "Sexual Dysfunction and Antidepressants," *Journal of Clinical Psychiatry* 57 (1996) [12, Intercom, the Experts Converse]: 1–12.

76. B. D. Bartlik, P. Kaplan, and H. S. Kaplan, "Psychostimulants Apparently Reverse Sexual Dysfunction Secondary to Selective Serotonin Re-Uptake Inhibitors [Prozac-type antidepressants]," *Journal of Sex and Marital Therapy* 21 (1995): 264–71.

77. R. T. Segraves, T. L. Thompson, and T. Wise, "Sexual Dysfunction and Antidepressants," *Journal of Clinical Psychiatry* 57 (1996) [12, Intercom, the Experts Converse]: 1–12.

78. Ibid., p. 8.

4

Bones Rattling Like Tuning Forks:
Startling New Information on Suicide and Violence

1. M. H. Teicher, C. Glod, and J. O. Cole, "Emergence of Intense Suicidal Preoccupation During Fluoxetine [Prozac] Treatment," *American Journal of Psychiatry* 147 (1990):

207–10. Teicher and Cole's patients all had complicated psychiatric histories. Some but not all of them were on additional medications. But, said Teicher and Cole, the timing of the suicidality and violence coincided with the patients' going on Prozac. The reaction subsided only when the Prozac was stopped. Moreover, in many subsequent cases, the patients did not have complicated psychiatric histories. In addition, as discussed later in the chapter, subsequent rechallenge studies have linked the suicidal and violent reaction even more closely to Prozac.

2. P. Masand, S. Gupta, and M. Dewan, "Suicidal Ideation Related to Fluoxetine [Prozac] Treatment," *New England Journal of Medicine* 324 (1991): 420.

3. H. Koizumi, "Fluoxetine [Prozac] and Suicidal Ideation," *Journal of the American Academy of Child and Adolescent Psychiatry* 30 (1991): 695; R. A. King, M. A. Riddle, P. B. Chappell, M. T. Hardin, G. M. Anderson, P. Lombroso, and L. Scahill, "Emergence of Self-Destructive Phenomena in Children and Adolescents During Fluoxetine [Prozac] Treatment," *Journal of the American Academy of Child and Adolescent Psychiatry* 30 (1991): 179–86.

4. M. J. Dewan and P. Masand, "Prozac and Suicide," *Journal of Family Practice* 33 (1991): 312.

5. K. Dasgupta, "Additional Cases of Suicidal Ideation Associated with Fluoxetine [Prozac]," *American Journal of Psychiatry* 147 (1990): 1570; L. A. Papp and J. M. Gorman, "Suicidal Preoccupation During Fluoxetine [Prozac] Treatment," *American Journal of Psychiatry* 147 (1990): 1380.

6. J. J. Mann and S. Kapur, "The Emergence of Suicidal Ideation and Behavior During Antidepressant Pharmacotherapy," *Archives of General Psychiatry* 48 (1991): 1027–33.

7. W. Creaney, I. Murray, and D. Healy, "Antidepressant [Prozac and Luvox]-Induced Suicidal Ideation," *Human Psychopharmacology* 6 (1991): 329–32.

8. *Lancet*, "5-HT Blockers [serotonin boosters] and All That," Editorial, August 11, 1990, p. 345.

9. J. Cornwell, *The Power to Harm: Mind, Medicine, and Murder on Trial* (New York: Viking, 1996), p. 154.

10. G. Cowley, "The Promise of Prozac," cover story, *Newsweek*, March 26, 1990, p. 38.

11. N. Varchaver, "Lilly's Phantom Verdict," *American Lawyer*, September 1995, pp. 74–83.

12. Associated Press, "Shannon Widow Sues Drug Company," *Variety*, January 30, 1991; N. Angier, "Suicidal Behavior Tied Again to Drug," *New York Times*, February 7, 1991, p. B15.

13. P. Kramer, *Listening to Prozac* (New York: Viking, 1993), p. 318.

14. A. D. Marcus, "Murder Trials Introduce Prozac Defense," *Wall Street Journal*, February 7, 1991, p. B1.

15. N. Angier, "Eli Lilly Facing Million-Dollar Suits on Its Antidepressant Drug Prozac," *New York Times*, August 16, 1990, p. B13; J. Cornwell, *The Power to Harm: Mind, Medicine, and Murder on Trial* (New York: Viking, 1996).

16. A. D. Marcus and W. Lambert, "Eli Lilly to Pay Costs of Doctors Sued After They Prescribe Prozac," *Wall Street Journal*, June 6, 1991, p. B5; A. D. Marcus, "Prozac Firm Fights Drug's Use as Defense," *Wall Street Journal*, April 9, 1991, p. B8; M. Mitka, "Drug Maker to Defend Physicians Sued over Prozac," *American Medical News*, June 24, 1991, p. 14.

17. C. Breitner, "The Hazard of Amphetamine Medication," *Psychosomatics* 6 (1965): 217–19; P. G. Schube, M. C. McManamy, C. E. Trapp, and A. Myerson, "The Effect of Benzedrine [an amphetamine] Sulphate on Certain Abnormal Mental States," *American Journal of Psychiatry* 94 (1937): 27–32.

18. This well-known clinical phenomenon was discussed at the FDA hearing on Prozac's safety. See Transcript of the Food and Drug Administration, Psychopharmacological Drugs Advisory Committee, Thirty-fourth Meeting, September 20, 1991, Department of Health and Human Services, Public Health Service, Food and Drug Administration, Rockville, Maryland, which can be obtained from the FDA through the Freedom of Information Act. See also M. H. Teicher, C. A. Glod, and J. O. Cole, "Antidepressant Drugs and the Emergence of Suicidal Tendencies," *Drug Safety* 8 (1993): 186–212 (see page 188 for the discussion of antidepressants "energising" patients and putting them at increased risk).

19. M. H. Teicher, C. Glod, and J. O. Cole, "Emergence of Intense Suicidal Preoccupation During Fluoxetine [Prozac] Treatment," *American Journal of Psychiatry* 147 (1990): 207–10.

20. *Lancet,* "5-HT Blockers [serotonin boosters] and All That," Editorial, August 11, 1990, p. 345.

21. Public Citizen's petition for revision of fluoxetine (Prozac) labeling. Memo from Dr. Sidney Wolfe and Dr. Ida Hellander of the Public Citizen Health Research Group to Dr. David Kessler, Commissioner of the Food and Drug Administration, May 23, 1991. See also Reuters, "Warning on Suicide in Prozac Use Is Sought," *New York Times,* May 24, 1991.

22. G. D. Tollefson, "Fluoxetine [Prozac] and Suicidal Ideation," *American Journal of Psychiatry* 147 (1990): 1691–92.

23. Transcript of the Food and Drug Administration, Psychopharmacological Drugs Advisory Committee, September 20, 1991, p. 189. Department of Health and Human Services, Public Health Service, Food and Drug Administration, Rockville, Maryland. Obtained through the Freedom of Information Act.

24. T. Burton, "Panel Finds No Credible Evidence to Tie Prozac to Suicides and Violent Behavior," *Wall Street Journal,* September 23, 1991, p. B4.

25. R. Behar, "The Thriving Cult of Greed and Power," cover story, *Time,* May 6, 1991.

26. T. Burton, "Panel Finds No Credible Evidence to Tie Prozac to Suicides and Violent Behavior," *Wall Street Journal,* September 23, 1991, p. B4.

27. *Physicians' Desk Reference (PDR)* (Montvale, N.J.: Medical Economics, 1999), pp. 924–28.

28. Ibid., pp. 2443–50 (Zoloft) and 3078–82 (Paxil).

29. A liquid form of Prozac was available, but it is roughly twice the cost of the already expensive capsules, greatly limiting its use. Moreover, many doctors were not aware the liquid form was available.

30. A. J. Rothschild and C. A. Locke, "Re-exposure to Fluoxetine [Prozac] After Serious Suicide Attempts by Three Patients: The Role of Akathisia [agitation]," *Journal of Clinical Psychiatry* 52 (1991): 491–93. One of Rothschild's patients was on other psychiatric medications, but these were not drugs that would be expected to contribute to the drug-induced agitation and suicidality, which appeared only when the Prozac was restarted. His other patients were not on any other medication.

31. T. Van Putten and S. R. Marder, "Behavioral Toxicity of Antipsychotic [major tranquilizer] Drugs," *Journal of Clinical Psychiatry* 48 (1987)[9, suppl.]: 13–19; T. Van Putten, "Why Do Schizophrenic Patients Refuse to Take Their Drugs?," *Archives of General Psychiatry* 31 (1974): 67–72; T. Van Putten, L. R. Mutalipassi, and M. D. Malkin, "Phenothiazine [major tranquilizer]-Induced Decompensation," *Archives of General Psychiatry* 30 (1974): 102–5; T. Van Putten, "The Many Faces of Akathisia [agitation]," *Comprehensive Psychiatry* 16 (1975): 43–47.

32. M. K. Shear, A. Frances, and P. Weiden, "Suicide Associated with Akathisia [agitation] and Depot Fluphenazine [a major tranquilizer] Treatment," *Journal of Clinical Psychopharmacology* 3 (1983): 235–36; R. E. Drake and J. Ehrlich, "Suicide Attempts Associated with Akathisia [agitation]," *American Journal of Psychiatry* 142 (1985): 499–501.

33. T. Van Putten, L. R. Mutalipassi, and M. D. Malkin, "Phenothiazine [major tranquilizer]-Induced Decompensation," *Archives of General Psychiatry* 30 (1974): 102–5. L. B. Kalinowsky, "Appraisal of the 'Tranquilizers' [now called "major tranquilizers"] and Their Influence on Other Somatic Treatments in Psychiatry," *American Journal of Psychiatry* 115 (1958): 294–300.

34. T. Van Putten, "Why Do Schizophrenic Patients Refuse to Take Their Drugs?," *Archives of General Psychiatry* 31 (1974): 67–72.

35. Ibid., p. 71.

36. W. C. Wirshing, T. Van Putten, J. Rosenberg, S. Marder, D. Ames, and T. Hicks-Gray, "Fluoxetine [Prozac], Akathisia [agitation] and Suicidality: Is There a Causal Connection?," *Archives of General Psychiatry* 49 (1992): 580–81. Some but not all of Van Putten and Wirshing's patients were on other medications, but in every case the suicidality coincided with going on Prozac.

37. M. S. Hamilton and L. A. Opler, "Akathisia [agitation], Suicidality, and Fluoxetine [Prozac]," *Journal of Clinical Psychiatry* 53 (1992): 401–6.

38. D. Healy, Declaration of David Healy, M.D., in *Susan Forsyth, et al. v. Eli Lilly, et al.* Case No. 95-00185 ACK, United States District Court for the District of Hawaii, pp. 15–16. See Healy's discussion of Lilly's explanation for the disappearance of akathisia [agitation] in later clinical studies.

39. Internal Eli Lilly document. Draft package insert [the official information that would be inserted into the package with the drug, appear in official publications like the *Physicians' Desk Reference,* and be reproduced in advertisements] for Prozac. 1983, p. 2. Plaintiff's exhibit No. 4 in *Susan Forsyth, et al. v. Eli Lilly, et al.* Case No. 95-00185 ACK, United States District Court for the District of Hawaii. As in previous chapters, I am using the word "adrenaline" for both adrenaline and the closely related noradrenaline (also called epinephrine and norepinephrine, respectively), because "adrenaline" is the term well known to a nontechnical audience. Noradrenaline—or norepinephrine—is the form found in the brain.

40. Internal Eli Lilly document. Memo from Dr. R. F. Bergstrom to Dr. D. S. Dobbs. Re: Package insert [the official information] for fluoxetine [Prozac]. August 24, 1983, p. 2. The memo contains comments from Dr. Bergstrom and a Dr. Lemberger. Plaintiff's exhibit No. 4 in *Susan Forsyth, et al. v. Eli Lilly, et al.* Case No. 95-00185 ACK, United States District Court for the District of Hawaii.

41. C. Beasley, "Fluoxetine [Prozac]-Dopaminergic [Dopamine] Interaction Data," *Journal of Clinical Psychiatry* 55 (1994): 77–78.

42. Conflict of Interest Statement for the Psychopharmacologic Drugs Advisory Committee, September 20, 1991. Department of Health and Human Services, Public Health Service, Food and Drug Administration, Rockville, Maryland. Obtained through the Freedom of Information Act.

43. Dunner's having been a principal investigator in one of Lilly's major clinical studies of Prozac was not specifically divulged in the minutes of the hearing. Instead, his relationship to a number of pharmaceutical companies was described as an "interest in Sandoz, Burroughs-Wellcome, American Home Products, including Wyeth Labs [manufacturer of Effexor] and A. H. Robbins, Eli Lilly [manufacturer of Prozac], Pfizer [manufacturer of Zoloft], Ciba-Geigy, Warner-Lambert, including Parke-Davis [manufacturer of Celexa], SmithKline Beecham [manufacturer of Paxil], and Bristol-Myers Squibb [manufacturer of Serzone]." See Transcript of the Food and Drug Administration, Psychopharmacological Drugs Advisory Committee, September 20, 1991, p. 11. Department of Health and Human Services, Public Health Service, Food and Drug Administration, Rockville, Maryland. Obtained from the FDA through the Freedom of Information Act. A separate document, a summary Conflict of Interest Statement for the Psychopharmacologic Drugs Advisory Committee, September 20, 1991, also obtained through the Freedom of Information Act, lists Dunner's conflicts in the same abbreviated way. In addition to this summary statement, each advisory committee member had to fill out an individual waiver form, which may provide more details on the specifics of their relationships to pharmaceutical companies. Unfortunately, the FDA is no longer able to release the individual waivers after protests that this was an invasion of the individuals' privacy. Dunner is listed as a principal investigator in one of the major clinical studies Eli Lilly submitted to the FDA to win approval to market Prozac in the Summary Basis of Approval NDA 18-936 [Eli Lilly's New Drug Application for Prozac], October 3, 1988, p. 21. Department of Health and Human Services, Food and Drug Administration, Rockville, Maryland. Obtained through the Freedom of Information Act.

44. Montgomery requested that his role as a principal investigator in a Prozac study be announced at the hearing for the record. See Transcript of the Food and Drug Administration, Psychopharmacological Drugs Advisory Committee, September 20, 1991, p. 11. Department of Health and Human Services, Public Health Service, Food and Drug Administration, Rockville, Maryland. Obtained through the Freedom of Information Act.

45. Conflict of Interest Statement for the Psychopharmacologic Drugs Advisory Committee, September 20, 1991. Department of Health and Human Services, Public Health Service, Food and Drug Administration. Obtained through the Freedom of Information Act.

46. Transcript of the Food and Drug Administration, Psychopharmacological Drugs Advisory Committee, September 20, 1991. Department of Health and Human Services, Public Health Service, Food and Drug Administration, Rockville, Maryland. Obtained through the Freedom of Information Act.

47. Ibid, p. 140. Other quotes in the paragraph are on pages 147 and 157.

48. Ibid., p. 233.

49. Ibid., p. 209.

50. Ibid., p. 273.

51. Ibid, p. 196. See also J. Fawcett, "Suicide Risk Factors in Depressive Disorders and in Panic Disorder," *Journal of Clinical Psychiatry* 53 (1992) [3, suppl.]: 9–13; J. Fawcett, "Targeting Treatment in Patients with Mixed Symptoms of Anxiety and Depression," *Journal of Clinical Psychiatry* 51 (1990) [11, suppl.]: 40–43.

52. Transcript of the Food and Drug Administration, Psychopharmacological Drugs Advisory Committee, September 20, 1991, pp. 278–79. Department of Health and Human Services, Public Health Service, Food and Drug Administration, Rockville, Maryland. Obtained through the Freedom of Information Act.

53. Ibid., p. 287.

54. M. Fava and J. Rosenbaum, "Suicidality and Fluoxetine [Prozac]: Is There a Relationship?," *Journal of Clinical Psychiatry* 52 (1991): 108–11. Fava and Rosenbaum are psychopharmacologists at the Massachusetts General Hospital and Harvard Medical School with extensive ties to the pharmaceutical industry to which they consult, are on advisory boards, receive grants, or honoraria. The pharmaceutical companies one or both of them have ties to include most of the manufacturers of the new antidepressants of the past decade, including Eli Lilly (Prozac), Pfizer (Zoloft), SmithKline Beecham (Paxil), Forest Labs (Celexa), Bristol-Myers Squibb (Serzone), Wyeth-Ayerst (Effexor), Organon (Remeron), and Glaxo Wellcome (Wellbutrin). See Faculty disclosure statements, Massachusetts General Hospital, Harvard Medical School Psychopharmacology Courses, October 25–27, 1996, and October 17–19, 1997. Fava and Rosenbaum's original analysis of their data was cited by Lilly and drug proponents as evidence that Prozac is not associated with a higher incidence of suicidality than other antidepressants. But Teicher's re-analysis of Fava and Rosenbaum's data showed that patients on Prozac were "at least 3-fold more likely to develop new suicidal ideation than those treated" with older antidepressants. Teicher eventually published his re-evaluations of Fava and Rosenbaum's data. In addition, other experts have seconded Teicher's re-analysis. See note 61 below.

55. Transcript of the Food and Drug Administration, Psychopharmacological Drugs Advisory Committee, September 20, 1991, p. 220. Department of Health and Human Services, Public Health Service, Food and Drug Administration, Rockville, Maryland. Obtained through the Freedom of Information Act.

56. T. Burton, "Panel Finds No Credible Evidence to Tie Prozac to Suicides and Violent Behavior," *Wall Street Journal,* September 23, 1991, p. B4.

57. Transcript of the Food and Drug Administration, Psychopharmacological Drugs Advisory Committee, September 20, 1991, p. 322. Department of Health and Human Services, Public Health Service, Food and Drug Administration, Rockville, Maryland. Obtained through the Freedom of Information Act.

58. Ibid, p. 331.

59. A. D. Marcus and W. Lambert, "Eli Lilly to Pay Costs of Doctors Sued After They Prescribe Prozac," *Wall Street Journal,* June 6, 1991, p. B5.

60. D. J. Graham, Internal FDA memo, September 11, 1990, on the subject of Sponsor's [Lilly's] ADR submission on fluoxetine [Prozac] dated July 17, 1990. Department of Health and Human Services, Public Health Service, Food and Drug Administration, Center for Drug Evaluation and Research, Rockville, Maryland. Obtained through the Freedom of Information Act.

61. Teicher eventually published the information that he had tried to show to the committee. See M. H. Teicher, C. A. Glod, and J. O. Cole, "Antidepressant Drugs and the Emergence of Suicidal Tendencies," *Drug Safety* 8 (1993): 186–212 (see page 200). The data Teicher re-evaluated were originally published by Drs. Maurizio Fava and Jerrold Rosenbaum. See note 54 above. Fava and Rosenbaum's original analysis of their data was cited by Lilly and drug proponents as evidence that Prozac is not associated with a higher incidence of suicidality than other antidepressants. But Teicher's re-analysis of Fava and Rosenbaum's data showed patients on Prozac were "at least 3-fold more likely to develop new suicidal ideation than those treated" with older antidepressants. In addition to Graham at the FDA, others who have seconded Teicher's re-evaluation of Fava and Rosenbaum's data are: J. J. Mann and S. Kapur, "The Emergence of Suicidal Ideation

and Behavior During Antidepressant Pharmacotherapy," *Archives of General Psychiatry* 48 (1991): 1027–33 (see page 1029) and D. Healy, Declaration of David Healy, M.D., in *Susan Forsyth, et al. v. Eli Lilly, et al.* Case No. 95-00185 ACK, United States District Court for the District of Hawaii (see pages 32–33). For critiques of Lilly's use of their clinical studies of Prozac to argue that the drug is not associated with a higher incidence of suicidality, see M. H. Teicher, C. A. Glod, and J. O. Cole, "Antidepressant Drugs and the Emergence of Suicidal Tendencies," *Drug Safety* 8 (1993): 186–212 (see pages 201–3); D. Healy and W. Creaney, "Fluoxetine [Prozac] and Suicide," *British Medical Journal* 303 (1991): 1058–59; and I. Oswald, "Fluoxetine [Prozac] and Suicide," *British Medical Journal* 303 (1991): 1058. Another study often cited by drug advocates as evidence that Prozac is not associated with a higher incidence of suicidality is S. S. Jick, A. D. Dean, and H. Jick, *British Medical Journal* 310 (1995): 215–18. But for a re-evaluation of the data in the Jick study, see D. Healy, Declaration of David Healy, M.D., in *Susan Forsyth, et al. v. Eli Lilly, et al.* Case No. 95-00185 ACK, United States District Court for the District of Hawaii (see pages 20–28). For one of the most concise critiques of why large databases are not useful in studying a phenomenon like drug-induced suicidality emerging in a small percentage of patients on a drug, see W. C. Wirshing, T. Van Putten, J. Rosenberg, S. Marder, D. Ames, and T. Hicks-Gray, "Fluoxetine [Prozac] Akathisia [agitation] and Suicidality: Is There a Causal Connection?," *Archives of General Psychiatry* 49 (1992): 580–81.

62. Internal Eli Lilly memo from Dr. L. Thompson to A. Weinstein, P. Keohane, M. Talbott, and R. Zerbe, February 7, 1999. Plaintiff's exhibit No. 97 in *Susan Forsyth, et al. v. Eli Lilly, et al.* Case No. 95-00185 ACK, United States District Court for the District of Hawaii.

63. Internal Eli Lilly memo from Dr. L. Thompson to A. Weinstein, February 7, 1990. Plaintiff's exhibit No. 98 in *Susan Forsyth, et al. v. Eli Lilly, et al.* Case No 95-00185 ACK, United States District Court for the District of Hawaii.

64. Internal Eli Lilly memo from Dr. L. Thompson to R. Thompson, A. Weinstein, R. Zerbe, and P. Roffey, November 5, 1990. Plaintiff's exhibit No. 116 in *Susan Forsyth, et al. v. Eli Lilly, et al.* Case No. 95-00185 ACK, United States District Court for the District of Hawaii.

65. Internal Eli Lilly memo from Dr. L. Thompson to A. Weinstein, February 7, 1990. Plaintiff's exhibit No. 98 in *Susan Forsyth, et al. v. Eli Lilly, et al.* Case No. 95-00185 ACK, United States District Court for the District of Hawaii.

66. Internal Eli Lilly memo from Dr. L. Thompson to M. Perelman, R. Zerbe, M. Talbott, D. Masica, M. Amundson, P. Reid, and R. Goss, July 18, 1990. Plaintiff's exhibit No. 104 in *Susan Forsyth, et al. v. Eli Lilly, et al.* Case No. 95-00185 ACK, United States District Court for the District of Hawaii.

67. Internal Eli Lilly memo from Dr. L. Tompson to M. Perelman, R. Zerbe, A. Weinstein, M. Talbott, and R. Goss, September 12, 1990. Plaintiff's exhibit No. 109 in *Susan Forsyth, et al. v. Eli Lilly, et al.* Case No. 95-00185 ACK, United States District Court for the District of Hawaii.

68. P. Breggin, *Talking Back to Prozac* (New York: St. Martin's Press, 1994), pp. 168–70.

69. T. Moore, *Prescription for Disaster* (New York: Simon & Schuster, 1998), pp. 138–52.

70. N. Varchaver, "Lilly's Phantom Verdict," *American Lawyer,* September 1995, pp. 74–83.

71. The transcript of the Wesbecker trial is entitled *Joyce Fentress* [the first of 27 plaintiffs, i.e. the victims and survivors], *et al. v. Shea Communications* [the owner of Standard Gravure, Wesbecker's employer, and the first of a number of defendants, including Eli Lilly, which was the only defendant in the actual trial], *et. al.* Case Number 90CI6033, the Jefferson County Circuit Courthouse, Archives, 514 West Liberty Street, Louisville, Kentucky.

72. J. Cornwell, *The Power to Harm: Mind, Medicine, and Murder on Trial* (New York: Viking, 1996), p. 182.

73. The transcript of the Wesbecker trial, quoted in Cornwell, p. 160.

74. Ibid., p. 161.

75. P. Kramer, *Listening to Prozac* (New York: Viking, 1993), p. 321.

76. J. Cornwell, *The Power to Harm: Mind, Medicine, and Murder on Trial* (New York: Viking, 1996), pp. 159–60.

77. The transcript of the Wesbecker trial, quoted in Cornwell, p. 182.
78. Ibid, pp. 199–201.
79. Ibid, pp. 147–48.
80. Ibid, pp. 182, 235.
81. Ibid., p. 198.
82. Internal Eli Lilly memo from C. Bouchy to L. Thompson, A. Weinstein, and R. Zerbe, November 13, 1990. Plaintiff's exhibit No. 117 in *Susan Forsyth, et al. v. Eli Lilly, et al.* Case No. 95-00185 ACK, United States District Court for the District of Hawaii.
83. The transcript of the Wesbecker trial, quoted in Cornwell, p. 199.
84. Ibid, p. 198.
85. Ibid., p. 200.
86. Ibid., pp. 231–34.
87. Ibid., p. 242.
88. D. Nelkin, *Selling Science* (New York: W. H. Freeman, 1995), p. 139.
89. P. Shenon, "Lilly Pleads Guilty to Oraflex Charges," *New York Times,* August 22, 1985, p. A16.
90. J. Davidson and C. Phillips, "Eli Lilly Admits It Failed to Inform U.S. of Deaths, Illnesses Tied to Oraflex Drug," *Wall Street Journal,* August 22, 1985.
91. J. Cornwell, *The Power to Harm: Mind, Medicine, and Murder on Trial* (New York: Viking, 1996), p. 47.
92. *Los Angeles Times,* "FDA: Scientists Failed to Disclose Hepatitis Drug's Risks." Reprinted in the *Boston Sunday Globe,* May 15, 1994, p. 25.
93. Ibid.
94. Ibid.
95. N. Varchaver, "Lilly's Phantom Verdict," *American Lawyer,* September 1995, pp. 74–83.
96. The transcript of the Wesbecker trial, quoted in J. Cornwell, p. 242.
97. N. Varchaver, "Lilly's Phantom Verdict," *American Lawyer,* September 1995, pp. 74–83.
98. The transcript of the Wesbecker trial, quoted in Cornwall, pp. 268–69.
99. Ibid., pp. 268–69.
100. Ibid., p. 269. For technical legal reasons, only the Oraflex and not the fialuridine evidence was allowed.
101. N. Varchaver, "Lilly's Phantom Verdict," *American Lawyer,* September 1995, pp. 74–83.
102. Ibid.
103. Report of the Friend of the Court [the Office of the Attorney General of Kentucky] in *Joyce Fentress et al. v. Shea Communications et al.* [the official name of the Wesbecker trial], March 4, 1997.
104. N. Varchaver, "Lilly's Phantom Verdict," *American Lawyer,* September 1995, pp. 74–83.
105. This was a point of disagreement between the judge and Lilly in the attorney general's investigation. For a good description of how the attorneys for the survivors and Lilly "misled the judge repeatedly about the agreement both by implication and by explicit misstatements," see ibid.
106. Ibid.
107. J. Cornwell, *The Power to Harm: Mind, Medicine, and Murder on Trial* (New York: Viking, 1996), p. 285.
108. Ibid. The *Indianapolis News* is quoted on p. 287.
109. Cited in N. Varchaver, "Lilly's Phantom Verdict," *American Lawyer,* September 1995, pp. 74–83.
110. J. Cornwell, *The Power to Harm: Mind, Medicine, and Murder on Trial* (New York: Viking, 1996), p. 286.
111. Ibid, p. 56.
112. Ibid, p. 286.
113. N. Varchaver, "Lilly's Phantom Verdict," *American Lawyer,* September 1995, pp. 74–83.
114. Ibid.
115. J. Davidson and C. Phillips, "Eli Lilly Admits It Failed to Inform U.S. of Deaths, Illnesses Tied to Oraflex Drug," *Wall Street Journal,* August 22, 1985.
116. Report of the Friend of the Court [the Office of the Attorney General of Kentucky] in *Joyce Fentress, et al. v. Shea Communications, et al.* [the official name of the Wesbecker trial], March 4, 1997.

117. Court's Motion Pursuant to Civil Rule 60.01 and Notice, *Joyce Fentress, et al. v. Shea Communications, et al.* [the official name of the Wesbecker trial], April 19, 1985. Jefferson Circuit Court, Division 1. No. 90CI06033.
118. N. Varchaver, "Lilly's Phantom Verdict," *American Lawyer,* September 1995, pp. 74–83.
119. *Potter v. Eli Lilly and Company,* Supreme Court of Kentucky No. 926 S.W.2d 449. Opinion of the Court by Justice Wintersheimer, May 23, 1996.
120. J. Cornwell, *The Power to Harm: Mind, Medicine, and Murder on Trial* (New York: Viking, 1996), p. 296.
121. Ibid., p. 298.
122. Ibid., p. 271.
123. Ibid., p. 272.
124. N. Varchaver, "Lilly's Phantom Verdict," *American Lawyer,* September 1995, pp. 74–83.
125. J. Cornwell, *The Power to Harm: Mind, Medicine, and Murder on Trial* (New York: Viking, 1996), p. 167.
126. *Potter v. Eli Lilly and Company,* Supreme Court of Kentucky No. 926 S.W.2d 449. Opinion of the Court by Justice Wintersheimer, May 23, 1996.
127. Report of the Friend of the Court [the Office of the Attorney General of Kentucky] in *Joyce Fentress, et al. v. Shea Communications, et al.* [the official name of the Wesbecker trial], March 4, 1997.
128. Ibid. See also N. Varchaver, "Lilly's Phantom Verdict," *American Lawyer,* September 1995, pp. 74–83.
129. N. Varchaver, "Lilly's Phantom Verdict," *American Lawyer,* September 1995, pp. 74–83.
130. Corrected judgment, *Joyce Fentress, et al. v. Shea Communications, et al.* [the official name of the Wesbecker trial], March 24, 1997. Jefferson Circuit Court, Div. 5. Case Number 90-CI6033.
131. J. Cornwell, *The Power to Harm: Mind, Medicine, and Murder on Trial* (New York: Viking, 1996), p. 299.
132. Ibid., pp. 205–13.
133. Eli Lilly's Expert Witnesses Disclosures in *Joyce Fentress, et al. v. Shea Communications, et al.* [the official name of the Wesbecker trial], Case Number 90CI6033, the Jefferson Circuit Courthouse, Archives, 514 West Liberty Street, Louisville, Kentucky, pp. 4–6.
134. D. Healy, Declaration of David Healy, M.D., in *Susan Forsyth, et al. v. Eli Lilly, et al.* Case No. 95-00185 ACK, United States District Court for the District of Hawaii, pp. 25–27.
135. Internal Eli Lilly memo from A. Weinstein to C. Beasley, V. Bryson, R. Cage, R. Clarke, R. Luedke, R. Matricaria, M. Perelman, S. Taurel, L. Thompson, R. Thompson, and R. Zerbe, April 8, 1992. Plaintiff's exhibit No. 144 in *Susan Forsyth, et al. v. Eli Lilly, et al.* Case Number 95-00185 ACK, United States District Court for the District of Hawaii.
136. J. Cornwell, *The Power to Harm: Mind, Medicine, and Murder on Trial* (New York: Viking, 1996), pp. 59–70.
137. Ibid, p. 3.
138. Ibid, p. 1.
139. Ibid., p. 85.
140. Ibid., p. 70.
141. Wesbecker received other diagnoses in addition to depression, including borderline personality disorder and manic depressive illness. But see Chapter 5 for a discussion of these types of diagnoses in a psychopharmacology setting if a patient's psychosocial circumstances are not adequately factored into the equation. See in particular the discussion of the "case" of Hamlet.
142. J. Cornwell, *The Power to Harm: Mind, Medicine, and Murder on Trial* (New York: Viking, 1996), p. 5.
143. For some time, Wesbecker had also been on lithium and Valium-type medication. After Wesbecker's death, the coroner reported that his blood contained only Prozac and lithium in levels doctors normally prescribe. See ibid., p. 39. Valium-type medication would have mitigated Prozac-induced agitation. Since it did not appear in his blood, Wesbecker was apparently not taking this medication at the time of the shootings.
144. Ibid., p. 185.
145. Ibid., p. 7.
146. Report of the Friend of the Court [the Office of the Attorney General of Kentucky] in

Joyce Fentress, et al. v. Shea Communications, et al. [the official name of the Wesbecker trial], March 4, 1997. See also N. Varchaver, "Lilly's Phantom Verdict," *American Lawyer,* September 1995, pp. 74–83.

147. Faculty disclosure statements, Harvard Medical School/Massachusetts General Hospital Conferences on Psychopharmacology, October 25–27, 1996, and October 17–19, 1997.
148. M. H. Pollack, "Management of Antidepressant and Lithium Induced Side Effects," talk given at the Harvard Medical School/Massachusetts General Hospital Conference on Psychopharmacology, October 17–19, 1997.
149. Transcript of the Food and Drug Administration, Psychopharmacological Drugs Advisory Committee, September 20, 1991, p. 285. Department of Health and Human Services, Public Health Service, Food and Drug Administration, Rockville, Maryland. Obtained through the Freedom of Information Act.
150. P. Kramer, *Listening to Prozac* (New York: Viking, 1993), p. 321.
151. *Physicians' Desk Reference (PDR)* (Montvale, N.J.: Medical Economics, 1999), pp. 924–28 (Prozac), 2443–50 (Zoloft), 3078–82 (Paxil), and 3121–24 (Luvox).
152. W. Creaney, I. Murray, and D. Healy, "Antidepressant [Prozac and Luvox]-Induced Suicidal Ideation," *Human Psychopharmacology* 6 (1991): 329–32.
153. H. Koizumi, "Fluoxetine [Prozac] and Suicidal Ideation," *Journal of the American Academy of Child and Adolescent Psychiatry* 30 (1991): 695. R. A. King, M. A. Riddle, P. B. Chappell, M. T. Hardin, G. M. Anderson, P. Lombroso, and L. Scahill, "Emergence of Self-Destructive Phenomena in Children and Adolescents During Fluoxetine [Prozac] Treatment," *Journal of the American Academy of Child and Adolescent Psychiatry* 30 (1991): 179–86.
154. M. H. Teicher, C. Glod, and J. O. Cole, follow-up to their original article "Emergence of Intense Suicidal Preoccupation During Fluoxetine [Prozac] Treatment," *American Journal of Psychiatry* 147 (1990): 1380.

5
Behind-the-Scenes Forces:
Understanding the Prozac Phenomenon

1. I. Elkin, M. T. Shea, J. T. Watkins, S. D. Imber, S. M. Sotsky, J. F. Collins, D. R. Glass, P. A. Pilkonis, W. R. Leber, J. P. Docherty, S. J. Fiester, and M. B. Parloff, "National Institute of Mental Health Treatment of Depression Collaborative Research Program: General Effectiveness of Treatments," *Archives of General Psychiatry* 46 (1989): 971–82; S. D. Hollon, R. J. DeRubeis, M. D. Evans, M. J. Wiemer, M. J. Garvey, W. M. Grove, and V. B. Tuason, "Cognitive Therapy and Pharmacotherapy for Depression, Singly and in Combination," *Archives of General Psychiatry* 49 (1992): 774–81.
2. I. M. Blackburn, K. M. Eunson, and S. Bishop, "A Two-Year Naturalistic Follow-up of Depressed Patients Treated with Cognitive Therapy, Pharmacotherapy, and a Combination of Both," *Journal of Affective Disorders* 10 (1986): 67–75.
3. I. M. Marks, R. P. Swinson, M. Basoglu, K. Kuch, H. Noshirvani, G. O'Sullivan, P. T. Lelliott, M. Kirby, G. McNamee, S. Sengun, and K. Wickwire, "Alprazolam [Xanax, a Valium-type antianxiety agent] and Exposure Alone and Combined in Panic Disorder with Agoraphobia," *British Journal of Psychiatry* 162 (1993): 776–87; G. A. Fava, M. Zielezny, G. Savron, and S. Grandi, "Long-Term Effects of Behavioural Treatment for Panic Disorder with Agoraphobia," *British Journal of Psychiatry* 166 (1995): 87–92.
4. *Journal of Geriatric Psychiatry and Neurology* 7 (1994) [suppl. 1]: S1–S68.
5. H. Woelk, O. Kapoula, S. Lehrl, K. Schroter, and P. Weinholz, "Double-Blind Study: Kava Special Extract Versus Benzodiazepines [Valium-type antianxiety agents] in Treatment of Patients Suffering from Anxiety," *Zeitschrift für Allgemeinmedizin* 69 (1993): 271–77; H. Dressing et al., "Insomnia: Are Valerian/Balm Combinations of Equal Value to Benzodiazepines [Valium-type sleeping pills]?," *Therapiewoch* 42 (1992): 726–36.
6. R. Baldessarini, "Psychopharmacology: Where Have We Been; Where Are We; Where Are We Going?," Keynote address, Harvard Medical School/Massachusetts General Hospital Conference on Psychopharmacology, October 16–18, 1998.
7. L. L. Judd, "The Clinical Course of Unipolar Major Depressive Disorders," *Archives of General Psychiatry* 54 (1997): 989–91.

8. American Psychiatric Association, *Diagnostic and Statistical Manual of Mental Disorders (DSM)*, 4th edition (Washington: American Psychiatric Association, 1994).

9. P. Kramer, *Listening to Prozac* (New York: Viking, 1993), p. 166.

10. J. C. Bennett and F. Plum, eds., *Cecil Textbook of Medicine*, 20th edition (Philadelphia: W. B. Saunders, 1996), p. 1258.

11. B. J. Caroll, G. C. Curtis, and J. Mendels, "Neuroendocrine Regulation in Depression," *Archives of General Psychiatry* 33 (1976): 1039–44.

12. R. J. Baldessarini and G. W. Arana, "Does the Dexamethasone Suppression Test [DST] Have Clinical Utility in Psychiatry?," *Journal of Clinical Psychiatry* 46 (1985) [2, section 2]: 25–29.

13. J. J. Schildkraut, "The Catecholamine [adrenaline] Hypothesis of Affective Disorders [depression]," *American Journal of Psychiatry* 122 (1965): 509–22. As in previous chapters, I use the well-recognized term "adrenaline" for both adrenaline and the closely related noradrenaline (also called epinephrine and norepinephrine, respectively), because "adrenaline" is the term well known to a nontechnical audience. Noradrenaline—norepinephrine—is the form found in the brain and the one whose metabolites Schildkraut was measuring in the urine.

14. J. J. Schildkraut, "Norepinephrine [adrenaline] Metabolites as Biochemical Criteria for Classifying Depressive Disorders and Predicting Responses to Treatment: Preliminary Findings," *American Journal of Psychiatry* 130 (1973): 695–98.

15. H. M. van Praag, *"Make-Believes" in Psychiatry* (New York: Bruner/Mazel, 1993).

16. H. M. van Praag, J. Korf, and J. Puite, "5-Hydroxyindoleacetic Acid [5-HIAA] Levels in the Cerebrospinal Fluid of Depressive Patients Treated with Probenecid," *Nature* 225 (1970): 1259–60.

17. M. Asberg, L. Traskman, and P. Thoren, "5-HIAA in the Cerebrospinal Fluid: A Biochemical Suicide Predictor?," *Archives of General Psychiatry* 33 (1976): 1193–97.

18. E. F. Coccaro, "Central Serotonin and Impulsive Aggression," *British Journal of Psychiatry* 155 (1989) [suppl. 8]: 52–62.

19. H. M. van Praag, *"Make-Believes" in Psychiatry* (New York: Brunner/Mazel, 1993), p. 158.

20. J. A. Egeland, D. S. Gerhard, D. L. Pauls, J. N. Sussex, K. K. Kidd, C. R. Allen, A. M. Hostetter, and D. E. Housman, "Bipolar Affective [manic-depressive] Disorders Linked to DNA Markers on Chromosome 11," *Nature* 325 (1987): 783–87.

21. The retraction in *Nature* appeared almost two years after publication of the original study: J. R. Kelsoe, E. I. Ginns, J. A. Egeland, D. S. Gerhard, A. M. Goldstein, S. J. Bale, D. L. Pauls, R. T. Long, K. K. Kidd, G. Conte, D. E. Housman, and S. M. Paul, "Reevaluation of the Linkage Relationship Between Chromosome 11p Loci and the Gene for Bipolar Affective [manic-depressive] Disorder in the Old Order Amish," *Nature* 342 (1989): 238–43.

22. R. Lewontin, *Biology as Ideology* (New York: HarperPerennial, 1991), p. 96.

23. Ibid., p. 32.

24. Ibid., p. 96.

25. R. Lewontin, "The Dream of the Human Genome," *New York Review of Books*, May 28, 1992, pp. 31–40.

26. R. Lewontin, *Biology as Ideology* (New York: HarperPerennial, 1991), p. 57.

27. Ibid., p. 71.

28. L. L. Havens, personal communication.

29. P. Kramer, *Listening to Prozac* (New York: Viking, 1993), pp. 110–12.

30. Ibid., pp. 113–14.

31. J. Hooper, "A New Germ Theory," *Atlantic Monthly*, February 1999, pp. 41–53.

32. E. C. Azmitia and P. M. Whitaker-Azmitia, "Awakening the Sleeping Giant: Anatomy and Plasticity of the Brain Serotonergic System," *Journal of Clinical Psychiatry* 52 (1991) [12, suppl.]: 4–16.

33. A. Nierenberg, "Antidepressants: Current Issues and New Drugs," talk given at the Harvard Medical School/Massachusetts General Hospital Conference on Psychopharmacology, October 17–19, 1997.

34. J. Rosenbaum, "The Drug Treatment of Resistant Depression: Reviewing the Options," talk given at the Harvard Medical School/Massachusetts General Hospital Conference on Psychopharmacology, October 17–19, 1997.

35. A. Weil and W. Rosen, *From Chocolate to Morphine: Everything You Need to Know About Mind-Altering Drugs* (Boston: Houghton Mifflin, 1993), p. 48.

36. Good examples of Eli Lilly's claims for the scientific proof of Prozac's safety and efficacy are the transcript of the FDA hearing on Prozac's safety on September 20, 1991, and their defense of the drug during the Joseph Wesbecker trial in 1994, both of which are discussed in Chapter 4.

37. R. J. Baldessarini, "Drugs and the Treatment of Psychiatric Disorders: Depression and Mania," in J. G. Hardman and L. E. Limbird, eds., *Goodman and Gilman's The Pharmacological Basis of Therapeutics*, 9th edition (New York: McGraw-Hill, 1996), p. 436.

38. Ibid.

39. D. Healy, *The Antidepressant Era* (Cambridge, Mass.: Harvard University Press, 1997), p. 76.

40. W.W.K. Zung, "A Self-Rating Depression Scale," *Archives of General Psychiatry* 12 (1965): 63–70; M. Hamilton, "A Rating Scale for Depression," *Journal of Neurology, Neurosurgery, and Psychiatry* 23 (1960): 56–62.

41. W. S. Appleton, *Prozac and the New Antidepressants* (New York: Plume, 1997), pp. 36–37.

42. Ibid., p. 37.

43. R. P. Greenberg and S. Fisher, "Examining Antidepressant Effectiveness: Findings, Ambiguities, and Some Vexing Puzzles," in S. Fisher and R. P. Greenberg, eds., *The Limits of Biological Treatments for Psychological Distress: Comparisons with Psychotherapy and Placebo* (Hillsdale, N.J.: Erlbaum, 1989), pp. 1–37.

44. *Treatment of Depression—Newer Pharmacotherapies*, Summary, Evidence Report/Technology Assessment: No. 7, March 1999 (Rockville, Md.: Agency for Health Care Policy and Research, 1999).

45. J. Margraf, A. Ehlers, W. T. Roth, D. B. Clark, J. Sheikh, W. S. Agras and C. B. Taylor, "How 'Blind' Are Double-Blind Studies?," *Journal of Consulting and Clinical Psychology* 59 (1991): 184–87.

46. R. Thompson, "Side Effects and Placebo Amplification," *British Journal of Psychiatry* 140 (1982): 64–68.

47. R. P. Greenberg, F. R. Bornstein, M. D. Greenberg, and S. Fisher, "A Meta-Analysis of Antidepressant Outcome Under 'Blinder' Conditions," *Journal of Consulting and Clinical Psychology* 60 (1992): 664–69.

48. R. L. Fisher and S. Fisher, "Antidepressants for Children: Is Scientific Support Necessary?," *Journal of Nervous and Mental Disease* 184 (1996): 99–102.

49. E. D. Pellegrino, "Commentary: Clinical Judgment, Scientific Data, and Ethics: Antidepressant Therapy in Adolescents and Children," *Journal of Nervous and Mental Disease* 184 (1996): 106–8.

50. J. M. Cott and A. Fugh-Berman, "Is St. John's Wort *(Hypericum perforatum)* an Effective Antidepressant?," *Journal of Nervous and Mental Disease* 186 (1998): 500–501.

51. R. Whitaker, "Lure of Riches Fuels Testing," part 3 of a series entitled "Doing Harm: Research on the Mentally Ill," *Boston Globe*, November 17, 1998, pp. 1, A34–35.

52. Ibid.

53. Summary Basis of Approval NDA 18-936 [Eli Lilly's New Drug Application for Prozac], October 3, 1988, p. 21. Department of Health and Human Services, Public Health Service, Food and Drug Administration, Rockville Maryland. Obtained through the Freedom of Information Act.

54. M. J. Grinfeld, "Ex-Profs Charged in Psych Department Studies Scandal," *Psychiatric Times*, April 1997, pp. 1, 3–5.

55. R. Whitaker, "Lure of Riches Fuels Testing," part 3 of a series entitled "Doing Harm: Research on the Mentally Ill," *Boston Globe*, November 17, 1998, pp. 1, A34–35.

56. Ibid.

57. M. J. Grinfeld, "Ex-Profs Charged in Psych Department Studies Scandal," *Psychiatric Times*, April 1997, pp. 1, 3–5.

58. R. Whitaker, "Lure of Riches Fuels Testing," part 3 of a series entitled "Doing Harm: Research on the Mentally Ill," *Boston Globe*, November 17, 1998, pp. 1, A34–35.

59. R. J. Salin-Pascual, M. Rosas, A. Jimenez-Genchi, B. L. Rivera-Meza, and V. Delgado-

Parra, "Antidepressant Effect of Transdermal Nicotine Patches in Nonsmoking Patients with Major Depression," *Journal of Clinical Psychiatry* 57 (1996): 387–89.

60. D. Healy, Declaration of David Healy, M. D., in *Susan Forsyth, et al. v. Eli Lilly, et al.* Case No. 95-00185 ACK, United States District Court for the District of Hawaii, p. 4.

61. C. T. Gualtieri, "Paradoxical Effects of Fluoxetine [Prozac]," *Journal of Clinical Psychopharmacology* 11 (1991): 393–94.

62. R. S. Schwartz, "Mood Brighteners, Affect Tolerance, and the Blues," *Psychiatry* 54 (1991): 397–403.

63. C. Medawar, "The Antidepressant Web," *International Journal of Risk & Safety in Medicine* 10 (1997): 75–126.

64. N. S. Kline, "Monoamine Oxidase Inhibitors: An Unfinished Picaresque Tale," in F. J. Ayd and B. Blackwell, eds., *Discoveries in Biological Psychiatry* (Philadelphia: J. B. Lippincott, 1970).

65. P. Kramer, *Listening to Prozac* (New York: Viking, 1993), p. 162.

66. T. W. Rall, "Central Nervous System Stimulants," in A. G. Gilman, L. S. Goodman, and A. Gilman, eds., *Goodman and Gilman's The Pharmacological Basis of Therapeutics*, 6th edition (New York: Macmillan, 1980), pp. 592–607. See also L. Grinspoon and P. Hedblom, *The Speed Culture* (Cambridge: Harvard University Press, 1975), pp. 62–95.

67. F. Gardner, "Prozac 'Abuse,'" *Anderson Valley Advertiser* (Boonville, California), February 23, 1994, p. 5.

68. L. Grinspoon and P. Hedblom, *The Speed Culture* (Cambridge, Mass.: Harvard University Press, 1975), pp. 20, 51.

69. C. M. Beasley, M. E. Sayler, J. C. Bosomworth, and J. F. Wernicke, "High-Dose Fluoxetine [Prozac]: Efficacy and Activating-Sedating Effects in Agitated and Retarded Depression," *Journal of Clinical Psychopharmacology* 11 (1991): 166–74; C. M. Beasley, M. E. Sayler, A. M. Weiss, and J. H. Potvin, "Fluoxetine [Prozac]: Activating and Sedating Effects at Multiple Fixed Doses," *Journal of Clinical Psychopharmacology* 12 (1992): 328–33.

70. J. A. Bodkin, R. A. Lasser, J. D. Wines, D. M. Gardner, and R. J. Baldessarini, "Combining Serotonin Reuptake Inhibitors [Prozac-type antidepressants] and Bupropion [Wellbutrin] in Partial Responders to Antidepressant Monotherapy," *Journal of Clinical Psychiatry* 58 (1997): 137–45. See also T. R. Green, "Bupropion [Wellbutrin] for SSRI [Prozac-type antidepressant]-Induced Fatigue," *Journal of Clinical Psychiatry* 54 (1997): 174.

71. R. Kapit, Safety Review of NDA 18-936 [Eli Lilly's New Drug Application for Prozac], March 28, 1986, p. 5. Department of Health and Human Services, Public Health Service, Food and Drug Administration, Rockville, Maryland. Obtained through the Freedom of Information Act.

72. M. J. Grinfeld, "Gag Rules Wane, but Hidden Managed Care Restraints Linger," *Psychiatric Times*, December 1996, pp. 1, 22.

73. *Health Care Plan Design and Cost Trends: 1988 Through 1997*, a report by the Hay Group for the National Association of Psychiatric Health Systems, the Association of Behavioral Group Practices, and the National Alliance for the Mentally Ill. See also M. J. Grinfeld, "Discrimination Yields Decline in Mental Health Benefits," *Psychiatric Times*, July 1998, p. 8.

74. M. J. Grinfeld, "Protecting Prozac," *California Lawyer*, December 1998, pp. 36–40, 79. See also E. J. Pollock, "Managed Care's Focus on Psychiatric Drugs Alarms Many Doctors," *Wall Street Journal*, December 1, 1995, p. 1, A11.

75. W. H. Rogers, K. B. Wells, L. S. Meredith, R. Sturm, and M. A. Burnam, "Outcomes for Adult Outpatients with Depression Under Prepaid or Fee-for-Service Financing," *Archives of General Psychiatry* 50 (1993): 517–25.

76. D. Kong, "Doctors Fault Service Access: Mental Health Care Is Concern," *Boston Globe*, October 16, 1997.

77. B. Strauch, "Use of Antidepression Medicine for Young Patients Has Soared," *New York Times*, August 10, 1997, p. 1.

78. J. V. O'Neill, "Managed Care Lawsuit Going Forward," *NASW [National Association of Social Workers] News*, September 1999, pp. 1, 10.

79. A. Pham, "Drug Costs Put Strain on Health Insurers, May Force Change for Managed Care," *Boston Globe*, March 18, 1998, p. 1, A20.

80. D. Blumenthal, E. G. Campbell, M. S. Anderson, N. Causina, and K. S. Louis, "Withholding Research Results in Academic Life Science: Evidence from a National Survey of Faculty," *Journal of the American Medical Association* 277 (1997): 1224–28.

81. B. J. Dong, W. W. Hauck, J. G. Gambertoglio, L. Gee, J. R. White, J. L. Bubp, and F. S. Greenspan, "Bioequivalence of Generic and Brand-Name Levothyroxine Products in the Treatment of Hypothyroidism," *Journal of the American Medical Association* 277 (1997): 1205–13.

82. I. M. Marks, R. P. Swinson, M. Basoglu, K. Kuch, H. Noshirvani, G. O'Sullivan, P. T. Lelliott, M. Kirby, G. McNamee, S. Sengun, and K. Wickwire, "Alprazolam [Xanax, a Valium-type antianxiety agent] and Exposure Alone and Combined in Panic Disorder with Agoraphobia," *British Journal of Psychiatry* 162 (1993): 776–87.

83. I. M. Marks, R. P. Swinson, M. Basoglu, H. Noshirvani, K. Kuch, G. O'Sullivan, and P. T. Lelliott, "Reply to Comment on the London/Toronto Study," *British Journal of Psychiatry* 162 (1993): 790–94.

84. M. Leonard, "Children Are the Hot New Market for Antidepressants. But Is This How to Make Them Feel Better?," *Boston Globe*, May 25, 1997, pp. D1, D5; B. Strauch, "Use of Antidepression Medicine for Young Patients Has Soared," *New York Times*, August 10, 1997, p. 1.

85. *Physicians' Desk Reference (PDR)* (Montvale, N.J.: Medical Economics, 1999), p. 2078.

86. A. J. Zametkin, "Attention-Deficit Disorder: Born to Be Hyperactive?," *Journal of the American Medical Association* 273 (1995): 1871–74.

87. J. Avorn, M. Chen, and R. Hartley, "Scientific Versus Commercial Sources of Influence on the Prescribing Behavior of Physicians," *American Journal of Medicine* 73 (1982): 4–8.

88. Quoted in R. Whitaker, "Lure of Riches Fuels Testing," part 3 of a series entitled "Doing Harm: Research on the Mentally Ill," *Boston Globe*, November 17, 1998, pp. 1, A34–35.

89. D. Kong and A. Bass, "Case at Brown Leads to Review, NIMH Studies Tighter Rules on Conflicts," *Boston Globe*, October 8, 1999, pp. B1, B5.

90. C. D. Chambers, K. A. Johnson, L. M. Dick, R. J. Felix, and K. L. Jones, "Birth Outcomes in Pregnant Women Taking Fluoxetine [Prozac]," *New England Journal of Medicine* 335 (1996): 1010–15.

91. *New York Times*, "Questions Raised About Prozac in Pregnancy," October 3, 1996.

92. Health Wire, Indianapolis, Indiana, "Medical Experts Dispute Findings in NEJM [New England Journal of Medicine] Study." UPI-data. October 4, 1996.

93. L. Cohen, Faculty disclosure statement, Harvard Medical School/Massachusetts General Hospital Conference on Psychopharmacology, October 25–27, 1996.

94. The statement of Lilly's financial support can be found in the fine print of promotional material for National Depression Screening Day, such as their poster "Facing the Day" prominently displayed on college campuses or their 1998 Registration Information and Registration Form. It is difficult to tell from the promotional material what, if any, other pharmaceutical companies or organizations provide financial support. Material such as the poster "Facing the Day" lists only Eli Lilly's support. Other promotional material lists a number of professional organizations—such as the American Association of General Hospital Psychiatrists, Charter Behavioral Health Systems, and Columbia Behavioral Health Services—who are described as "supporters" of National Depression Screening Day. This may mean that they just endorse the screening, since Eli Lilly is listed separately for specifically providing financial support in the form of an "educational grant."

95. D. Healy, *The Antidepressant Era* (Cambridge, Mass.: Harvard University Press, 1997), p. 198.

96. Ibid., p. 190.

97. R. Baldessarini, "Psychopharmacology: Where Have We Been; Where Are We; Where Are We Going?," Keynote address at the Massachusetts General Hospital/Harvard Medical School Conference on Psychopharmacology, October 16, 1998.

98. T. Moore, "Hard to Swallow," *The Washingtonian*, December 1997, pp. 69–71, 140–145.

99. J. R. Hoffman and M. Wilkes, "Direct to Consumer Advertising of Prescription Drugs, An Idea Whose Time Should Not Come," *British Medical Journal* 318 (1999): 1301–2.

100. M. S. Wilkes, B. H. Doblin, and M. F. Shapiro, "Pharmaceutical Advertisements in Lead-

ing Medical Journals: Experts' Assessments," *Annals of Internal Medicine* 116 (1992): 912–19.

101. D. A. Kessler, "Addressing the Problem of Misleading Advertising," *Annals of Internal Medicine* 116 (1992): 950–51.
102. Effexor advertisement, *New York Times,* January 27, 1997, p. B14. The same ad appears in professional journals. See also *Journal of Clinical Psychiatry* 57 (1996): 543.
103. Zoloft advertisement, *Journal of Clinical Psychiatry* 57 (1996): 355, 360.
104. Prozac advertisement, *Parade,* September 28, 1997, pp. 20–22.
105. G. Fava and E. Tomba, "The Use of Antidepressant Drugs: Some Reasons for Concern," *International Journal of Risk & Safety in Medicine* 11 (1998): 271–74.

6

Unraveling Depression:
Stifled Anger and Sadness

1. I. Elkin, M. T. Shea, J. T. Watkins, S. D. Imber, S. M. Sotsky, J. F. Collins, D. R. Glass, P. A. Pilkonis, W. R. Leber, J. P. Docherty, S. J. Fiester, and M. B. Parloff, "National Institute of Mental Health Treatment of Depression Collaborative Research Program: General Effectiveness of Treatments," *Archives of General Psychiatry* 46 (1989): 971–82.
2. I. M. Blackburn, S. Bishop, A.I.M. Glen, L. J. Whalley, and J. E. Christie, "The Efficacy of Cognitive Therapy in Depression: A Treatment Trial Using Cognitive Therapy and Pharmacotherapy, Each Alone and in Combination," *British Journal of Psychiatry* 139 (1981): 181–89; A. J. Rush, A. T. Beck, M. Kovacs, and S. D. Hollon, "Comparative Efficacy of Cognitive Therapy and Pharmacotherapy in the Treatment of Depressed Outpatients," *Cognitive Therapy and Research* 1 (1977): 17–37; M. M. Weissman, B. A. Prusoff, A. DiMascio, C. Neu, M. Goklaney, and G. L. Klerman, "The Efficacy of Drugs and Psychotherapy in the Treatment of Acute Depressive Episodes," *American Journal of Psychiatry* 136 (1979): 555–58; M. E. Thase, A. D. Simons, J. Cahalane, J. McGeary, and T. Harden, "Severity of Depression and Response to Cognitive Behavior Therapy," *American Journal of Psychiatry* 148 (1991): 784–89; R. B. Jarrett, M. Schaffer, D. McIntire, A. Witt-Browder, D. Kraft, and R. C. Risser, "Treatment of Atypical Depression with Cognitive Therapy or Phenelzine," *Archives of General Psychiatry* 56 (1999): 431–37; I. M. Blackburn and R. G. Moore, "Controlled Acute and Follow-up Trial of Cognitive Therapy and Pharmacotherapy in Out-Patients with Recurrent Depression," *British Journal of Psychiatry* 171 (1997): 328–34.
3. S. D. Hollon, R. J. DeRubeis, M. D. Evans, M. J. Wiemer, M. J. Garvey, W. M. Grove, and V. B. Tuason, "Cognitive Therapy and Pharmacotherapy for Depression, Singly and in Combination," *Archives of General Psychiatry* 49 (1992): 774–81.
4. Two points are not fully resolved by the research because of contradictory results in different studies. In the NIMH study, when the patients were divided into those who were more severely depressed versus those who were less so, there was "some, but not a great deal" of evidence that medication is more effective in the short term for the more severely depressed. But this was not true in the Minnesota study: There were no differences between therapy and drugs "even among the more severely depressed outpatients." Because of the contradictory results in these and other studies, this point is not fully settled. When one looks at the full spectrum of patients, however, psychotherapy and drugs are comparable. The other point not fully resolved is whether or not a combination of psychotherapy and drugs has some benefit, at least for some subgroups of patients, such as those who are hospitalized or more depressed. Here again the results of different studies are contradictory. As described in the previous chapter, all of these kinds of studies have serious limitations. The psychotherapy, in particular, is compromised by having to be one or another type of therapy; most often cognitive therapy or interpersonal therapy because these have been standardized. In clinical practice, clinicians often use a mix of approaches and try one after another until something works. By contrast, those patients receiving medications are not really receiving just the drug. In the NIMH study, the medication patients received "support and encouragement and direct advice if necessary" in weekly meetings that the researchers described as a "minimal supportive therapy." Thus, medication patients were receiving a combination of medica-

tion with some therapy. Given these methodological problems, I have presented the most general findings in the studies. These general findings are consistent with my own experience in clinical practice. Moreover, as discussed later in the chapter, repeated follow-up studies have demonstrated that the beneficial effects of psychotherapy are longer-lasting than those of drugs. When viewed from this long-range perspective, the unresolved issues in research on short-term treatment become even less important.

5. J. T. Watkins, W. R. Leber, S. D. Imber, J. F. Collins, I. Elkin, P. A. Pilkonis, S. M. Sotsky, M. T. Shea, and D. R. Glass, "Temporal Course of Change in Depression," *Journal of Consulting and Clinical Psychology* 61 (1993): 858–64; A. DiMascio, M. M. Weissman, B. A. Prusoff, C. Neu, M. Zwilling, and G. L. Klerman, "Differential Symptom Reduction by Drugs and Psychotherapy in Acute Depression," *Archives of General Psychiatry* 36 (1979): 1450–56.

6. J. Greenwald, "Herbal Healing," cover story, *Time,* November 23, 1998, pp. 58–69; R. L. Hoffman, "Nature's Answer to Prozac," *Greatlife,* January 1998, pp. 29–31.

7. S. E. Ewing, "St. John's Wort as an Antidepressant," *McLean Hospital Psychiatric Update* 1 (1998): 1–2.

8. H. M. Zal, "St. John's Wort and the Treatment of Depressive Disorders," *Hospital Physician,* September 1998, pp. 19–41.

9. H. Sommer and G. Harrer, "Placebo-Controlled Double-Blind Study Examining the Effectiveness of a Hypericum [St. John's wort] Preparation in 105 Mildly Depressed Patients," *Journal of Geriatric Psychiatry and Neurology* 7 (1994) [suppl. 1]: S9–S11; W. D. Hubner, S. Lande, and H. Podzuweit, "Hypericum [St. John's wort] Treatment of Mild Depressions with Somatic Symptoms," *Journal of Geriatric Psychiatry and Neurology* 7 (1994) [suppl. 1]: S12–S14; K. D. Hansgen, J. Vesper, and M. Ploch, "Multicenter Double-Blind Study Examining the Antidepressant Effectiveness of the Hypericum [St. John's wort] Extract LI 160," *Journal of Geriatric Psychiatry and Neurology* 7 (1994) [suppl. 1]: S15–S18.

10. *Journal of Geriatric Psychiatry and Neurology* 7 (1994) [suppl. 1]: S1–S68.

11. G. Harrer and V. Schulz, "Clinical Investigation of the Antidepressant Effectiveness of Hypericum [St. John's wort]," *Journal of Geriatric Psychiatry and Neurology* 7 (1994) [suppl. 1]: S6–S8.

12. E. U. Vorbach, W. D. Hubner, and K. H. Arnoldt, "Effectiveness and Tolerance of the Hypericum [St. John's wort] Extract LI 160 in Comparison with Imipramine [a prescription antidepressant often used as the standard against which new antidepressants are tested]: Randomized Double-Blind Study with 135 Outpatients," *Journal of Geriatric Psychiatry and Neurology* 7 (1994) [suppl. 1]: S19–S23.

13. H. Sommer and G. Harrer, "Placebo-Controlled Double-Blind Study Examining the Effectiveness of a Hypericum [St. John's wort] Preparation in 105 Mildly Depressed Patients," *Journal of Geriatric Psychiatry and Neurology* 7 (1994) [suppl. 1]: S9–S11.

14. W. D. Hubner, S. Lande, and H. Podzuweit, "Hypericum [St. John's wort] Treatment of Mild Depressions with Somatic Symptoms," *Journal of Geriatric Psychiatry and Neurology* 7 (1994) [suppl. 1]: S12–S14.

15. M. A. Jenike, Editorial, *Journal of Geriatric Psychiatry and Neurology* 7 (1994) [suppl. 1]: S1.

16. K. Linde, G. Ramirez, C. D. Mulrow, A. Pauls, W. Weidenhammer, and D. Melchart, "St. John's Wort for Depression—An Overview and Meta-analysis of Randomized Clinical Trials," *British Medical Journal* 313 (1996): 253–58.

17. S. Bratman, *St. John's Wort and Depression* (Rocklin, Calif.: Prima Publishing, 1999), p. 74.

18. P. A. De Smet and W. A. Nolen, "St. John's Wort as an Antidepressant: Longer Term Studies Are Needed Before It Can Be Recommended in Major Depression," *British Medical Journal* 313 (1996): 241.

19. T. Stephens, "Physical Activity and Mental Health in the United States and Canada: Evidence from Four Population Surveys," *Preventive Medicine* 17 (1988): 35–47; T. C. Camacho, R. E. Roberts, N. B. Lazarus, G. A. Kaplan, and R. D. Cohen, "Physical Activity and Depression: Evidence from the Alameda County Study," *American Journal of Epidemiology* 134 (1991): 220–31; J. P. Foreyt, R. L. Brunner, G. K. Goodrick, S. T. St. Jeor, and G. D. Miller, "Psychological Correlates of Reported Physical Activity in Normal-

Weight and Obese Adults: The Reno Diet-Heart Study," *International Journal of Obesity* 19 (1995) [suppl. 4]: S69–S72; C. E. Ross and D. Hayes, "Exercise and Psychologic Well-Being in the Community," *American Journal of Epidemiology* 127 (1988): 762–71.

20. J. H. Greist, M. H. Klein, R. R. Eischens, J. Faris, A. S. Gurman, and W. P. Morgan, "Running as a Treatment for Depression," *Comprehensive Psychiatry* 20 (1979): 41–54; E. W. Martinsen, "The Role of Aerobic Exercise in the Treatment of Depression," *Stress Medicine* 3 (1987): 93–100; T. C. North, P. McCullagh, and Z. V. Tran, "Effect of Exercise on Depression," *Exercise and Sport Sciences Reviews* 18 (1990): 379–415; D. M. Landers, "The Influence of Exercise on Mental Health," *President's Council on Physical Fitness and Sports Research Digest* 2 (1997): 2–8.

21. M. T. Shea, I. Elkin, S. D. Imber, S. M. Sotsky, J. T. Watkins, J. F. Collins, P. A. Pilkonis, E. Beckham, D. R. Glass, R. T. Dolan, and M. B. Parloff, "Course of Depressive Symptoms Over Follow-up, Findings from the National Institute of Mental Health Treatment of Depression Collaborative Research Program," *Archives of General Psychiatry* 49 (1992): 782–87.

22. M. D. Evans, S. D. Hollon, R. J. DeRubeis, J. M. Piasecki, W. M. Grove, M. J. Garvey, and V. B. Tuason, "Differential Relapse Following Cognitive Therapy and Pharmacotherapy for Depression," *Archives of General Psychiatry* 49 (1992): 802–8.

23. I. M. Blackburn, K. M. Eunson, and S. Bishop, "A Two-Year Naturalistic Follow-up of Depressed Patients Treated with Cognitive Therapy, Pharmacotherapy and a Combination of Both," *Journal of Affective Disorders* 10 (1986): 67–75.

24. M. Kovacs, A. J. Rush, A. T. Beck, and S. D. Hollon, "Depressed Outpatients Treated with Cognitive Therapy or Pharmacotherapy: A 1-Year Follow-up," *Archives of General Psychiatry* 38 (1981): 33–39; A. D. Simons, G. E. Murphy, J. L. Levine, and R. D. Wetzel, "Cognitive Therapy and Pharmacotherapy for Depression: Sustained Improvement Over 1 Year," *Archives of General Psychiatry* 43 (1986): 43–48; I. M. Blackburn and R. G. Moore, "Controlled Acute and Follow-up Trial of Cognitive Therapy and Pharmacotherapy in Out-Patients with Recurrent Depression," *British Journal of Psychiatry* 171 (1997): 328–34; G. A. Fava, C. Rafanelli, S. Grandi, S. Conti, and P. Belluardo, "Prevention of Recurrent Depression with Cognitive Behavioral Therapy," *Archives of General Psychiatry* 55 (1998): 816–20.

25. G. A. Fava, S. Grandi, M. Zielezny, C. Rafanelli, and R. Canestrari, "Four-Year Outcome for Cognitive Behavioral Treatment of Residual Symptoms in Major Depression," *American Journal of Psychiatry* 153 (1996): 945–47.

26. G. A. Fava, C. Rafanelli, S. Grandi, S. Conti, and P. Belluardo, "Prevention of Recurrent Depression with Cognitive Behavioral Therapy," *Archives of General Psychiatry* 55 (1998): 816–20.

27. An example of a strong drug proponent who advocates chronic maintenance administration of antidepressant medication is Dr. Martin Keller, professor and chairman of the department of psychiatry at Brown University. Keller has published numerous research articles, many of them coauthored with other psychopharmacologists who take a similar position on the treatment of depression. Appearing in prestigious medical and psychiatric journals, Keller's articles have the appearance of impartial academic publications. Yet, as described in Chapter 5, the October 8, 1999, *Boston Globe* revealed that "Keller earned a total of $842,000 last year [1998], according to financial records, and more than half of his income came . . . from pharmaceutical companies whose drugs he touted in medical journals and at conferences." For example, while publishing articles specifically endorsing Zoloft for the chronic treatment of depression, Keller received $218,000 in 1998 alone from Zoloft's manufacturer, Pfizer. "At the same time," continued the *Boston Globe*, "Keller was receiving millions of dollars in funding from the National Institute of Mental Health for research on depression and ways to treat it." The *Boston Globe* said Keller cited his NIMH-funded research on depression in an article in which he made claims on behalf of drugs like Zoloft. See D. Kong and A. Bass, "Case at Brown Leads to Review, NIMH Studies Tighter Rules on Conflicts," *Boston Globe,* October 8, 1999, pp. B1, B5.

28. "Mental Health: Does Therapy Help?," *Consumer Reports,* November 1995, pp. 734–39.

7
Surmounting Anxiety:
Training for Elevators, a Patient's Story

1. I. M. Marks, R. P. Swinson, M. Basoglu, K. Kuch, H. Noshirvani, G. O'Sullivan, P. T. Lelliot, M. Kirby, G. McNamee, S. Sengun, and K. Wickwire, "Alprazolam [Xanax, a Valium-type antianxiety agent] and Exposure Alone and Combined in Panic Disorder with Agoraphobia," *British Journal of Psychiatry* 162 (1993): 776–87.

2. H. Cass and T. McNally, *Kava: Nature's Answer to Stress, Anxiety, and Insomnia* (Rocklin, Calif.: Prima Publishing, 1998), p. 68.

3. Ibid., p. 67.

4. C. Kilham, *Kava: Medicine Hunting in Paradise* (Rochester, Vt.: Park Street Press, 1996), p. 99.

5. H. Cass and T. McNally, *Kava: Nature's Answer to Stress, Anxiety, and Insomnia* (Rocklin, Calif.: Prima Publishing, 1998), p. 93.

6. H. P. Volz and M. Kieser, "Kava-Kava Extract WS 1490 Versus Placebo in Anxiety Disorders: A Randomized Placebo-Controlled 25-Week Outpatient Trial," *Pharmacopsychiatry* 30 (1997): 1–5.

7. E. Lehmann, E. Kinzler, and J. Friedemann, "Efficacy of a Special Kava Extract *(Piper methysticum)* in Patients with States of Anxiety, Tension and Excitedness of Non-mental Origin—A Double-Blind Placebo-Controlled Study of Four Weeks Treatment," *Phytomedicine* 3 (1996): 113–19; V. G. Warnecke, "Psychosomatic Dysfunctions in the Female Climacteric: Clinical Effectiveness and Tolerance of Kava Extract WS 1490," *Fortschritte de Medizin* 109 (1991): 119–22.

8. M. T. Murray, *Stress, Anxiety, and Insomnia* (Rocklin, Calif.: Prima Publishing, 1995), p. 135.

9. H. Woelk, O. Kapoula, S. Lehrl, K. Schroter, and P. Weinholz, "Double-Blind Study: Kava Special Extract Versus Benzodiazepines [Valium-type antianxiety agents] in Treatment of Patients Suffering from Anxiety," *Zeitschrift für Allgemeinmedizin* 69 (1993): 271–77.

10. H. Cass and T. McNally, *Kava: Nature's Answer to Stress, Anxiety, and Insomnia* (Rocklin, Calif.: Prima Publishing, 1998), p. 139.

11. D. Tenney, *Kava Kava, Valerian and Other Nervine Herbs* (Pleasant Grove, Utah: Woodland Publishing, 1997), p. 9.

12. Personal communication, *United States Pharmacopoeia.* See *U.S. Pharmacopoeia, Number 12* (Rockville, Md.: United States Pharmacopoeial Convention, 1936), p. 428; *National Formulary, Ninth Edition* (Washington: American Pharmaceutical Association, 1950), p. 45. Note that valerian will be officially listed again in the year 2000 edition of the now combined *U.S. Pharmacopoeia/National Formulary.* See *USP [U.S. Pharmacopoeia] 24 NF [National Formulary] 19* (Rockville, Md.: United States Pharmacopoeial Convention, 2000), pp. 2533, 2534. St. John's wort is also again listed. Kava is in the process of being evaluated.

13. A. Weil, *Spontaneous Healing* (New York: Knopf, 1995), p. 261.

14. P. D. Leathwood, F. Chauffard, E. Heck, and R. Munoz-Box, "Aqueous Extract of Valerian Root *(Valeriana officinalis L.)* Improves Sleep Quality in Man," *Pharmacology, Biochemistry, and Behavior* 17 (1982): 65–71.

15. E. U. Vorbach, R. Gortelmayer, and J. Bruning, "Therapie von Insomnien: Wirksamkeit und Vertraglichkeit eines Baldrian-Praparates," *Psychopharmakotherapie* 3 (1996): 109–115. Considered one of the best studies of valerian, the Vorbach study is not yet readily available in English translation. A detailed summary appears in V. Schulz, R. Hansel, and V. Tyler, *Rational Phytotherapy* (Berlin: Springer, 1998), pp. 78–80.

16. H. Dressing, et al., "Insomnia: Are Valerian/Balm Combinations of Equal Value to Benzodiazepines [Valium-type sleeping pills]?," *Therapiewoch* 42 (1992): 726–36.

17. A. Fugh-Berman and J. M. Cott, "Dietary Supplements and Natural Products as Psychotherapeutic Agents," *Psychosomatic Medicine* 61 (1999): 712–28.

18. I. M. Marks, R. P. Swinson, M. Basoglu, K. Kuch, H. Noshirvani, G. O'Sullivan, P. T. Lelliott, M. Kirby, G. McNamee, S. Sengun, and K. Wickwire, "Alprazolam [Xanax, a Valium-type antianxiety agent] and Exposure Alone and Combined in Panic Disorder with Agoraphobia," *British Journal of Psychiatry* 162 (1993): 776–87.

19. I. Marks, J. Greist, M. Basoglu, H. Noshirvani, and G. O'Sullivan, "Comment on the Second Phase of the Cross-National Collaborative Panic Study," *British Journal of Psychiatry* 160 (1992): 202–5.

20. F. H. Wilhelm and W. T. Roth, "Acute and Delayed Effects of Alprazolam [Xanax, a Valium-type Antianxiety Agent] on Flight Phobics During Exposure," *Behavior Research and Therapy* 35 (1997): 831–41.

21. D. Barlow et al., personal communication. Paper pending publication. The results of this study were presented in a symposium at the November 1998 Annual Convention of the Association for Advancement of Behavior Therapy in Washington, D.C. Because the study was planned before the Prozac group became established for anxiety, the antidepressant used was one of the older tricyclics, imipramine. The Prozac group have since become widely established for anxiety and are considered comparable to imipramine in their effectiveness.

22. J. C. Beckham, S. R. Vrana, J. G. May, D. J. Gustafson, and G. R. Smith, "Emotional Processing and Fear Measurement Synchrony as Indicators of Treatment Outcome in Fear of Flying," *Journal of Behavior Therapy and Experimental Psychiatry* 21 (1990): 153–162.

23. M. Basoglu, "Pharmacological and Behavioural Treatment of Panic Disorder," *Psychotherapy and Psychosomatics* 58 (1992): 57–59.

24. G. McNamee, G. O'Sullivan, P. Lelliott, and I. Marks, "Telephone-Guided Treatment for Housebound Agoraphobics with Panic Disorder: Exposure vs. Relaxation," *Behavior Therapy* 20 (1989): 491–97.

25. C. Kilic, H. Noshirvani, M. Basoglu, and I. Marks, "Agoraphobia and Panic Disorder: 3.5 Years After Alprazolam [Xanax] and/or Exposure Treatment," *Psychotherapy and Psychosomatics* 66 (1997): 175–78.

26. G. A. Fava, M. Zielezny, G. Savron, and L. Grandi, "Long-Term Effects of Behavioral Treatment for Panic Disorder with Agoraphobia," *British Journal of Psychiatry* 166(1995): 87–92.

8

Conquering Addictions:
Substance Abuse, Sexual Addictions, and Eating Disorders

1. D. Mura, "A Male Grief: Notes on Pornography and Addiction," in M. S. Kimmel, ed., *Men Confront Pornography* (New York: Meridian, 1990), pp. 123–41.

2. K. Chernin, *The Hungry Self* (New York: Perennial Library, 1985), pp. xiv–xvi.

EPILOGUE
Effecting Personal Change

1. C. Medawar, "The Antidepressant Web," *International Journal of Risk & Safety in Medicine* 10 (1997): 75–126.

2. G. Dukes, Editorial, *International Journal of Risk & Safety in Medicine* 10 (1997): 67–69.

3. As in previous chapters, I use the term "adrenaline" for both adrenaline and the closely related noradrenaline—also known as epinephrine and norepinephrine, respectively—because "adrenaline" is well known to a nontechnical audience. Noradrenaline, or norepinephrine, is the form found in the brain.

4. J. Stringer, "Sepracor, Eli Lilly Pen Prozac Deal," *Mass High Tech,* December 14–20, 1998, p. 7.

5. The parent compound of Redux is fenfluramine. The chemical name for Redux is "dexfenfluramine," or "right-fenfluramine."

INDEX

ABOUT THE AUTHOR

Joseph Glenmullen, M.D., is a clinical instructor in psychiatry at Harvard Medical School, is on the staff of the Harvard University Health Services, and is in private practice in Harvard Square. He is the author of the widely applauded book *Sexual Mysteries: Tales of Psychotherapy*, a collection of ten fascinating cases ranging from sexual addictions to sexual abuse, with a foreword by Robert Coles. A graduate of Brown University and Harvard Medical School, Dr. Glenmullen lives with his wife and children in Cambridge, Massachusetts, and can be found on the Web at www.glenmullen.com.